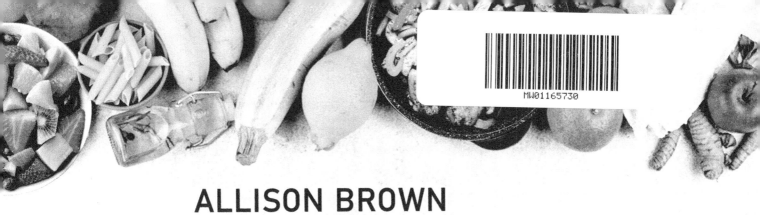

ALLISON BROWN

THE COMPLETE
DASH
DIET
COOKBOOK

1000+ LOW SODIUM, FLAVORFUL RECIPES TO LOWER
BLOOD PRESSURE. *INCLUDING A 8-WEEK MEAL PLAN*

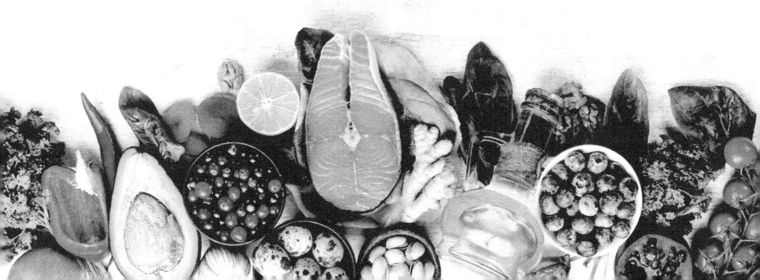

Table of Contents

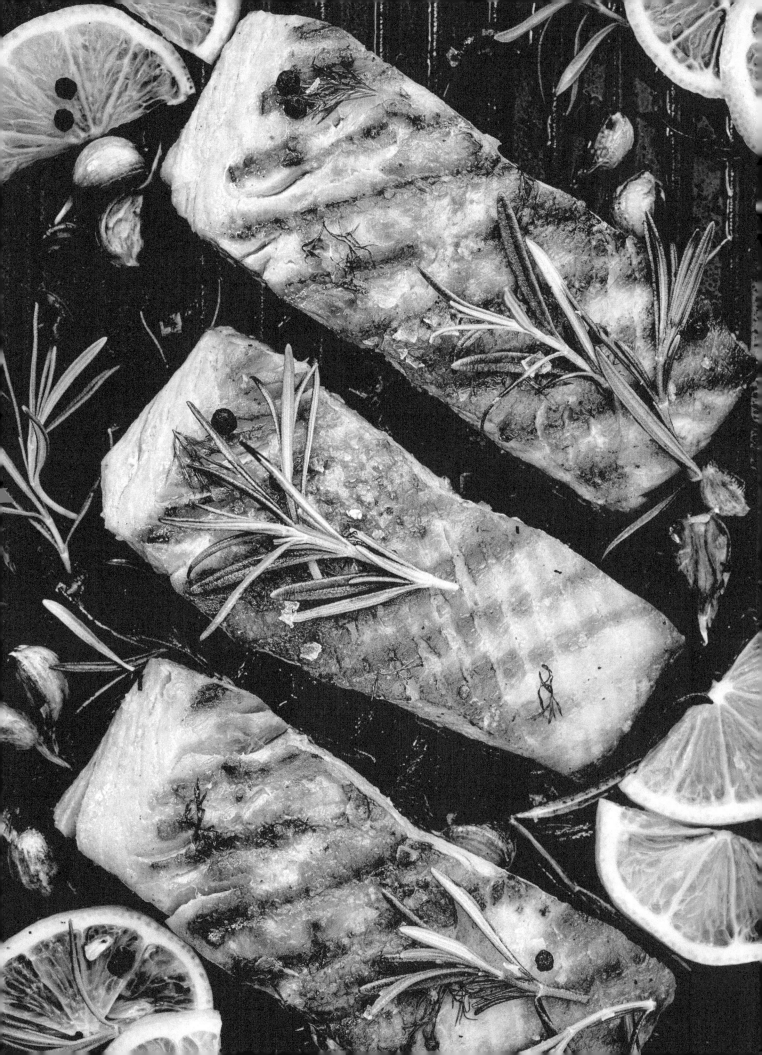

Introduction

If you want to lose or simply maintain your current weight, the Dash diet has proven time and time again to be the most effective method available. This plan is based on a list of foods that should make up the bulk of your diet.

Fruits, vegetables, lean meats such as chicken, turkey or fish and low-fat dairy products such as milk or yogurt are the key ingredients of this diet. The Dash diet is also known as one of the cleanest "diets" out there because there are few restrictions. All you have to do is eat things in moderation and avoid processed foods.

The Dash diet focuses on minimizing the levels of sodium in your diet, hence the name "Dash." It was developed by the National Heart, Lung, and Blood Institute in the late 1990s to help people with high blood pressure. The Dietary Approaches to Stop Hypertension is an excellent strategy for losing weight, improving heart health and overall health. The Dash diet, created by Dr. Marjorie Haynes, has been on the market for over 20 years and is a very popular diet.

DASH is a registered trademark of the National Heart, Lung, and Blood Institute.

It stands for Dietary Approaches to Stop Hypertension. It was created to demonstrate the effect of a plant-based diet in lowering blood pressure.

It is an eating plan that has been shown to help lower blood pressure levels, reduce the risk of heart disease, control diabetes and maintain a healthy weight.

The DASH is a very balanced diet created from the National Dietary Recommendations. It is a low-fat, low-sodium, low-cholesterol diet, rich in fiber, potassium and magnesium; all ingredients have been shown to be helpful in lowering blood pressure.

The DASH diet is a very simple concept. You won't have to give up many of the foods you already love; it's very easy to fit into your daily routine, and you can eat without any side effects. What makes this diet different from others is that it is a healthy program that has been initially created and tested for a specific purpose to be very effective in lowering blood pressure.

This regime has been around for a while and has been proven time and time again to be one of the most effective methods for weight loss. In the past, it was used as a plan to help people with epilepsy lose weight, but recently it has become popular. This diet plan can help you lose pounds quickly by eliminating or severely limiting your sugar and carbohydrate intake.

It is also a low-carb diet, so you don't have to worry about going crazy eating starchy foods like potatoes, rice or bread. As long as you are eating whole, natural foods, you will see more noticeable results than ever before.

The good news is that this diet doesn't require you to give up your favorite foods altogether, just make better choices when you eat. It's especially designed for people who love the way they eat but struggle with their weight. You can still enjoy your favorite foods in moderation, making it easier to lose weight while still indulging.

It may seem like an impossible task to cut out all junk food or processed foods, but if you follow this plan to the letter, it will help you lose weight and improve your overall health in no time.

Chapter I. Strategies for Limiting or Replacing Sodium

One of the best ways to improve and preserve your health over time is to decrease the amount of sodium, or salt, in your diet.
In recent years, doctors have begun advising people who suffer from high blood pressure to limit their daily intake to no more than 2,300 milligrams (2.3 grams) or one teaspoon.

From the latest statistics, Americans consume at least 50% more sodium than the recommended amounts daily. Diets high in sodium increase blood pressure levels, leading to damaging kidney function, creating kidney failure.
Below you can find 11 strategies to reduce or replace sodium in your recipes.

1. Use fresh herbs to season your dishes, such as parsley, thyme, basil, rosemary, marjoram. For example, fresh basil contains only 4 mg of sodium per 100 g, parsley 56 mg/100 g, and thyme 9 mg/ 100 g. The extra flavor these herbs will give to your dishes will compensate for the lower amounts of salt. Fresh herbs also have exceptional beneficial properties such as anti-inflammatory, digestive, antibacterial, and antioxidant actions.

2. Marinate your meat or fish before cooking; the use of ingredients such as lemon, lime, citrus fruits, together with oil (in low quantities) and aromatic herbs, will give an exceptional taste to your dishes without having to use extra sodium. We recommend marinating your ingredients at least 2 hours before cooking and compose marinades with three elements, one oily, one aromatic, and one acidic, in 3/1 parts. For example, use three parts olive oil and 1 part lemon along with a clove of garlic and parsley for a delicious marinade for fish. At the same time, you can substitute lemon for lime and add honey for a marinade for pork.

3. Use gomasio instead of salt! This condiment is used in the macrobiotic tradition on sesame seeds (goma) and whole sea salt (shio). The original recipe requires from 7 to 20 parts of sesame seeds and one amount of salt. Its use drastically lowers sodium intake. It is recommended to use it raw at the end of preparing dishes and be rich in nutrients such as Omega 3, Omega 6, phosphor, iron, and calcium. Do not use gomasio if you are allergic to sesame!
4. Use fresh meat instead of sausages such as ham, salami, bacon, bresaola. Sausages contain very high amounts of salt, so they must be absolutely eliminated from your diet. Fresh meat naturally includes a part of sodium; therefore, it will be delicious without adding extra salt. Instead, you can use the marinades we have just described.
5. Read carefully the labels of the foods you buy;, behind statements such as "low sodium" hides a pitfall, the product is low in sodium but high in potassium, which in high doses is dangerous for the heart. Also, observe the position of the ingredients and the quantity because if sodium is in the first five ingredients of the list, it means that such food is rich in salt.

6. Do not use canned foods, which are added with extra salt. If you can't give up canned foods, remember not to use the preserving liquid, but rinse the contents very well with water. We recommend using frozen ingredients instead of canned food, such as peas, beans, spinach, asparagus, artichokes.

7. Eliminate aged cheeses, which are incredibly high in sodium. Cheddar contains over 600 mg/100 g, Parmigiano 1,500 mg/100 g, Provolone 900 mg/100 g. Instead, it is better to use fresh cheeses such as ricotta, but always in small quantities, as they are rich in fats.

8. Do not use ready-made sauces such as ketchup, mayonnaise, mustard, but try to make delicious homemade sauces, combining Greek yogurt, olive oil, chives, or Greek yogurt, lemon juice, olive oil, and garlic.

9. Train your taste buds by gradually decreasing the amount of salt in your dishes. It will take 6 to 8 weeks to train your palate for new flavors. After this period, if you go back to eating salt-rich dishes, you will find them almost disgusting.
10. Use little tricks, such as not bringing a salt shaker to the table, to avoid further salting your dishes, removing the temptation from the beginning!

11. Use vegetables already rich in sodium to season or flavor your dishes; celery, artichokes, spinach, raw carrots, beets are naturally sapid and can be used to replace sodium in your recipes, enriching your dishes with additional flavors and nutrients.

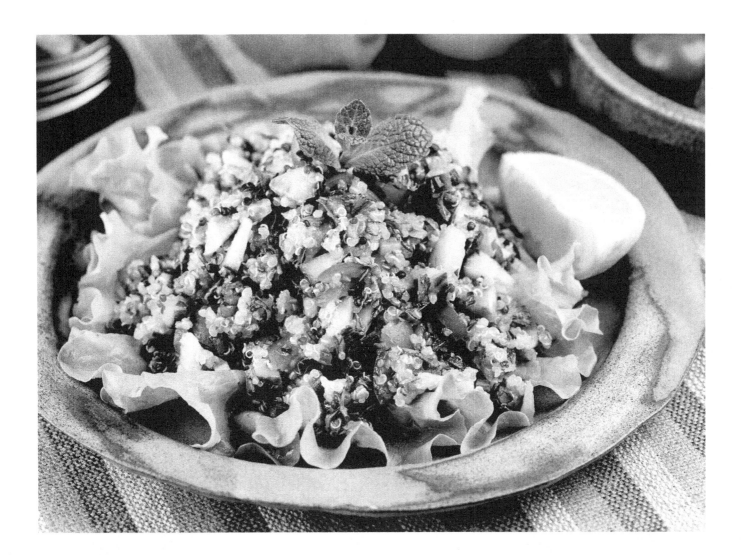

Chapter 2. Foods to Prefer, Limit and Avoid in the Dash Diet + Shopping List

Foods to Prefer

Here are some foods that you should have, but remember that nothing is good in excess.

- Vegetables (4 to 5 servings a day.)
- Fruits (4 to 5 servings a day.)
- Lean meats (2 or less daily servings)
- Poultry skinless (2 or less daily servings)
- Fish (2 or less daily servings)
- No fat dairy products (2-3 daily servings)
- Low fat dairy products (2-3 daily servings)
- Nuts, seeds and legumes (4 to 5 servings a week)
- Grains (6 to 8 servings a day.)

Foods to Avoid

These foods you should try to limit as much as possible, and it would be better if you could cut them out of your diet all together.

- Salt
- High fat dairy products
- Salted nuts
- Sugary beverages
- Processed food
- Animal based fats (in excess)

How Much Is a Serving

Vegetables

- 1 cup raw leafy green vegetable as salad or spinach.
- 1/2 cup raw or cooked vegetables
- 1/2 cup low-sodium vegetable juice

Fat-free or low-fat dairy products

- 1 cup low-fat or fat-free milk
- 1 cup fat-free or low-fat yogurt
- 1 1/2 ounces fat-free or low-fat cheese

Grains

- 1 slice bread (preferably whole wheat)
- 1 ounce dry cereal (preferably whole grain)
- 1/2 cup cooked cereal, pasta or rice (preferably whole grain)

Fruits

- 1 medium size fruit
- 1/4 cup dried fruit
- 1/2 cup fresh or frozen fruit
- 1/2 cup 100% fruit juice

Lean meats, fish and poultry

- 1 ounce cooked lean meat, fish or skinless poultry
- 1 egg
- 2 egg whites

Fats and oils

- 1 tsp. margarine
- 1 tsp. vegetable oil
- 1 tsb. mayonnaise
- 2 tsp. low-fat salad dressing
- **Nuts, seeds and legumes**
- 1/3 cup nuts
- 2 tsp. peanut butter
- 2 tsp. seeds
- 1/2 cup cooked legumes (dried beans or peas)

Sweets and added sugars

- 1 tsp. sugar
- 1 tsp. jelly or jam
- 1/2 cup sorbet
- 1 cup sugar-sweetened lemonade

Shopping List

Fruits

Tart, sweet, soft, crunchy, thin, huge; fruits are one of those unique food groups that offer a huge variety to tempt your taste buds and keep you healthy and fit. They are a beneficial component of the dash diet and are the easiest to prepare. They are an important source of minerals, magnesium, potassium, fiber and other nutrients. Fruits are generally low in fat, excluding coconuts and avocados.

According to the dash diet, you should eat more fruit than the average American. If you are not a fruit fan, fruit juices can also be helpful. Read the product label to make sure it is 100% fruit juice, because only then will you get the true nutrition from the juice. Avoid consuming drinks, labeled as fruit cocktails, or fruit drinks, as they often have added sugars and can increase your calorie intake.

Your daily diet should include at least 4 to 5 servings of fruit. A single serving includes:

- One medium-sized or a half cup of fruit
- Half cup of pure fruit juice

Vegetables

Have you ever had Italian food that didn't have tomato sauce? Or Chinese food that didn't have broccoli and onions? Vegetables lend color, texture and, of course, a special flavor to your favorite cuisines. Rich in nutrients such as potassium, fiber and magnesium, vegetables are low in fat, sodium and calories, which is why they are a key element of the dash diet.

Your daily diet should include at least 4 to 5 servings of vegetables. A single serving includes:

- Half cup of cooked vegetable, such as broccoli, kale, spinach, cauliflower, etc.
- One cup of fresh leafy vegetables, such as lettuce or spinach
- Three-fourth cup of vegetable juice
- Half potato or 1/4 cup of mashed potato
- Half cup of tomato sauce

Dairy Foods

While dairy products have been a vital part of our daily diet since ancient times, the dash diet emphasizes their importance even more, as they are a great source of protein, calcium and vitamin D. Still, it should be remembered that they can be high in saturated fat, so it is always good to choose fat-free or low-fat dairy products. This will give you huge health benefits without increasing your fat intake.

Your daily diet should have at least 3 servings of dairy products. A single serving includes:

- One cup of 2 percent low-fat milk, 1 percent low-fat milk, or skim milk
- 1/3 cup of non-fat milk powder
- One cup of low-fat or non-fat cottage cheese
- One cup of non-fat or low-fat yogurt
- Half cup of non-fat or low-fat frozen yogurt
- 1/4 cups of non-fat or low-fat cheeses, such as ricotta and cheddar

Grains

We mean everything from bread, cereals, pasta, rice, bagels, and tortillas by grains.

Your daily diet should have at least 6 servings of grain. A single serving includes:

- One slice of whole-wheat bread
- 1/4 cup dry cereal
- Half cup cooked pasta, rice, or cereal

Poultry, Lean Meat and Fish

Meat is a great source of B vitamins, protein, zinc and iron. However, even lean meats contain large amounts of cholesterol and fat, so it is best not to make them the mainstay of your diet. When following the dash diet plan, you can reduce your usual meat portions and replace them with vegetables and fruits.

Your diet should have at least 5 servings of lean meat, fish and poultry. A single serving includes:

- 1/4 cup cooked seafood, lean meat, or skinless poultry
- One egg

Sweets and Desserts

The dash diet doesn't let you crave those tempting sweet-smelling desserts you can't do without. You don't need to banish them at all. Instead, consume them in limited quantities.

You should have 4 or fewer servings of sweets and desserts per week. A single serving includes:

- One tablespoon of sugar, jam, or jelly
- Half cup sorbet
- One cup lemonade

Legumes, Nuts, and Seeds

This is an important food group of the dash diet, as it offers you some delicious and healthy options. Having lentils, peas, almonds, beans, sunflower seeds and many other healthy foods, this family supports your physical and mental health with protein, potassium, magnesium and fiber. In addition, they are a rich source of phytochemicals. These plant-based compounds keep you protected from cardiovascular disease and certain types of cancer.

Since these foods have a higher amount of calories, they should be consumed in limited quantities.

Legumes, nuts and seeds should be consumed at least 4 times per week. A single serving includes:

- 1/3 cup nuts
- Half cup cooked peas or beans
- Two tablespoons of seeds

Fats and Oils

Wondering why this family of foods is part of the dash diet? Well, your body needs some fats and oils to absorb vitamins and keep your immune system strong. However, overconsumption of fats can increase your chances of developing diabetes, obesity and heart disease.

The dash diet maintains a healthy balance and restricts total fat to less than 27% of daily calories. In addition, it focuses on the consumption of monosaturated fats.

The daily diet should include at least 2 servings of oils and fats. A single serving includes:

- Two tablespoons of salad dressing
- One tablespoon of mayonnaise
- One teaspoon of soft margarine

Tips at Mealtime

Reduce meat consumption. Cook stews and casseroles with about two-thirds of the meat called for in the recipe, and add more whole-grain pasta, bulgur, tofu, brown rice or vegetables.

Make lower-fat substitutions. Swap full-fat dairy products for fat-free or reduced-fat versions.

Be careful with broth. You can prepare onions, mushrooms or other vegetables in a small low-sodium broth inside a nonstick skillet. A small amount of healthy oil (such as olive oil) may be a better choice, as even low-sodium broth can contain a lot of sodium.

Give it more flavor. Enhance flavor without adding fat or salt by using Sodium free broth, garlic powder or garlic, lemon, ginger, peppers, onions, flavored vinegars, spices or herbs. The use of spices can enhance the flavor of the food even if you do not add salt or fat to the food. Spices and herbs such as onions, vinegar, pepper, lemon, ginger and garlic can add natural flavor to your food. Spices such as rosemary, cayenne pepper, chili, cilantro, dill, cinnamon, etc., can saturate the flavor and make even unsalted foods more delicious. Make your food colorful.

Use healthy cooking methods. Even if you can't cook your food using a deep fryer, you can still cook delicious dishes. The thing is, there are many healthy cooking methods you can use to cook your food. In addition to boiling and roasting, you have the option of poaching, steaming, pan frying, baking and sautéing your food.

Rinse your ingredients. This tip refers to canned foods, such as beans and vegetables. Before using them, deliberately washing them with water can remove excess salt.

Use water when making broth. You should avoid using prepared broths to make soup because they can contain large amounts of sodium. Instead, you can use water or make your own broth. To make a delicious broth suitable for the DASH diet, you can put mushrooms, onions, carrots and other vegetables and simmer for an hour to bring out the best flavor in the broth.

Rinse canned foods. Canned vegetables are a quick way to buy vegetables, prepare them and have them last you. They are perfectly fine to eat as part of the DASH diet. However, the juice from the can carries a lot of excess salt. Get rid of most of this excess by simply rinsing the vegetables with water before eating them.

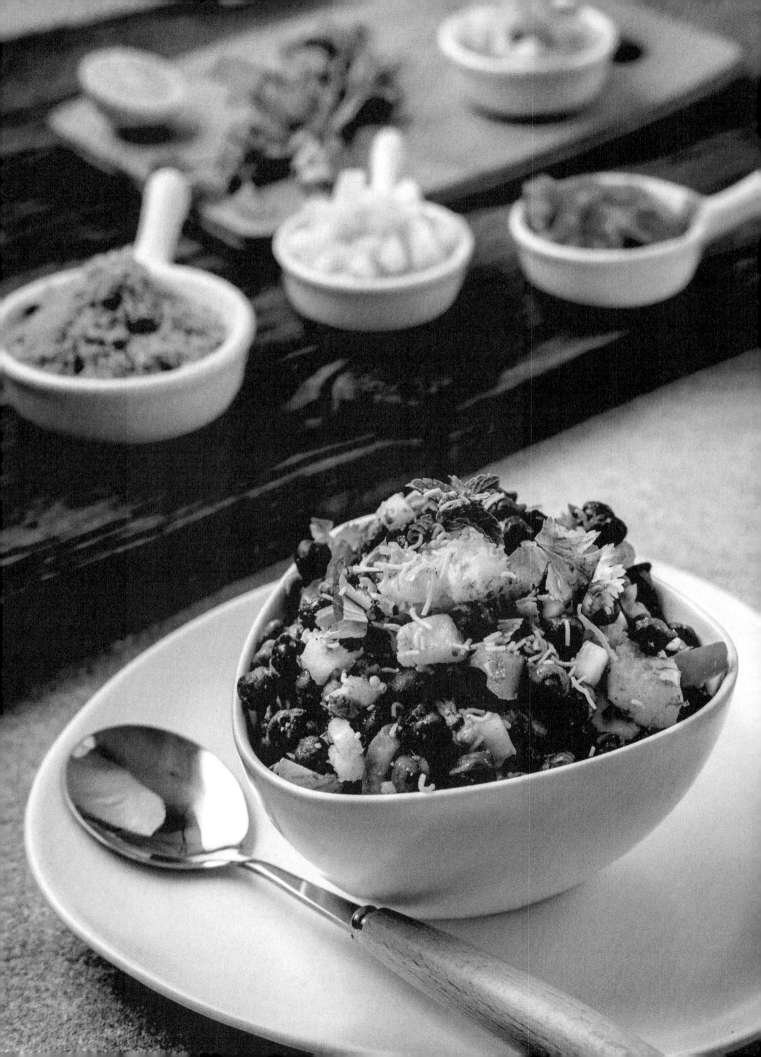

Chapter 3. Mix Spices/Herbs, Marinades

1. Chicken Rub

Preparation Time: 10 minutes
Cooking Time: 0 minutes
Servings: ¼ cup
Ingredients:
- 1¼ teaspoons garlic powder
- ½ teaspoon onion powder
- ½ teaspoon freshly ground black pepper
- ½ teaspoon ground chipotle chili pepper
- ½ teaspoon smoked paprika
- ¼ teaspoon dried oregano leaves
- ¼ teaspoon mustard powder
- ¼ teaspoon cayenne pepper

Directions:
1. In a small airtight container or zip-top bag, combine the garlic powder, onion powder, black pepper, chipotle pepper, paprika, oregano, mustard, and cayenne. Close the container and shake to mix. The unused rub will keep in an airtight container for months.

Nutrition:
Calories: 20, Carbs: 5g, Protein: 1g, Potassium: 123mg, Sodium: 53mg.

2. Dill Seafood Rub

Preparation Time: 10 minutes
Cooking Time: 0 minutes
Servings: ¼ cup
Ingredients:
- 2 tablespoons dried dill weed
- 1 tablespoon garlic powder
- 1½ teaspoons lemon pepper

Directions:
1. Combine the dill, garlic powder, and lemon pepper in a small airtight container or zip-top bag. Close the container and shake to mix. The unused rub will keep in an airtight container for months.

Nutrition:
Calories: 20, Carbs: 5g, Protein: 1g, Potassium: 113mg, Sodium: 53mg.

3. Cajun Rub

Preparation Time: 10 minutes
Cooking Time: 0 minutes
Servings: ¼ cup

Ingredients:
- 1 teaspoon freshly ground black pepper
- 1 teaspoon onion powder
- 1 teaspoon garlic powder
- 1 teaspoon sweet paprika
- ½ teaspoon cayenne pepper
- ½ teaspoon red pepper flakes
- ½ teaspoon dried oregano leaves
- ½ teaspoon dried thyme
- ½ teaspoon smoked paprika

Directions:
1. In a small airtight container or zip-top bag, combine the black pepper, onion powder, garlic powder, sweet paprika, cayenne, red pepper flakes, oregano, thyme, and smoked paprika. Close the container and shake to mix. The unused rub will keep in an airtight container for months.

Nutrition:
Calories: 20, Carbs: 5g, Protein: 1g, Potassium: 125mg, Sodium: 53mg.

4. Sweet and Spicy Cinnamon Rub

Preparation Time: 10 minutes
Cooking Time: 0 minutes
Servings: ¼ cup
Ingredients:
- 2 tablespoons light brown sugar
- 1 teaspoon garlic powder
- 1 teaspoon onion powder
- 1 teaspoon sweet paprika
- ½ teaspoon freshly ground black pepper
- ½ teaspoon cayenne pepper
- ½ teaspoon dried oregano leaves
- ½ teaspoon ground ginger
- ½ teaspoon ground cumin
- ¼ teaspoon smoked paprika
- ¼ teaspoon ground cinnamon
- ¼ teaspoon ground coriander
- ¼ teaspoon chili powder

Directions:
1. In a small airtight container or zip-top bag, combine the brown sugar, garlic powder, onion powder, sweet paprika, black pepper, cayenne, oregano, ginger, cumin, smoked paprika, cinnamon, coriander, and chili powder. Close the container and shake to mix. The unused rub will keep in an airtight container for months.

Nutrition:
Calories: 10, Carbs: 6g, Protein: 1g, Potassium: 103mg, Sodium: 53mg.

5. Burger Shake

Preparation Time: 10 minutes
Cooking Time: 0 minutes
Servings: ¼ cup
Ingredients:
- 1 teaspoon garlic powder
- 1 teaspoon dried minced onion
- 1 teaspoon onion powder
- 1 teaspoon freshly ground black pepper
- ½ teaspoon sweet paprika
- ¼ teaspoon mustard powder
- ¼ teaspoon celery seed

Directions:
1. In a small airtight container or zip-top bag, combine the salt, garlic powder, minced onion, onion powder, black pepper, sweet paprika, mustard powder, and celery seed. Close the container and shake to mix. The unused burger shake will keep in an airtight container for months.

Nutrition:
Calories: 10, Carbs: 6g, Protein: 1g, Potassium: 113mg, Sodium: 23mg.

6. Tea Injectable

Preparation Time: 10 minutes
Cooking Time: 0 minutes
Servings: 2 cups
Ingredients:
- ¼ cup favorite spice rub or shake
- 2 cups water

Directions:
1. Place the rub in a standard paper coffee filter and tie it up with kitchen string to seal.
2. In a small pot over high heat, bring the water to a boil.
3. Drop the filter into the boiling water and remove the pot from

the heat. Let it steep for 30 minutes.

4. Remove and discard the filter. Discard any unused tea.

Nutrition:
Calories: 10, Carbs: 6g, Protein: 1g, Sodium: 63mg, Potassium: 123mg.

7. Garlic Butter Injectable

Preparation Time: 10 minutes
Cooking Time: 0 minutes
Servings: ¼ cup
Ingredients:
- 16 tablespoons (2 sticks) butter
- 1½ tablespoons garlic powder

Directions:
1. In a small skillet over medium heat, melt the butter.
2. Stir in the garlic powder until well mixed. Use immediately.

Nutrition:
Calories: 10, Carbs: 6g, Protein: 1g, Sodium: 53mg, Potassium: 123mg.

8. Easy Teriyaki Marinade

Preparation Time: 10 minutes
Cooking Time: 0 minutes
Servings: 1 cup
Ingredients:
- ¼ cup water
- ¼ cup soy sauce
- ¼ cup Worcestershire sauce
- 2 garlic cloves, sliced

Directions:
1. In a small bowl, whisk the water, soy sauce, Worcestershire sauce, and garlic until combined. Refrigerate any unused marinade in an airtight container for 2 or 3 days.

Nutrition:
Calories: 10, Carbs: 6g, Protein: 1g, Sodium: 63mg, Potassium: 123mg.

9. Lemon Butter Mop for Seafood

Preparation Time: 10 minutes
Cooking Time: 0 minutes
Servings: ¼ cup
Ingredients:
- 8 tablespoons (1 stick) butter
- Juice of 1 small lemon
- 1½ teaspoons garlic powder

- 1½ teaspoons dried dill weed

Directions:
1. In a small skillet over medium heat, melt the butter.
2. Stir in the lemon juice, garlic powder, and dill, stirring until well mixed. Use immediately.

Nutrition:
Calories: 10, Carbs: 6g, Protein: 1g, Sodium: 43mg, Potassium: 133mg.

10. Worcestershire Mop and Spritz

Preparation Time: 10 minutes
Cooking Time: 0 minutes
Servings: 1 cup
Ingredients:
- ½ cup water
- ½ cup Worcestershire sauce
- 2 garlic cloves, sliced

Directions:
1. In a small bowl, stir together the water, Worcestershire sauce, and garlic until mixed. Transfer to a spray bottle for spritzing. Refrigerate unused spritz for up to 3 days and use for all types of meats.

Nutrition:
Calories: 20, Carbs: 9g, Protein: 5g, Sodium: 63mg, Potassium: 123mg.

11. Chimichurri

Preparation Time: 10 minutes
Cooking Time: 5 minutes
Servings: 8
Ingredients:
- 1/2 yellow bell pepper, deseeded and finely chopped
- 1 green chili pepper, deseeded and finely chopped
- Juice and zest of 1 lemon
- 1 cup olive oil
- 1/2 cup parsley, chopped
- 2 garlic cloves, grated
- pepper to taste

Directions:
1. Add all ingredients to a large mixing bowl. It can be mixed by hand or with an immersion blender. Mix until desired consistency is achieved.
2. It can be served over burgers, sandwiches, salads and more. It can be stored in the refrigerator for up to 5 days or for longer in the freezer.

Nutrition:

Total Fat: 25.3g, Sodium: 3mg, Fiber: 2g.

12. Vegan Raw Cashew Cheese Sauce

Preparation Time: 5 minutes
Cooking Time: 5 minutes
Servings: 6
Ingredients:
- 1 cup raw cashews, soaked in water for at least 3 hours before making the recipe
- 2 tablespoons olive oil
- 2 tablespoon nutritional yeast
- 1/4 teaspoon garlic powder
- 2 tablespoons fresh lemon juice
- 1/2 cup water

Directions:
1. To prepare cashews before making the sauce, boil 2 cups of water, turn off the heat and add cashews. This can be allowed to soak overnight. Rinse and strained cashews. Discard water.
2. Add all ingredients to a food processor and blend until a smooth consistency is achieved. It can be used to make pizzas, over roasted veggies, in lasagna, as a dip and more.

Nutrition:
Total Fat: 15.5g, Sodium: 34mg, Total carbohydrates: 9.23g, Protein: 5.1g.

13. Spicy Avocado Mayonnaise

Preparation Time: 10 minutes
Cooking Time: 10 minutes
Servings: 8
Ingredients:
- 2 ripe avocados, pitted and peeled
- 1/4 jalapeno pepper, minced
- 2 tablespoon lemon juice
- 1/2 teaspoon onion powder
- 2 tablespoons fresh cilantro, chopped

Directions:
1. Add all ingredients to a food processor and blender until a smooth creamy consistency is achieved.
2. The jalapeno peppers can be foregone if you prefer a cooler mayo. It can be enjoyed in sandwiches, on toast, as a topping, in veggie wraps and salads.

Nutrition:

Total Fat: 9.8g, Cholesterol: 0mg, Sodium: 23mg, Total carbohydrates: 4.6g, Dietary Fiber: 3.4g, Protein: 1g.

14. Green Coconut Butter

Preparation Time: 10 minutes
Cooking Time: 10 minutes
Servings: 8
Ingredients:
- 2 cups unsweetened shredded coconut
- 2 teaspoon matcha powder
- 1 tablespoon coconut oil

Directions:
1. Add shredded coconut to a food processor and blend for 5 minutes or until a smooth but runny consistency is achieved.
2. Add matcha powder and olive oil. Blend for 1 more minute.
3. It can be stored in an airtight container at room temperature for up to 2 weeks. This is a delicious fruit sauce and can be added to smoothies, on pancakes and toast.

Nutrition:
Total Fat: 5.2g, Cholesterol: 0mg, Sodium: 3mg, Total carbohydrates: 1.7g, Dietary Fiber: 1.2g, Protein: 0.7g.

15. Spiced Almond Butter

Preparation Time: 10 minutes
Cooking Time: 5 minutes
Servings: 10
Ingredients:
- 2 cups raw almond
- 1/8 teaspoon allspice
- 1/8 teaspoon cinnamon
- 1/8 teaspoon cardamom
- 1/8 teaspoon ground ginger
- 1/8 teaspoon ground cloves

Directions:
1. Place all ingredients in a food processor and blend until a smooth consistency is achieved. Makes a delicious fruit and veggie dip and can be added to smoothies, on toast, on pancakes and waffles.

Nutrition:
Total Fat: 9.5g, Cholesterol: 0mg, Sodium: 117mg, Total carbohydrates: 4.1g, Dietary Fiber: 2.4g, Protein: 4g, Sodium: 63mg. Potassium: 123mg.

16. Edamame Hummus

Preparation Time: 15 minutes
Cooking Time: 11 minutes
Servings: 5
Ingredients:
- 10 ounces frozen edamame pods
- 1 ripe avocado, peeled, pitted, and chopped roughly
- 1/2 cup fresh cilantro, chopped
- 1/4 cup scallion, chopped
- 1 jalapeño pepper
- 1 garlic clove, peeled
- 2–3 tablespoons fresh lime juice
- Salt and ground black pepper to taste
- 1/4 cup avocado oil
- 2 tablespoons fresh basil leaves

Directions:
1. In a small pot of boiling water, cook the edamame pods for 6–8 minutes.
2. Drain the edamame pods and let them cool completely.
3. Remove soybeans from the pods.
4. In a food processor, add edamame and remaining ingredients (except for oil) and pulse until mostly pureed.
5. While the motor is running, add the reserved oil and pulse until light and smooth.
6. Transfer the hummus into a bowl and serve with the garnishing of remaining basil leaves.

Nutrition:
Calories: 339, Total Fat: 33.8g, Saturated Fat: 4.3g, Cholesterol: 0mg, Sodium: 27mg, Total Carbs: 6.3g, Fiber: 3.1g, Sugar: 0.3g, Protein: 5.1g, Potassium: 125mg.

17. Beans Mayonnaise

Preparation Time: 10 minutes
Cooking Time: 2 minutes
Servings: 4
Ingredients:
- 1 (15-ounce) can white beans, drained and rinsed
- 2 tablespoons apple cider vinegar
- 1 tablespoon fresh lemon juice
- 2 tablespoons yellow mustard
- 2 garlic cloves, peeled
- 2 tablespoons aquafaba (liquid from the can of beans)

Directions:

1. In a food processor, add all ingredients (except for oil) and pulse until mostly pureed.
2. While the motor is running, add the reserved oil and pulse until light and smooth.
3. Transfer the mayonnaise into a container and refrigerate to chill before serving.

Nutrition:
Calories: 8, Total Fat: 1.1g, Saturated Fat: 0.1g, Cholesterol: 0mg, Sodium: 559mg, Total Carbs: 14.3g, Fiber: 4.1g, Sugar: 0.2g, Protein: 5.2g, Potassium: 234mg.

18. Cashew Cream

Preparation Time: 10 minutes
Cooking Time: 0 minutes
Servings: 5
Ingredients:
- 1 cup raw, unsalted cashews, soaked for 12 hours and drained
- 1/2 cup water
- 1 tablespoon nutritional yeast
- 1 teaspoon fresh lemon juice

Directions:
1. In a food processor, add all ingredients and pulse at high speed until creamy and smooth.
2. Serve immediately.

Nutrition:
Calories: 165, Total Fat: 12.8g, Saturated Fat: 2.5g, Cholesterol: 0mg, Sodium: 65mg, Total Carbs: 9.9g, Fiber: 1.3g, Sugar: 1.4g, Protein: 5.1g, Potassium: 323mg.

19. Lemon Tahini

Preparation Time: 15 minutes
Cooking Time: 0 minutes
Servings: 4
Ingredients:
- 1/4 cup fresh lemon juice
- 4 medium garlic cloves, pressed
- 1/2 cup tahini
- Pinch of ground cumin
- 6 tablespoons ice water

Directions:
1. In a medium bowl, combine the lemon juice and garlic and set aside for 10 minutes.
2. Through a fine-mesh sieve, strain the mixture into another medium bowl, pressing the garlic solids.
3. Discard the garlic solids.
4. In the lemon juice bowl, add the tahini and cumin. Whisk until well blended.
5. Slowly, add water, 2 tablespoons at a time, whisking well after each addition.

Nutrition:

Calories: 187, Total Fat: 16.3g, Saturated Fat: 2.4g, Cholesterol: 0mg, Sodium: 273mg, Total Carbs: 7.7g, Fiber: 2.9g, Sugar: 0.5g, Protein: 5.4g, Potassium: 123mg.

20. Fancy Taco Seasoning

Preparation Time: 10 minutes

Cooking Time: 0 minutes
Servings: 4
Ingredients:

- 1 tablespoon of chili powder
- ½ a teaspoon of garlic powder
- ½ a teaspoon of onion powder
- 1 and a ½ teaspoon of ground cumin
- 1 teaspoon of pepper
- ¼ teaspoon of crushed red pepper flakes
- ¼ teaspoon of dried oregano
- ½ a teaspoon of paprika

Directions:

1. Mix the ingredients mentioned above to prepare the Taco seasoning and use it as needed.

Nutrition:

Calories: 10, Carbs: 7g, Protein: 2g, Sodium: 163mg, Potassium: 123mg.

Chapter 4. Sauces and Dressings

21. Salsa Verde

Preparation Time: 10 minutes
Cooking Time: 5 minutes
Servings: 5
Ingredients:
- 4 tablespoons fresh cilantro, finely chopped
- 1/4 cup fresh parsley, finely chopped
- 2 garlic cloves, grated
- 2 teaspoon lemon juice
- 3/4 cup of olive oil
- 2 tablespoon small capers
- 1/2 teaspoon black pepper

Directions:
1. Add all ingredients to a large mixing bowl. It can be mixed by hand or with an immersion blender. Mix until desired consistency is achieved.
2. It can be served over burgers, sandwiches, salads and more. It can be stored in the refrigerator for up to 5 days or for longer in the freezer.

Nutrition:
Total Fat: 25.3g, Cholesterol: 0mg, Sodium: 475mg, Protein: 0.2g, Potassium 123mg.

22. Caramel Sauce

Preparation Time: 10 minutes
Cooking Time: 35 minutes
Servings: 8
Ingredients:
- 1/2 cup raw cashews
- 1/2 cup coconut cream, melted
- 10 drops liquid stevia
- 2 tablespoon vegan butter
- 3 teaspoon vanilla extract

Directions:
1. Preheat your oven to 325 degrees F.
2. Place nuts on a greased baking tray and toast for 20 minutes or until lightly golden and crunchy.
3. Allow the nuts to cool slightly and add them to a food processor and blend to a slightly lumpy consistency.
4. Add remaining ingredients and blend until a smooth and creamy consistency is achieved. Do not over blend or the coconut cream will become separated from the rest of the ingredients

5. It can be stored in a glass, airtight container in the refrigerator if not being served immediately. To reheat the caramel to make it more flow able, add to a saucepan and gently warm on low heat. It can be served with your favorite keto vegan treats, such as ice cream.

Nutrition:
Total Fat: 9.8g, Cholesterol: 0mg, Sodium: 29mg, Total carbohydrates: 4.6g, Sodium: 103mg, Potassium: 123mg.

23. Pecan Butter

Preparation Time: 10 minutes
Cooking Time: 10 minutes
Servings: 8
Ingredients:
- 3 cups pecans, soaked well at least 3 hours, rinsed, strained and dried

Directions:
1. Add the pecans to a food processor and blend until a smooth and creamy consistency is achieved. Scrape down the sides of the bowl when necessary.
2. Transfer to a Mason jar and store in the refrigerator. It can be stored in the refrigerator for several months. Makes a great spread on toast and sandwiches and a great fruit and veggie dip.

Nutrition:
Total Fat: 25g, Cholesterol: 0mg, Sodium: 0mg, Total carbohydrates: 5g, Potassium 235mg.

24. Vegan Ranch Dressing

Preparation Time: 5 minutes
Cooking Time: 10 minutes
Servings: 3
Ingredients:
- 1 cup vegan mayo
- 1 1/2 cup coconut milk
- 2 scallions
- 2 garlic cloves, peeled
- 1 cup fresh dill
- 1 teaspoon garlic powder
- pepper to taste

Directions:

1. Add scallion, fresh dill and garlic cloves to a food processor and pulse until finely chopped.
2. Add the rest of the ingredients and blend until a smooth, creamy consistency is achieved. Makes a great creamy salad dressing. Store in the refrigerator.

Nutrition:
Total Fat: 11.9g, Cholesterol: 0mg, Sodium: 50mg, Fiber: 4g, Potassium 187mg.

25. Vegan Ketchup

Preparation Time: 35 minutes
Cooking Time: 11 minutes
Servings: 12
Ingredients:
1/8 t of the following:
- Mustard powder
- Cloves, ground
- 1/4 t. paprika
- 1/2 t. garlic powder
- 3/4 t. onion powder
- 3 tablespoons. apple cider vinegar
- 1/4 c. powdered monk fruit
- 1 c. water
- 6 oz. tomato paste

Directions:
1. In a little saucepan, whisk together all the ingredients.
2. Cover the pan and bring to low heat and simmer for 30 minutes, stirring occasionally.
3. Once reduced, add to the blender and puree until it's a smooth consistency.

Nutrition:
Calories: 13, Carbohydrates: 2g, Proteins: 0g, Fats: 0g, Sodium: 24mg, Potassium: 123mg.

26. Avocado Hummus

Preparation Time: 5 minutes
Cooking Time: 5 minutes
Servings: 6
Ingredients:
- 1 tablespoon cilantro, finely chopped
- 1/8 t. cumin
- 1 clove garlic

- 3 tablespoons. lime juice

1 1/2 tablespoon. of the following:
- Tahini
- Olive oil
- 2 avocados, medium cored & peeled
- 15 oz. chickpeas, drained
- pepper to taste

Directions:
1. In a food processor, add garlic, lime juice, tahini, olive oil, chickpeas, and pulse until combined.
2. Add cumin and avocados and blend until smooth consistency, approximately 2 minutes.
3. Add pepper to taste.

Nutrition:
Calories: 310, Carbohydrates: 26g, Proteins: 8g, Fats: 20g, Sodium: 63mg, Potassium: 345mg.

27. Guacamole with Tomato

Preparation Time: 5 minutes
Cooking Time: 5 minutes
Servings: 6
Ingredients:
3 tablespoons of the following:
- Tomato, diced
- Onion, diced

2 tablespoons of the following:
- Cilantro, chopped
- Jalapeno juice
- 1/4 t. garlic powder
- 1/2 lime, squeezed
- 2 big avocados
- 1 jalapeno, diced

Directions:
1. Using a molcajete, crush the diced jalapenos until soft.
2. Add the avocados to the molcajete.
3. Squeeze the lime juice from ½ of the lime on top of the avocados.
4. Add the jalapeno juice, garlic, and salt and mix until smooth.
5. Once smooth, add in the onion, cilantro, and tomato and stir to incorporate.

Nutrition:
Calories: 127, Carbohydrates: 9.3g, Proteins: 2.4g, Fats: 10.2g, Sodium: 53mg, Potassium: 113mg.

28. Vegan Mayo

Preparation Time: 5 minutes
Cooking Time: 5 minutes

Servings: 6
Ingredients:
1/2 c. of the following:
- Extra virgin olive oil
- Almond milk, unsweetened
- 1/4 t. xanthan gum
- Pinch of white pepper, ground
- 1 t. Dijon mustard
- 2 t. apple cider vinegar

Directions:
1. In a blender, place milk, pepper, mustard, and vinegar.
2. Turn the blender to high speed and slowly add xanthan and then the olive oil.
3. Remove from the blender and allow cooling for 2 hours in the refrigerator.
4. During cooling, the mixture will thicken.

Nutrition:
Calories: 160.4, Carbohydrates: 0.2g, Proteins: 0g, Fats: 18g, Sodium: 23mg, Potassium: 189mg.

29. Peanut Sauce

Preparation Time: 10 minutes
Cooking Time: 10 minutes
Servings: 4
Ingredients:
- 1/2 t. Thai red curry paste

1 t. of the following:
- Coconut oil
- Soy sauce
- Chili garlic sauce
- 1 tablespoon sweetener of your choice
- 1/3 c. coconut milk
- 1/4 c. peanut butter, smooth

Directions:
1. Using a microwave-safe dish, add the peanut butter and heat for about 30 seconds.
2. Whisk into the peanut butter, soy sauce, sweetener, and chili garlic, then set to the side.
3. Warm a little saucepan over medium heat and add oil.
4. Cook the Thai red curry paste until fragrant, then add to a microwave-safe bowl.
5. Continuously stir the peanut mixture as you add the coconut milk. Stir until well-combined.
6. Enjoy at room temperature or warmed.

Nutrition:
Calories: 151, Carbohydrates: 4g, Proteins: 4g, Fats: 13g, Sodium: 63mg, Potassium: 123mg.

30. Tasty Ranch Dressing/Dip

Preparation Time: 45 minutes
Cooking Time: 45 minutes
Servings: 16
Ingredients:
- 1/2 c. soy milk, unsweetened
- 1 tablespoon dill, chopped
- 2 t. parsley, chopped
- 1/4 t. black pepper

1/2 t. of the following:
- Onion powder
- Garlic powder
- 1 c. vegan mayonnaise

Directions:
1. In a medium bowl, whisk all the ingredients together until smooth. If dressing is too thick, add 1/4 tablespoon of soy milk at a time until the desired consistency.
2. Transfer to an airtight container or jar and refrigerate for 1 hour.
3. Serve over leafy greens or as a dip.

Nutrition:
Calories: 93, Carbohydrates: 0g, Proteins: 0g, Fats: 9g, Sodium: 63mg, Potassium: 100mg.

31. Creamy Avocado Cilantro Lime Dressing

Preparation Time: 5 minutes
Cooking Time: 0 minutes
Servings: 2
Ingredients:
- 1 avocado, diced
- ½ cup water
- ¼ cup cilantro leaves
- ¼ cup fresh lime or lemon juice (about 2 limes or lemons)
- ½ teaspoon ground cumin

Directions:
1. Put all the ingredients in a blender (high-speed blenders work best for this), and pulse until well combined. Taste and adjust the seasoning as needed. It is best served within 1 day.

Nutrition:
Calories: 94, Fat: 7.4g, Carbs: 5.7g, Protein: 1.1g, Fiber: 3.5g, Sodium: 63mg, Potassium 176mg.

32. Maple Dijon Dressing

Preparation Time: 5 minutes
Cooking Time: 0 minutes

Servings: 1
Ingredients:
- ¼ cup apple cider vinegar
- 2 teaspoons Dijon mustard
- 2 tablespoons maple syrup
- 2 tablespoons low-sodium vegetable broth
- ¼ teaspoon black pepper

Directions:
1. Mix the apple cider vinegar, Dijon mustard, maple syrup, vegetable broth, and black pepper in a resealable container until well incorporated.
2. The dressing can be refrigerated for up to 5 days.

Nutrition:
Calories: 82, Fat: 0.3g, Carbs: 19.3g, Protein: 0.6g, Fiber: 0.7g, Sodium: 53mg, Potassium: 67mg.

33. Avocado-Chickpea Dip

Preparation Time: 15 minutes
Cooking Time: 0 minutes
Servings: 2
Ingredients:
- 1 (15-ounce / 425-g) can cooked chickpeas, drained and rinsed
- 2 large, ripe avocados, chopped
- ¼ cup red onion, finely chopped
- 1 tablespoon Dijon mustard
- 1 to 2 tablespoons lemon juice
- 2 teaspoons chopped fresh oregano
- 1/2 teaspoon garlic clove, finely chopped

Directions:
1. In a medium bowl, mash the cooked chickpeas with a potato masher or the back of a fork, or until the chickpeas pop open (a food processor works best for this).
2. Stir in the remaining ingredients and continue to mash until completely smooth.
3. Place in the refrigerator to chill until ready to serve.

Nutrition:
Calories: 101, Fat: 1.9g, Carbs: 16.2g, Protein: 4.7g, Fiber: 4.6g, Sodium: 63mg, Potassium: 155mg.

34. Beer "Cheese" Dip

Preparation Time: 10 minutes
Cooking Time: 7 minutes
Servings: 3
Ingredients:

- ¾ cup water
- ¾ cup brown ale
- ½ cup raw walnuts, soaked in hot water for at least 15 minutes, then drained
- ½ cup raw cashews, soaked in hot water for at least 15 minutes, then drained
- 2 tablespoons tomato paste
- 2 tablespoons fresh lemon juice
- 1 tablespoon apple cider vinegar
- ½ cup nutritional yeast
- ½ teaspoon sweet or smoked paprika
- 1 tablespoon arrowroot powder
- 1 tablespoon red miso

Directions:
1. Place the water, brown ale, walnuts, cashews, tomato paste, lemon juice, apple cider vinegar into a high-speed blender, and purée until thoroughly mixed and smooth.
2. Transfer the mixture to a saucepan over medium heat. Add the nutritional yeast, paprika, and arrowroot powder, and whisk well. Bring to a simmer for about 7 minutes, stirring frequently, or until the mixture begins to thicken and bubble.
3. Remove from the heat and whisk in the red miso. Let the dip cool for 10 minutes and refrigerate in an airtight container for up to 5 days.

Nutrition:
Calories: 113, Fat: 5.1g, Carbs: 10.4g, Protein: 6.3g, Fiber: 3.8g, Potassium 176mg, Sodium: 43mg.

35. Creamy Black Bean Dip

Preparation Time: 10 minutes
Cooking Time: 0 minutes
Servings: 3
Ingredients:
- 4 cups cooked black beans, rinsed and drained
- 2 tablespoons Italian seasoning
- 2 tablespoons minced garlic
- 2 tablespoon low-sodium vegetable broth
- 2 tablespoons onion powder
- 1 tablespoon lemon juice, or more to taste

Directions:
1. In a large bowl, mash the black beans with a potato masher or the back of a fork until mostly smooth.

2. Add the remaining ingredients to the bowl and whisk to combine.
3. Taste and add more lemon juice, if needed. Serve immediately or refrigerate for at least 30 minutes to better incorporate the flavors.

Nutrition:
Calories: 387, Fat: 6.5g, Carbs: 63.0g, Protein: 21.2g, Fiber: 16.0g, Sodium: 63mg, Potassium: 76mg.

36. Spicy and Tangy Black Bean Salsa

Preparation Time: 15 minutes
Cooking Time: 0 minutes
Servings: 3
Ingredients:
- 1 (15-ounce / 425-g) can cooked black beans, drained and rinsed
- 1 cup chopped tomatoes
- 1 cup corn kernels, thawed if frozen
- ½ cup cilantro or parsley, chopped
- ¼ cup finely chopped red onion
- 1 tablespoon lemon juice
- 1 tablespoon lime juice
- 1 teaspoon chili powder
- ½ teaspoon ground cumin
- ½ teaspoon regular or smoked paprika
- 1 medium clove garlic, finely chopped

Directions:
1. Put all the ingredients in a large bowl and stir with a fork until well incorporated.
2. Serve immediately, or chill for 2 hours in the refrigerator to let the flavors blend.

Nutrition:
Calories: 83, Fat: 0.5g, Carbs: 15.4g, Protein: 4.3g, Fiber: 4.6g, Sodium: 33mg, Potassium: 133mg.

37. Homemade Chimichurri

Preparation Time: 5 minutes
Cooking Time: 0 minutes
Servings: 1
Ingredients:
- 1 cup finely chopped flat-leaf parsley leaves
- Zest and juice of 2 lemons
- ¼ cup low-sodium vegetable broth

- 4 garlic cloves
- 1 teaspoon dried oregano

Directions:
1. Place all the ingredients into a food processor, and pulse until it reaches the consistency you like.
2. Refrigerate the chimichurri in an airtight container for up to 5 days. It's best served within 1 day.

Nutrition:
Calories: 19, Fat: 0.2g, Carbs: 3.7g, Protein: 0.7g, Fiber: 0.7g, Sodium: 63mg, Potassium: 28mg.

38. Cilantro Coconut Pesto

Preparation Time: 5 minutes
Cooking Time: 0 minutes
Servings: 2
Ingredients:
- 1 (13.5-ounce / 383-g) can unsweetened coconut milk
- 2 jalapeños, seeds and ribs removed
- 1 bunch cilantro, leaves only
- 1 tablespoon white miso
- 1-inch (2.5 cm) piece ginger, peeled and minced
- Water, as needed

Directions:

1. Pulse all the ingredients in a blender until creamy and smooth.
2. Thin with a little extra water as needed to reach your preferred consistency.
3. Store in an airtight container in the fridge for up to 2 days or in the freezer for 6 months.

Nutrition:
Calories: 141, Fat: 13.7g, Carbs: 2.8g, Protein: 1.6g, Fiber: 0.3g, Sodium: 23mg, Potassium: 67mg.

39. Fresh Mango Salsa

Preparation Time: 10 minutes
Cooking Time: 0 minutes
Servings: 6
Ingredients:
- 2 small mangoes, diced
- 1 red bell pepper, finely diced
- ½ red onion, finely diced
- Juice of ½ lime, or more to taste
- 2 tablespoon low-sodium vegetable broth
- Handful cilantro, chopped
- Freshly ground black pepper to taste

Directions:
1. Stir together all the ingredients in a large bowl until well incorporated.
2. Taste and add more lime juice or salt, if needed.

3. Store in an airtight container in the fridge for up to 5 days.

Nutrition:
Calories: 86, Fat: 1.9g, Carbs: 13.3g, Protein: 1.2g, Fiber: 0.9g, Sodium: 63mg, Potassium: 58mg.

40. Pineapple Mint Salsa

Preparation Time: 10 minutes
Cooking Time: 0 minutes
Servings: 3
Ingredients:
- 1 pound (454 g) fresh pineapple, finely diced and juices reserved
- 1 bunch mint, leaves only, chopped
- 1 minced jalapeño (optional)
- 1 white or red onion, finely diced

Directions:
1. In a medium bowl, mix the pineapple with its juice, mint, jalapeño (if desired), and onion, and whisk well.,
2. Refrigerate in an airtight container for at least 2 hours to better incorporate the flavors.

Nutrition:
Calories: 58, Fat: 0.1g, Carbs: 13.7g, Protein: 0.5g, Fiber: 1.0g, Sodium: 63mg, Potassium: 87mg.

Chapter 5. Juices and Smoothies

41. Chocolate and Peanut Butter Smoothie

Preparation Time: 5 minutes
Cooking Time: 0 minutes
Servings: 4
Ingredients:

- 1 tablespoon unsweetened cocoa powder
- 1 tablespoon peanut butter
- 1 banana
- 1 teaspoon maca powder
- ½ cup unsweetened soy milk
- ¼ cup rolled oats
- 1 tablespoon flaxseeds
- 1 tablespoon maple syrup
- 1 cup water

Directions:

1. Add all the ingredients to a blender, then process until the mixture is smooth and creamy. Add water or soy milk if necessary.
2. Serve immediately.

Nutrition:

Calories: 474, Fat: 16.0g, Carbs: 27.0g, Fiber: 18.0g, Protein: 13.0g, Sodium: 53mg, Potassium: 89mg.

42. Golden Milk

Preparation Time: 5 minutes
Cooking Time: 0 minutes
Servings: 4
Ingredients:

- ¼ teaspoon ground cinnamon
- ½ teaspoon ground turmeric
- ½ teaspoon grated fresh ginger
- 1 teaspoon maple syrup
- 1 cup unsweetened coconut milk
- Ground black pepper to taste
- 2 tablespoon water

Directions:

1. Combine all the ingredients in a saucepan. Stir to mix well.
2. Heat over medium heat for 5 minutes. Keep stirring during the heating.
3. Allow to cool for 5 minutes, then pour the mixture into a blender. Pulse until creamy and smooth. Serve immediately.

Nutrition:

Calories: 577, Fat: 57.3g, Carbs: 19.7g, Fiber: 6.1g, Protein: 5.7g,

Sodium: 45mg, Potassium: 364mg.

43. Mango Agua Fresca

Preparation Time: 5 minutes
Cooking Time: 0 minutes
Servings: 2
Ingredients:

- 2 fresh mangoes, diced
- 1½ cups water
- 1 teaspoon fresh lime juice
- Maple syrup to taste
- 2 cups ice
- 2 slices fresh lime for garnish
- 2 fresh mint sprigs for garnish

Directions:

1. Put the mangoes, lime juice, maple syrup, and water in a blender. Process until creamy and smooth.
2. Divide the beverage into two glasses, then garnish each glass with ice, lime slice, and mint sprig before serving.

Nutrition:

Calories: 230, Fat: 1.3g, Carbs: 57.7g, Fiber: 5.4g, Protein: 2.8g, Sodium: 53mg, Potassium: 143mg.

44. Light Ginger Tea

Preparation Time: 5 minutes
Cooking Time: 10 to 15 minutes
Servings: 2
Ingredients:

- 1 small ginger knob, sliced into four 1-inch chunks
- 4 cups water
- Juice of 1 large lemon
- Maple syrup to taste

Directions:

1. Add the ginger knob and water in a saucepan, then simmer over medium heat for 10 to 15 minutes.
2. Turn off the heat, then mix in the lemon juice. Strain the liquid to remove the ginger, then fold in the maple syrup and serve.

Nutrition:

Calories: 32, Fat: 0.1g, Carbs: 8.6g, Fiber: 0.1g, Protein: 0.1g, Sodium: 63mg, Potassium: 187mg.

45. Classic Switchel

Preparation Time: 5 minutes
Cooking Time: 0 minutes
Servings: 4
Ingredients:

- 1-inch piece ginger, minced
- 2 tablespoons apple cider vinegar
- 2 tablespoons maple syrup
- 4 cups water
- ¼ teaspoon sea salt, optional

Directions:

1. Combine all the ingredients in a glass. Stir to mix well.
2. Serve immediately or chill in the refrigerator for an hour before serving.

Nutrition:

Calories: 110, Fat: 0g, Carbs: 28.0g, Fiber: 0g, Protein: 0g, Sodium: 63mg, Potassium: 387mg.

46. Lime and Cucumber Electrolyte Drink

Preparation Time: 5 minutes
Cooking Time: 0 minutes
Servings: 4
Ingredients:

- ¼ cup chopped cucumber
- 1 tablespoon fresh lime juice
- 1 tablespoon apple cider vinegar
- 2 tablespoons maple syrup
- ¼ teaspoon sea salt, optional
- 4 cups water

Directions:

1. Combine all the ingredients in a glass. Stir to mix well.
2. Refrigerate overnight before serving.

Nutrition:

Calories: 114, Fat: 0.1g, Carbs: 28.9g, Fiber: 0.3g, Protein: 0.3g, Sodium: 63mg, Potassium: 123mg.

47. Easy and Fresh Mango Madness

Preparation Time: 5 minutes
Cooking Time: 0 minutes
Servings: 4

Ingredients:
- 1 cup chopped mango
- 1 cup chopped peach
- 1 banana
- 1 cup strawberries
- 1 carrot, peeled and chopped
- 1 cup water

Directions:
1. Put all the ingredients in a food processor, then blitz until glossy and smooth.
2. Serve immediately or chill in the refrigerator for an hour before serving.

Nutrition:
Calories: 376, Fat: 22.0g, Carbs: 19.0g, Fiber: 14.0g, Protein: 5.0g, Sodium: 53mg, Potassium: 103mg.

48. Simple Date Shake

Preparation Time: 10 minutes
Cooking Time: 0 minutes
Servings: 2
Ingredients:
- 5 Medjool dates, pitted, soaked in boiling water for 5 minutes
- ¾ cup unsweetened coconut milk
- 1 teaspoon vanilla extract
- ½ teaspoon fresh lemon juice
- ¼ teaspoon sea salt, optional
- 1½ cups ice

Directions:
1. Put all the ingredients in a food processor, then blitz until it has a milkshake and smooth texture.
2. Serve immediately.

Nutrition:
Calories: 380, Fat: 21.6g, Carbs: 50.3g, Fiber: 6.0g, Protein: 3.2g, Sodium: 63mg, Potassium: 189mg.

49. Beet and Clementine Protein Smoothie

Preparation Time: 10 minutes
Cooking Time: 0 minutes
Servings: 3
Ingredients:
- 1 small beet, peeled and chopped
- 1 clementine, peeled and broken into segments
- ½ ripe banana
- ½ cup raspberries
- 1 tablespoon chia seeds
- 2 tablespoons almond butter

- ¼ teaspoon vanilla extract
- 1 cup unsweetened almond milk
- 1/8 teaspoon fine sea salt, optional

Directions:
1. Combine all the ingredients in a food processor, then pulse on high for 2 minutes or until glossy and creamy.
2. Refrigerate for an hour and serve chilled.

Nutrition:
Calories: 526, Fat: 25.4g, Carbs: 61.9g, Fiber: 17.3g, Protein: 20.6g, Sodium: 69mg, Potassium: 352mg

50. Matcha Limeade

Preparation Time: 10 minutes
Cooking Time: 0 minutes
Servings: 4
Ingredients:
- 2 tablespoons matcha powder
- ¼ cup raw agave syrup
- 3 cups water, divided
- 1 cup fresh lime juice
- 3 tablespoons chia seeds

Directions:
1. Lightly simmer the matcha, agave syrup, and 1 cup of water in a saucepan over medium heat. Keep stirring until no matcha lumps.
2. Pour the matcha mixture into a large glass, add the remaining ingredients, and mix well.
3. Refrigerate for at least an hour before serving.

Nutrition:
Calories: 152, Fat: 4.5g, Carbs: 26.8g, Fiber: 5.3g, Protein: 3.7g, Sodium: 148mg, Potassium: 165mg.

51. Fruit Infused Water

Preparation Time: 5 minutes
Cooking Time: 0 minutes
Servings: 2
Ingredients:
- 3 strawberries, sliced
- 5 mint leaves
- ½ of orange, sliced
- 2 cups of water

Directions:
1. Divide fruits and mint between two glasses, pour in water, stir until just mixed, and refrigerate for 2 hours.
2. Serve straight away.

Nutrition:
Calories: 5.4, Fat: 0.1g, Carbs: 1.3g, Protein: 0.1g, Fiber: 0.4g, Sodium: 73mg, Potassium: 125mg.

52. Hazelnut and Chocolate Milk

Preparation Time: 5 minutes
Cooking Time: 0 minutes
Servings: 2
Ingredients:
- 2 tablespoons cocoa powder
- 4 dates, pitted
- 1 cup hazelnuts
- 3 cups of water

Directions:
1. Place all the ingredients in the order in a food processor or blender and then pulse for 2 to 3 minutes at high speed until smooth.
2. Pour the smoothie into two glasses and then serve.

Nutrition:
Calories: 120, Fat: 5g, Carbs: 19g, Protein: 2g, Fiber: 1g, Sodium: 34mg, Potassium: 755mg.

53. Banana Milk

Preparation Time: 5 minutes
Cooking Time: 0 minutes
Servings: 2
Ingredients:
- 2 dates
- 2 medium bananas, peeled
- 1 teaspoon vanilla extract, unsweetened
- 1/2 cup ice
- 2 cups of water

Directions:
1. Place all the ingredients in the order in a food processor or blender and then pulse for 2 to 3 minutes at high speed until smooth.
2. Pour the smoothie into two glasses and then serve.

Nutrition:
Calories: 79, Fat: 0g, Carbs: 19.8g, Protein: 0.8g, Fiber: 6g, Sodium: 53mg, Potassium: 234mg.

54. Apple, Carrot, Celery and Kale Juice

Preparation Time: 5 minutes
Cooking Time: 0 minutes
Servings: 2
Ingredients:
- 5 curly kale
- 2 green apples, cored, peeled, chopped
- 2 large stalks celery
- 4 large carrots, cored, peeled, chopped

Directions:
1. Process all the ingredients in the order in a juicer or blender and then strain it into two glasses.
2. Serve straight away.

Nutrition:
Calories: 183, Fat: 2.5g, Carbs: 46g, Protein: 13g, Fiber: 3g, Sodium: 63mg, Potassium: 186mg.

55. Sweet and Sour Juice

Preparation Time: 5 minutes
Cooking Time: 0 minutes
Servings: 2
Ingredients:
- 2 medium apples, cored, peeled, chopped
- 2 large cucumbers, peeled
- 4 cups chopped grapefruit
- 1 cup mint

Directions:
1. Process all the ingredients in the order in a juicer or blender and then strain it into two glasses.
2. Serve straight away.

Nutrition:
Calories: 90, Fat: 0g, Carbs: 23g, Protein: 0g, Fiber: 9g, Sodium: 63mg, Potassium: 286mg.

56. Green Lemonade

Preparation Time: 5 minutes
Cooking Time: 0 minutes
Servings: 2
Ingredients:
- 10 large stalks of celery, chopped
- 2 medium green apples, cored, peeled, chopped

- 2 medium cucumbers, peeled, chopped
- 2 inches' piece of ginger
- 10 stalks of kale, chopped
- 2 cups parsley

Directions:
1. Process all the ingredients in the order in a juicer or blender and then strain it into two glasses.
2. Serve straight away.

Nutrition:
Calories: 102.3, Fat: 1.1g, Carbs: 26.2g, Protein: 4.7g, Fiber: 8.5g, Sodium: 43mg, Potassium: 103mg.

57. Pineapple and Spinach Juice

Preparation Time: 5 minutes
Cooking Time: 0 minutes
Servings: 2
Ingredients:
- 2 medium red apples, cored, peeled, chopped
- 3 cups spinach
- ½ of a medium pineapple, peeled
- 2 lemons, peeled

Directions:
1. Process all the ingredients in the order in a juicer or blender and then strain it into two glasses.
2. Serve straight away.

Nutrition:
Calories: 131, Fat: 0.5g, Carbs: 34.5g, Protein: 1.7g, Fiber: 5g, Sodium: 63mg, Potassium: 198mg.

58. Strawberry, Blueberry and Banana Smoothie

Preparation Time: 5 minutes
Cooking Time: 0 minutes
Servings: 2
Ingredients:
- 1 tablespoon hulled hemp seeds
- ½ cup of frozen strawberries
- 1 small frozen banana
- ½ cup frozen blueberries
- 2 tablespoons cashew butter
- ¾ cup cashew milk, unsweetened

Directions:

1. Place all the ingredients in the order in a food processor or blender and then pulse for 2 to 3 minutes at high speed until smooth.
2. Pour the smoothie into two glasses and then serve.

Nutrition:
Calories: 334, Fat: 17g, Carbs: 46g, Protein: 7g, Fiber: 7g, Sodium: 63mg, Potassium: 285mg.

59. Mango, Pineapple and Banana Smoothie

Preparation Time: 5 minutes
Cooking Time: 0 minutes
Servings: 2
Ingredients:
- 2 cups pineapple chunks
- 2 frozen bananas
- 2 medium mangoes, destoned, cut into chunks
- 1 cup almond milk, unsweetened
- Chia seeds as needed for garnishing

Directions:
1. Place all the ingredients in the order in a food processor or blender and then pulse for 2 to 3 minutes at high speed until smooth.
2. Pour the smoothie into two glasses and then serve.

Nutrition:
Calories: 287, Fat: 1.2g, Carbs: 73.3g, Protein: 3.5g, Fiber: 8g, Sodium: 53mg, Potassium: 364mg.

60. Blueberry and Banana Smoothie

Preparation Time: 5 minutes
Cooking Time: 0 minutes
Servings: 2
Ingredients:
- 2 frozen bananas
- 2 cups frozen blueberries
- 2 cups almond milk, unsweetened
- 1/2 teaspoon or so cinnamon
- dash of vanilla extract

Directions:

1. Place all the ingredients in the order in a food processor or blender and then pulse for 2 to 3 minutes at high speed until smooth.
2. Pour the smoothie into two glasses and then serve.

Nutrition:
Calories: 244, Fat: 3.8g, Carbs: 51.5g, Protein: 4g, Fiber: 7.3g, Sodium: 63mg, Potassium: 113mg.

61. Chard, Lettuce and Ginger Smoothie

Preparation Time: 5 minutes
Cooking Time: 0 minutes
Servings: 2
Ingredients:
- 10 Chard leaves, chopped
- 1-inch piece of ginger, chopped
- 10 lettuce leaves, chopped
- ½ teaspoon black salt
- 2 pears, chopped
- 2 teaspoons coconut sugar
- ¼ teaspoon ground black pepper
- ¼ teaspoon salt
- 2 tablespoons lemon juice
- 2 cups of water

Directions:
1. Place all the ingredients in the order in a food processor or blender and then pulse for 2 to 3 minutes at high speed until smooth.
2. Pour the smoothie into two glasses and then serve.

Nutrition:
Calories: 514, Fat: 0g, Carbs: 15g, Protein: 4g, Fiber: 4g, Sodium: 63mg, Potassium: 375mg.

62. Red Beet, Pear and Apple Smoothie

Preparation Time: 5 minutes
Cooking Time: 0 minutes
Servings: 2
Ingredients:
- 1/2 of medium beet, peeled, chopped
- 1 tablespoon chopped cilantro
- 1 orange, juiced

- 1 medium pear, chopped
- 1 medium apple, cored, chopped
- 1/4 teaspoon ground black pepper
- 1/8 teaspoon rock salt
- 1 teaspoon coconut sugar
- 1/4 teaspoons salt
- 1 cup of water

Directions:
1. Place all the ingredients in the order in a food processor or blender and then pulse for 2 to 3 minutes at high speed until smooth.
2. Pour the smoothie into two glasses and then serve.

Nutrition:
Calories: 132, Fat: 0g, Carbs: 34g, Protein: 1g, Fiber: 5g, Sodium: 53mg, Potassium: 214mg.

63. Berry and Yogurt Smoothie

Preparation Time: 5 minutes
Cooking Time: 0 minutes
Servings: 2
Ingredients:
- 2 small bananas
- 3 cups frozen mixed berries
- 1 ½ cup cashew yogurt
- 1/2 teaspoon vanilla extract, unsweetened
- 1/2 cup almond milk, unsweetened

Directions:
1. Place all the ingredients in the order in a food processor or blender and then pulse for 2 to 3 minutes at high speed until smooth.
2. Pour the smoothie into two glasses and then serve.

Nutrition:
Calories: 326, Fat: 6.5g, Carbs: 65.6g, Protein: 8g, Fiber: 8.4g, Sodium: 53mg, Potassium: 324mg.

64. Chocolate and Cherry Smoothie

Preparation Time: 5 minutes
Cooking Time: 0 minutes
Servings: 2
Ingredients:
- 4 cups frozen cherries
- 2 tablespoons cocoa powder

- 1 scoop of protein powder
- 1 teaspoon maple syrup
- 2 cups almond milk, unsweetened

Directions:
1. Place all the ingredients in the order in a food processor or blender and then pulse for 2 to 3 minutes at high speed until smooth.
2. Pour the smoothie into two glasses and then serve.

Nutrition:
Calories: 324, Fat: 5g, Carbs: 75.1g, Protein: 7.2g, Fiber: 11.3g, Sodium: 63mg, Potassium: 644mg.

65. Strawberry and Chocolate Milkshake

Preparation Time: 5 minutes
Cooking Time: 0 minutes
Servings: 2
Ingredients:
- 2 cups frozen strawberries
- 3 tablespoons cocoa powder
- 1 scoop protein powder
- 2 tablespoons maple syrup
- 1 teaspoon vanilla extract, unsweetened
- 2 cups almond milk, unsweetened

Directions:
1. Place all the ingredients in the order in a food processor or blender and then pulse for 2 to 3 minutes at high speed until smooth.
2. Pour the smoothie into two glasses and then serve.

Nutrition:
Calories: 199, Fat: 4.1g, Carbs: 40.5g, Protein: 3.7g, Fiber: 5.5g, Sodium: 63mg, Potassium: 223mg.

66. Trope-Kale Breeze

Preparation Time: 5 minutes
Cooking Time: 0 minutes
Servings: 3 to 4 cups
Ingredients:
- 1 cup chopped pineapple (frozen or fresh)
- 1 cup chopped mango (frozen or fresh)

- ½ to 1 cup chopped kale
- ½ avocado
- ½ cup coconut milk
- 1 cup water or coconut water
- 1 teaspoon matcha green tea powder (optional)

Directions:
1. Purée everything in a blender until smooth, adding more water (or coconut milk) if needed.

Nutrition:
Calories: 566, Total Fat: 36g, Carbs: 66g, Fiber: 12g, Protein: 8g, Sodium: 46mg, Potassium: 123mg.

67. Overnight Oats on the Go

Preparation Time: 5 minutes
Cooking Time: 5 minutes or overnight
Servings: 1 serving
Ingredients:
Basic Overnight Oats
- ½ cup rolled oats, or quinoa flakes for gluten-free
- 1 tablespoon ground flaxseed, or chia seeds, or hemp hearts
- 1 tablespoon maple syrup or coconut sugar (optional)
- ¼ teaspoon ground cinnamon (optional)

Topping Options
- 1 apple, chopped, and 1 tablespoon walnuts
- 2 tablespoons dried cranberries and 1 tablespoon pumpkin seeds
- 1 pear, chopped, and 1 tablespoon cashews
- 1 cup sliced grapes and 1 tablespoon sunflower seeds
- 1 banana, sliced, and 1 tablespoon peanut butter
- 2 tablespoons raisins and 1 tablespoon hazelnuts
- 1 cup berries and 1 tablespoon unsweetened coconut flakes

Directions:
1. Mix the oats, flax, maple syrup, and cinnamon (if using) in a bowl or to-go container (a travel mug or short thermos works beautifully).
2. Pour enough cool water over the oats to submerge them and stir to combine. Leave to soak for a minimum of half an hour or overnight.
3. Add your choice of toppings.

Nutrition:
Calories: 244, Total Fat: 6g, Carbs: 30g, Fiber: 6g, Protein: 7g, Sodium: 63mg, Potassium: 325mg.

68. Zobo Drink

Preparation Time: 5 minutes
Cooking Time: 10 minutes
Servings: 8
Ingredients:
- 2 cups dried hibiscus petals (zobo leaves), rinsed
- Pineapple rind from 1 pineapple
- 1 cup of granulated sugar
- 1 tsp. fresh ginger, grated
- 10 cups of water

Directions:
1. Add water, ginger, and sugar into the pot and mix well.
2. Then add zobo leaves and pineapple rind.
3. Cover and cook on High for 10 minutes. Open and discard solids.
4. Chill and serve.

Nutrition:
Calories: 65, Carbs: 7g, Fat: 2.6g, Protein: 1.14g, Sodium: 63mg, Potassium: 434mg.

69. Basil Lime Green Tea

Preparation Time: 5 minutes
Cooking Time: 4 minutes
Servings: 8
Ingredients:
- 8 cups of filtered water
- 10 bags of green tea
- ¼ cup of honey
- A pinch of baking soda
- Lime slices to taste
- Lemon slices to taste
- Basil leaves to taste

Directions:
1. Add water, honey, and baking soda to the pot and mix. Add the tea bags and cover. Cook on High for 4 minutes. Open and serve with lime slices, lemon slices, and basil leaves.

Nutrition:
Calories: 32, Carbs: 8g, Fat: 0g, Protein: 0g, Sodium: 63mg, Potassium: 164mg.

70. Turmeric Coconut Milk

Preparation Time: 5 minutes
Cooking Time: 15 minutes
Servings: 8
Ingredients:
- 13.5 oz. coconut milk
- 3 cups of filtered water
- 2 tsp. turmeric powder
- 3 whole cloves
- 2 cinnamon sticks
- ½ tsp. ginger powder
- A pinch of pepper
- 2 tbsp. honey

Directions:
1. Place everything except the honey in the pot. Cover and cook on High for 15 minutes. Remove cloves and cinnamon sticks. Add honey, mix and serve.

Nutrition:
Calories: 42, Carbs: 9g, Fat: 0g, Protein: 0g, Sodium: 63mg, Potassium: 645mg.

71. Berry Lemonade Tea

Preparation Time: 5 minutes
Cooking Time: 12 minutes
Servings: 4
Ingredients:
- 3 tea bags
- 2 cups of natural lemonade
- 1 cup of frozen mixed berries
- 2 cups of water
- 1 lemon, sliced

Directions:
1. Put everything in the Instant Pot and cover. Cook on High for 12 minutes. Open, strain, and serve.

Nutrition:
Calories: 21, Carbs: 8g, Fat: 0.2g, Protein: 0.4g, Sodium: 53mg, Potassium: 87mg.

72. Swedish Glögg

Preparation Time: 5 minutes
Cooking Time: 15 minutes
Servings: 1
Ingredients:
- ½ cup of orange juice
- ½ cup of water
- 1 piece of ginger cut into ½ pieces

- 1 whole clove
- 1 opened cardamom pods
- 2 tbsps. orange zest
- 1 cinnamon stick
- 1 whole allspice
- 1 vanilla bean

Directions:
1. Add everything in the pot. Cover and cook on High for 15 minutes. Open and serve.

Nutrition:
Calories: 194, Carbs: 41g, Fat: 3g, Protein: 1.7g, Sodium: 63mg, Potassium: 244mg.

73. Kale Smoothie
Preparation Time: 5 minutes
Cooking Time: 0 minutes
Servings: 2
Ingredients:
- 2 cups chopped kale leaves
- 1 banana, peeled
- 1 cup frozen strawberries
- 1 cup unsweetened almond milk
- 4 Medjool dates, pitted and chopped

Directions:
1. Put all the ingredients in a food processor, then blitz until glossy and smooth.
2. Serve immediately or chill in the refrigerator for an hour before serving.

Nutrition:
Calories: 663, Fat: 10.0g, Carbs: 142.5g, Fiber: 19.0g, Protein: 17.4g, Sodium: 63mg, Potassium: 120mg.

74. Hot Tropical Smoothie
Preparation Time: 5 minutes
Cooking Time: 0 minutes
Servings: 4
Ingredients:
- 1 cup frozen mango chunks
- 1 cup frozen pineapple chunks
- 1 small tangerine, peeled and pitted
- 2 cups spinach leaves
- 1 cup coconut water
- ¼ teaspoon cayenne pepper, optional

Directions:
1. Add all the ingredients to a food processor, then blitz until the mixture is smooth and combine well.

2. Serve immediately or chill in the refrigerator for an hour before serving.

Nutrition:
Calories: 283, Fat: 1.9g, Carbs: 67.9g, Fiber: 10.4g, Protein: 6.4g, Sodium: 63mg, Potassium: 133mg.

75. Berry Smoothie
Preparation Time: 5 minutes
Cooking Time: 0 minutes
Servings: 4
Ingredients:
- 1 cup berry mix (strawberries, blueberries, and cranberries)
- 4 Medjool dates, pitted and chopped
- 1½ cups unsweetened almond milk, plus more as needed

Directions:
1. Add all the ingredients to a blender, then process until the mixture is smooth and well mixed.
2. Serve immediately or chill in the refrigerator for an hour before serving.

Nutrition:
Calories: 473, Fat: 4.0g, Carbs: 103.7g, Fiber: 9.7g, Protein: 14.8g, Sodium: 63mg, Potassium: 123mg.

76. Cranberry and Banana Smoothie
Preparation Time: 5 minutes
Cooking Time: 0 minutes
Servings: 4
Ingredients:
- 1 cup frozen cranberries
- 1 large banana, peeled
- 4 Medjool dates, pitted and chopped
- 1½ cups unsweetened almond milk

Directions:
1. Add all the ingredients to a food processor, then process until the mixture is glossy and well mixed.
2. Serve immediately or chill in the refrigerator for an hour before serving.

Nutrition:
Calories: 616, Fat: 8.0g, Carbs: 132.8g, Fiber: 14.6g, Protein: 15.7g, Sodium: 63mg, Potassium: 434mg.

77. Pumpkin Smoothie
Preparation Time: 5 minutes
Cooking Time: 0 minutes
Servings: 5
Ingredients:
- ½ cup pumpkin purée
- 4 Medjool dates, pitted and chopped
- 1 cup unsweetened almond milk
- ¼ teaspoon vanilla extract
- ¼ teaspoon ground cinnamon
- ½ cup ice
- Pinch ground nutmeg

Directions:
1. Add all the ingredients to a blender, then process until the mixture is glossy and well mixed.
2. Serve immediately.

Nutrition:
Calories: 417, Fat: 3.0g, Carbs: 94.9g, Fiber: 10.4g, Protein: 11.4g, Sodium: 63mg, Potassium: 433mg.

78. Super Smoothie
Preparation Time: 5 minutes
Cooking Time: 0 minutes
Servings: 4
Ingredients:
- 1 banana, peeled
- 1 cup chopped mango
- 1 cup raspberries
- ¼ cup rolled oats
- 1 carrot, peeled
- 1 cup chopped fresh kale
- 2 tablespoons chopped fresh parsley
- 1 tablespoon flaxseeds
- 1 tablespoon grated fresh ginger
- ½ cup unsweetened soy milk
- 1 cup water

Directions:
1. Put all the ingredients in a food processor, then blitz until glossy and smooth.
2. Serve immediately or chill in the refrigerator for an hour before serving.

Nutrition:
Calories: 550, Fat: 39.0g, Carbs: 31.0g, Fiber: 15.0g, Protein: 13.0g, Sodium: 63mg, Potassium: 44mg.

79. Kiwi and Strawberry Smoothie

Preparation Time: 5 minutes
Cooking Time: 0 minutes
Servings: 3
Ingredients:

- 1 kiwi, peeled
- 5 medium strawberries
- ½ frozen banana
- 1 cup unsweetened almond milk
- 2 tablespoons hemp seeds
- 2 tablespoons peanut butter
- 1 to 2 teaspoons maple syrup
- ½ cup spinach leaves
- Handful broccoli sprouts

Directions:

1. Put all the ingredients in a food processor, then blitz until creamy and smooth.
2. Serve immediately or chill in the refrigerator for an hour before serving.

Nutrition:

Calories: 562, Fat: 28.6g, Carbs: 63.6g, Fiber: 15.1g, Protein: 23.3g, Sodium: 63mg, Potassium: 34mg.

80. Banana and Chai Chia Smoothie

Preparation Time: 5 minutes
Cooking Time: 0 minutes
Servings: 3
Ingredients:

- 1 banana
- 1 cup alfalfa sprouts
- 1 tablespoon chia seeds
- ½ cup unsweetened coconut milk
- 1 to 2 soft Medjool dates, pitted
- ¼ teaspoon ground cinnamon
- 1 tablespoon grated fresh ginger
- 1 cup water
- Pinch ground cardamom

Directions:

1. Add all the ingredients to a blender, then process until the mixture is smooth and creamy. Add water or coconut milk if necessary.
2. Serve immediately.

Nutrition:

Calories: 477, Fat: 41.0g, Carbs: 31.0g, Fiber: 14.0g, Protein: 8.0g, Sodium: 63mg, Potassium: 320mg.

Chapter 6. Breakfast

81. Blueberry Waffles

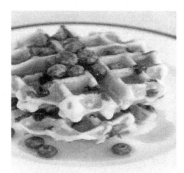

Preparation Time: 15 minutes
Cooking Time: 15 minutes
Servings: 8
Ingredients:

- 2 cups whole wheat flour
- 1 tablespoon baking powder
- 1 teaspoon ground cinnamon
- 2 tablespoons sugar
- 2 large eggs
- 3 tablespoons unsalted butter, melted
- 3 tablespoons nonfat plain Greek yogurt
- 1½ cups 1% milk
- 2 teaspoons vanilla extract
- 4 ounces blueberries
- Nonstick cooking spray
- ½ cup maple almond butter

Directions:

1. Preheat waffle iron. Mix the flour, baking powder, cinnamon, plus sugar in a large bowl. Mix the eggs, melted butter, yogurt, milk, and vanilla in a small bowl. Combine well.
2. Put the wet fixing to the dry mix and whisk until well combined. Do not over whisk; it's okay if the mixture has some lumps. Fold in the blueberries.
3. Grease the waffle iron with cooking spray. Then cook 1/3 cup of the batter until the waffles are lightly browned and slightly crisp. Repeat with the rest of the batter.
4. Place 2 waffles in each of 4 storage containers. Store the almond butter in 4 condiment cups. To serve, top each warm waffle with 1 tablespoon of maple almond butter.

Nutrition:
Calories: 647, Fat: 37g, Carbohydrates: 67g, Protein: 22g, Sodium: 156mg, Potassium: 123mg.

82. Apple Pancakes

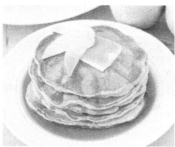

Preparation Time: 15 minutes
Cooking Time: 5 minutes
Servings: 16
Ingredients:

- ¼ cup extra-virgin olive oil, divided
- 1 cup whole wheat flour
- 2 teaspoons baking powder
- 1 teaspoon baking soda
- 1 teaspoon ground cinnamon
- 1 cup 1% milk
- 2 large eggs
- 1 medium Gala apple, diced
- 2 tablespoons maple syrup
- ¼ cup chopped walnuts

Directions:

1. Set aside 1 teaspoon of oil to use for greasing a griddle or skillet. In a large bowl, stir the flour, baking powder, baking soda, cinnamon, milk, eggs, apple, and the remaining oil.
2. Warm griddle or skillet on medium-high heat and coat with the reserved oil. Working in batches, pour in about ¼ cup of the batter for each pancake. Cook until browned on both sides.
3. Place 4 pancakes into each of 4 medium storage containers and the maple syrup in 4 small containers. Put each serving with 1 tablespoon of walnuts and drizzle with ½ tablespoon of maple syrup.

Nutrition:
Calories: 378, Fat: 22g, Carbohydrates: 39g, Protein: 10g, Sodium: 65mg, Potassium: 132mg.

83. Super-Simple Granola

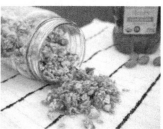

Preparation Time: 15 minutes
Cooking Time: 25 minutes
Servings: 8
Ingredients:

- ¼ cup extra-virgin olive oil
- ¼ cup honey
- ½ teaspoon ground cinnamon
- ½ teaspoon vanilla extract
- ¼ teaspoon salt
- 2 cups rolled oats
- ½ cup chopped walnuts
- ½ cup slivered almonds

Directions:

1. Preheat the oven to 350°F. Mix the oil, honey, cinnamon, vanilla, and salt in a large bowl. Add the oats, walnuts, and almonds. Stir to coat. Put the batter out onto the prepared sheet pan. Bake for 20 minutes. Let cool.

Nutrition:
Calories: 254, Fat: 16g, Carbohydrates: 25g, Fiber: 3.5g, Protein: 5g, Potassium: 163mg, Sodium: 73mg.

84. Savory Yogurt Bowls

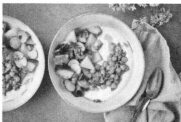

Preparation Time: 15 minutes
Cooking Time: 0 minutes

Servings: 4
Ingredients:
- 1 medium cucumber, diced
- ½ cup pitted Kalamata olives, halved
- 2 tablespoons fresh lemon juice
- 1 tablespoon extra-virgin olive oil
- 1 teaspoon dried oregano
- ¼ teaspoon freshly ground black pepper
- 2 cups nonfat plain Greek yogurt
- ½ cup slivered almonds

Directions:
1. In a small bowl, mix the cucumber, olives, lemon juice, oil, oregano, and pepper. Divide the yogurt evenly among 4 storage containers. Top with the cucumber-olive mix and almonds.

Nutrition:
Calories: 240, Fat: 16g, Carbohydrates: 10gm, Protein: 16g, Potassium: 353mg, Sodium: 350mg.

85. Energy Sunrise Muffins

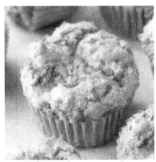

Preparation Time: 15 minutes
Cooking Time: 25 minutes
Servings: 16
Ingredients:
- Nonstick cooking spray
- 2 cups whole wheat flour
- 2 teaspoons baking soda
- 2 teaspoons ground cinnamon
- 1 teaspoon ground ginger
- ¼ teaspoon salt
- 3 large eggs
- ½ cup packed brown sugar
- 1/3 cup unsweetened applesauce
- ¼ cup honey
- ¼ cup vegetable or canola oil
- 1 teaspoon grated orange zest
- Juice of 1 medium orange
- 2 teaspoons vanilla extract
- 2 cups shredded carrots
- 1 large apple, peeled and grated

- ½ cup golden raisins
- ½ cup chopped pecans
- ½ cup unsweetened coconut flakes

Directions:
1. If you can fit two 12-cup muffin tins side by side in your oven, then leave a rack in the middle, and preheat the oven to 350°F.
2. Coat 16 cups of the muffin tins with cooking spray or line with paper liners. Mix the flour, baking soda, cinnamon, ginger, and salt in a large bowl. Set aside.
3. Mix the eggs, brown sugar, applesauce, honey, oil, orange zest, orange juice, and vanilla until combined in a medium bowl. Add the carrots and apple and whisk again.
4. Mix the dry and wet ingredients with a spatula. Fold in the raisins, pecans, and coconut. Mix everything once again, just until well combined. Put the batter into the prepared muffin cups, filling them to the top.
5. Bake within 20 to 25 minutes, or until a wooden toothpick inserted into the middle of the center muffin comes out clean (switching racks halfway through if baking on 2 racks). Cool for 5 minutes in the tins, then transfer to a wire rack to cool for an additional 5 minutes. Cool completely before storing in containers.

Nutrition:
Calories: 292, Fat: 14g, Carbohydrates: 42g, Protein: 5g, Sodium: 84mg, Potassium: 322mg.

86. Spinach, Egg, and Cheese Breakfast Quesadillas

Preparation Time: 15 minutes
Cooking Time: 15 minutes
Servings: 4
Ingredients:
- 1½ tablespoons extra-virgin olive oil
- ½ medium onion, diced
- 1 medium red bell pepper, diced
- 4 large eggs
- 1/8 teaspoon salt
- 1/8 teaspoon freshly ground black pepper
- 4 cups baby spinach
- ½ cup crumbled feta cheese
- Nonstick cooking spray

- 4 (6-inch) whole-wheat tortillas, divided
- 1 cup shredded part-skim low-moisture mozzarella cheese, divided

Directions:
1. Heat the oil over medium heat in a large skillet. Add the onion and bell pepper and sauté for about 5 minutes, or until soft.
2. Mix the eggs, salt, and black pepper in a medium bowl. Stir in the spinach and feta cheese. Put the egg batter in the skillet and scramble for about 2 minutes, or until the eggs are cooked. Remove from the heat.
3. Coat a clean skillet with cooking spray and add 2 tortillas. Place one-quarter of the spinach-egg mixture on one side of each tortilla. Sprinkle each with ¼ cup of mozzarella cheese. Fold the other halves of the tortillas down to close the quesadillas and brown for about 1 minute.
4. Turn over and cook again in a minute on the other side. Repeat with the remaining 2 tortillas and ½ cup of mozzarella cheese. Cut each quesadilla in half or wedges. Divide among 4 storage containers or reusable bags.

Nutrition:
Calories: 453, Fat: 28g, Carbohydrates: 28g, Fiber: 4.5g, Protein: 23g, Potassium: 205mg, Sodium: 837mg.

87. Simple Cheese and Broccoli Omelets

Preparation Time: 15 minutes
Cooking Time: 10 minutes
Servings: 4
Ingredients:
- 3 tablespoons extra-virgin olive oil, divided
- 2 cups chopped broccoli
- 8 large eggs
- ¼ cup 1% milk
- ½ teaspoon freshly ground black pepper
- 8 tablespoons shredded reduced-fat Monterey Jack cheese, divided

Directions:
1. In a nonstick skillet, heat 1 tablespoon of oil over medium-high flame. Add the broccoli and sauté, occasionally stirring, for 3 to 5 minutes, or until the

broccoli turns bright green. Scrape into a bowl.
2. Mix the eggs, milk, plus pepper in a small bowl. Wipe out the skillet and heat ½ tablespoon of oil. Add one-quarter of the egg mixture and tilt the skillet to ensure an even layer. Cook for 2 minutes and then add 2 tablespoons of cheese and one-quarter of the broccoli. Use a spatula to fold into an omelet.
3. Repeat step 3 with the remaining 1½ tablespoons of oil, remaining egg mixture, 6 tablespoons of cheese, and remaining broccoli to make a total of 4 omelets. Divide into 4 storage containers.

Nutrition:
Calories: 292, Fat: 23g, Carbohydrates: 4g, Fiber: 1g, Protein: 18g, Potassium: 308mg, Sodium: 282mg.

88. Creamy Avocado and Egg Salad Sandwiches

Preparation Time: 15 minutes
Cooking Time: 15 minutes
Servings: 4
Ingredients:
- 2 small avocados, halved and pitted
- 2 tablespoons nonfat plain Greek yogurt
- Juice of 1 large lemon
- ¼ teaspoon salt
- ½ teaspoon freshly ground black pepper
- 8 large eggs, hardboiled, peeled, and chopped
- 3 tablespoons finely chopped fresh dill
- 3 tablespoons finely chopped fresh parsley
- 8 whole wheat bread slices (or your choice)

Directions:
1. Scoop the avocados into a large bowl and mash. Mix in the yogurt, lemon juice, salt, and pepper. Add the eggs, dill, and parsley and combine.
2. Store the bread and salad separately in 4 reusable storage bags and 4 containers and assemble the night before or serving. To serve, divide the mixture evenly among 4 bread slices and top with the other slices to make sandwiches.

Nutrition:

Calories: 488, Fat: 22g, Carbohydrates: 48g, Fiber: 8g, Protein: 23g, Potassium: 469mg, Sodium: 597mg.

89. Breakfast Hash

Preparation Time: 15 minutes
Cooking Time: 25 minutes
Servings: 4
Ingredients:
- Nonstick cooking spray
- 2 large sweet potatoes, ½-inch cubes
- 1 scallion, finely chopped
- ¼ teaspoon salt
- ½ teaspoon freshly ground black pepper
- 8 ounces extra-lean ground beef (96% or leaner)
- 1 medium onion, diced
- 2 garlic cloves, minced
- 1 red bell pepper, diced
- ¼ teaspoon ground cumin
- ¼ teaspoon paprika
- 2 cups coarsely chopped kale leaves
- ¾ cup shredded reduced-fat Cheddar cheese
- 4 large eggs

Directions:
1. Grease a large skillet with cooking spray and heat over medium heat. Add the sweet potatoes, scallion, salt, and pepper. Sauté for 10 minutes, stirring often.
2. Add the beef, onion, garlic, bell pepper, cumin, and paprika. Sauté, frequently stirring, for about 4 minutes, or until the meat browns. Add the kale to the skillet and stir until wilted. Sprinkle with the Cheddar cheese.
3. Make four wells in the hash batter and crack an egg into each. Cover and let the eggs cook until the white is fully cooked and the yolk is to your liking. Divide into 4 storage containers.

Nutrition:
Calories: 323, Fat: 15g, Carbohydrates: 23g, Fiber: 4g, Protein: 25g, Potassium: 676mg, Sodium: 587mg.

90. Hearty Breakfast Casserole

Preparation Time: 15 minutes
Cooking Time: 30 minutes
Servings: 4
Ingredients:
- Nonstick cooking spray
- 1 large green bell pepper, diced
- 8 ounces Cremini mushrooms, diced
- ½ medium onion, diced
- 3 garlic cloves, minced
- 1 large sweet potato, grated
- 1 cup baby spinach
- 12 large eggs
- 3 tablespoons 1% milk
- 1 teaspoon mustard powder
- 1 teaspoon paprika
- 1 teaspoon freshly ground black pepper
- ½ teaspoon salt
- ½ cup shredded reduced-fat Colby-Jack cheese

Directions:
1. Preheat the oven to 350°F. Grease at a 9-by-13-inch baking dish with cooking spray. Coat a large skillet with cooking spray and heat over medium heat. Add the bell pepper, mushrooms, onion, garlic, and sweet potato.
2. Sauté, frequently stirring, for 3 to 4 minutes, or until the onion is translucent. Add the spinach and continue to sauté while stirring until the spinach has wilted. Remove, then set aside to cool slightly.
3. Mix the eggs, milk, mustard powder, paprika, black pepper, and salt in a large bowl. Add the sautéed vegetables. Put the batter into the prepared baking dish.
4. Bake for 30 minutes. Remove from the oven, sprinkle with the Colby-Jack cheese, return to the oven, and bake again within 5 minutes to melt the cheese. Divide into 4 storage containers.

Nutrition:
Calories: 378, Fat: 25g, Carbohydrates: 17g, Fiber: 3g, Protein: 26g, Potassium: 717mg, Sodium: 658mg.

91. Creamy Apple-Avocado Smoothie

Preparation Time: 15 minutes
Cooking Time: 0 minutes

Servings: 2
Ingredients:
- ½ medium avocado, peeled and pitted
- 1 medium apple, chopped
- 1 cup baby spinach leaves
- 1 cup nonfat vanilla Greek yogurt
- ½ to 1 cup of water
- 1 cup ice
- Freshly squeezed lemon juice (optional)

Directions:
1. Blend all the fixing using a blender, and blend until smooth and creamy. Put a squeeze of lemon juice on top if desired and serve immediately.

Nutrition:
Calories: 200, Fat: 7g, Sodium: 56mg, Potassium: 378mg. Carbohydrates: 27g, Fiber: 5g, Sugars: 20g, Protein: 10g.

92. Strawberry, Orange, and Beet Smoothie

Preparation Time: 5 minutes
Cooking Time: 0 minutes
Servings: 2
Ingredients:
- 1 cup nonfat milk
- 1 cup of frozen strawberries
- 1 medium beet, cooked, peeled, and cubed
- 1 orange, peeled and quartered
- 1 frozen banana, peeled and chopped
- 1 cup nonfat vanilla Greek yogurt
- 1 cup ice

Directions:
1. In a blender, combine all the fixings, and blend until smooth. Serve immediately.

Nutrition:
Calories: 266, Fat: 0g, Cholesterol: 7mg, Sodium: 104mg, Carbohydrates: 51g, Fiber: 6g, Sugars: 34g, Protein: 15g, Potassium: 231mg.

93. Blueberry-Vanilla Yogurt Smoothie

Preparation Time: 5 minutes
Cooking Time: 0 minutes
Servings: 2
Ingredients:
- 1½ cups frozen blueberries

- 1 cup nonfat vanilla Greek yogurt
- 1 frozen banana, peeled and sliced
- ½ cup nonfat or low-fat milk
- 1 cup ice

Directions:
1. In a blender, combine all the fixing listed, and blend until smooth and creamy. Serve immediately.

Nutrition:
Calories: 228, Fat: 1g, Sodium: 63mg, Potassium: 470mg, Carbohydrates: 45g, Fiber: 5g, Sugars: 34g, Protein: 12g.

94. Cereal with Cranberry-Orange Twist

Preparation Time: 5 minutes
Cooking Time: 0 minutes
Servings: 1
Ingredients:
- ½ c. water
- ½ c. orange juice
- 1/3 c. oat bran
- ¼ c. dried cranberries
- Sugar
- Milk

Directions:
1. In a bowl, combine all ingredients. For about 2 minutes, microwave the bowl, then serve with sugar and milk. Enjoy!

Nutrition:
Calories: 220 , Fat:2.4 g, Carbs:43.5 g,Protein:6.2 g ,Sugars:8 g ,Sodium:1 mg

95. Red Velvet Pancakes with Cream Cheese Topping

Preparation Time: 15 minutes
Cooking Time: 10 minutes
Servings: 2
Ingredients:
Cream Cheese Topping:

- 2 oz. Cream cheese
- 3 tbsps. Yogurt
- 3 tbsps. Honey
- 1 tbsp. Milk

Pancakes:

- ½ c. Whole wheat Flour
- ½ c. all-purpose flour
- 2¼tsps. Baking powder

- ½ tsp. Unsweetened Cocoa powder
- ¼ tsp. Salt
- ¼ c. Sugar
- 1 large Egg
- 1 c. + 2 tbsps. Milk
- 1 tsp. Vanilla
- 1 tsp. Red paste food coloring

Directions:
2. Combine all your topping ingredients in a medium bowl, and set aside. Add all your pancake ingredients in a large bowl and fold until combined. Set a greased skillet over medium heat to get hot.
3. Add ¼ cup of pancake batter onto the hot skillet and cook until bubbles begin to form on the top. Flip and cook until set. Repeat until your batter is done well. Add your toppings and serve.

Nutrition:
Calories: 231 , Protein 7g, Carbs 43g , Fat 4g, Sodium 0mg

96. Avocado Cup with Egg

Preparation Time: 5 minutes
Cooking Time: 0 minutes
Servings: 4
Ingredients:

- 4 tsp. parmesan cheese
- 1 chopped stalk scallion
- 4 dashes pepper
- 4 dashes paprika
- 2 ripe avocados
- 4 medium eggs

Directions:
1. Preheat oven to 375 0F. Slice avocadoes in half and discard the seed. Slice the rounded portions of the avocado to make it level and sit well on a baking sheet.
2. Place avocadoes on a baking sheet and crack one egg in each hole of the avocado. Season each egg evenly with pepper and paprika. Bake within 25 minutes or until eggs is cooked to your liking. Serve with a sprinkle of parmesan.

Nutrition:
Calories: 206 ,Fat:15.4 g , Carbs:11.3 g , Protein:8.5 g,Sugars:0.4 g , Sodium:21 mg

97. Greek Yogurt Oat Pancakes

Preparation Time: 15 minutes
Cooking Time: 10 minutes
Servings: 2
Ingredients:

- 6 egg whites (or ¾ cup liquid egg whites)
- 1 cup rolled oats
- 1 cup plain nonfat Greek yogurt
- 1 medium banana, peeled and sliced
- 1 teaspoon ground cinnamon
- 1 teaspoon baking powder

Directions:

1. Blend all the listed fixing using a blender. Heat a griddle over medium heat. Spray the skillet with nonstick cooking spray.
2. Put 1/3 cup of the mixture or batter onto the griddle. Allow to cook and flip when bubbles on the top burst, about 5 minutes. Cook again within a minute until golden brown. Repeat with the remaining batter. Divide between two serving plates and enjoy.

Nutrition:

Calories: 318, Fat: 4g, Sodium: 467mg, Potassium: 634mg, Carbohydrates: 47g, Fiber: 6g, Sugars: 13g, Protein: 28g.

98. Scrambled Egg and Veggie Breakfast Quesadillas

Preparation Time: 15 minutes
Cooking Time: 15 minutes
Servings: 2
Ingredients:

- 2 eggs
- 2 egg whites
- 2 to 4 tablespoons nonfat or low-fat milk
- ¼ teaspoon freshly ground black pepper
- 1 large tomato, chopped
- 2 tablespoons chopped cilantro
- ½ cup canned black beans, rinsed and drained
- 1½ tablespoons olive oil, divided
- 4 corn tortillas
- ½ avocado, peeled, pitted, and thinly sliced

Directions:

1. Mix the eggs, egg whites, milk, and black pepper in a bowl. Using an electric mixer, beat until smooth. To the same bowl, add the tomato, cilantro, and black beans, and fold into the eggs with a spoon.
2. Heat half of the olive oil in a medium pan over medium flame. Add the scrambled egg mixture and cook for a few minutes, stirring, until cooked through. Remove from the pan.
3. Divide the scrambled eggs mixture between the tortillas, layering only on one half of the tortilla. Top with avocado slices and fold the tortillas in half.
4. Heat the remaining oil over medium flame and add one of the folded tortillas to the pan. Cook within 1 to 2 minutes on each side or until browned. Repeat with remaining tortillas. Serve immediately.

Nutrition:

Calories: 445, Fat: 24g, Sodium: 228mg, Potassium: 614mg, Carbohydrates: 42g, Fiber: 11g, Sugars: 2g, Protein: 19g.

99. Stuffed Breakfast Peppers

Preparation Time: 15 minutes
Cooking Time: 45 minutes
Servings: 4
Ingredients:

- 4 bell peppers (any color)
- 1 (16-ounce) bag frozen spinach
- 4 eggs
- ¼ cup shredded low-fat cheese (optional)
- Freshly ground black pepper

Directions:

1. Preheat the oven to 400°F. Line a baking dish with aluminum foil. Cut the tops off the pepper, then discard the seeds. Discard the tops and seeds. Put the peppers in the baking dish and bake for about 15 minutes.
2. While the peppers bake, defrost the spinach and drain off the excess moisture. Remove the peppers, then stuff the bottoms evenly with the defrosted spinach.
3. Crack an egg over the spinach inside each pepper. Top each egg with a tablespoon of the cheese (if using) and season with black pepper to taste. Bake within 15 to 20 minutes, or until the egg whites are set and opaque.

Nutrition:

Calories: 136, Fat: 5g, Sodium: 131mg, Potassium: 576mg, Carbohydrates: 15g, Protein: 11g.

100. Sweet Potato Toast Three Ways

Preparation Time: 15 minutes
Cooking Time: 25 minutes
Servings:
Ingredients:

- 1 large sweet potato, unpeeled

Topping Choice #1:

- 4 tablespoons peanut butter
- 1 ripe banana, sliced
- Dash ground cinnamon

Topping Choice #2:

- ½ avocado, peeled, pitted, and mashed
- 2 eggs (1 per slice)

Topping Choice #3:

- 4 tablespoons nonfat or low-fat ricotta cheese
- 1 tomato, sliced
- Dash black pepper

Directions:

1. Slice the sweet potato lengthwise into ¼-inch thick slices. Place the sweet potato slices in a toaster on high for about 5 minutes or until cooked through.
2. Repeat multiple times, if necessary, depending on your toaster settings. Top with your desired topping choices and enjoy.

Nutrition:

Calories: 137, Fat: 0g, Sodium: 17mg, Potassium: 265mg, Carbohydrates: 32g, Fiber: 4g, Sugars: 0g, Protein: 2g.

101. Apple-Apricot Brown Rice Breakfast Porridge

Preparation Time: 15 minutes
Cooking Time: 8 minutes
Servings: 4
Ingredients:

- 3 cups cooked brown rice
- 1¾ cups nonfat or low-fat milk

- 2 tablespoons lightly packed brown sugar
- 4 dried apricots, chopped
- 1 medium apple, cored and diced
- ¾ teaspoon ground cinnamon
- ¾ teaspoon vanilla extract

Directions:
1. Combine the rice, milk, sugar, apricots, apple, and cinnamon in a medium saucepan. Boil it on medium heat, lower the heat down slightly and cook within 2 to 3 minutes. Turn it off, then stir in the vanilla extract. Serve warm.

Nutrition:
Calories: 260, Fat: 2g, Sodium: 50mg, Potassium: 421mg, Carbohydrates: 57g, Fiber: 4g, Sugars: 22g, Protein: 7g.

102. Carrot Cake Overnight Oats

Preparation Time: overnight
Cooking Time: 2 minutes
Servings: 1
Ingredients:
- ½ cup rolled oats
- ½ cup plain nonfat or low-fat Greek yogurt
- ½ cup nonfat or low-fat milk
- ¼ cup shredded carrot
- 2 tablespoons raisins
- ½ teaspoon ground cinnamon
- 1 to 2 tablespoons chopped walnuts (optional)

Directions:
1. Mix all the fixings in a lidded jar, shake well, and refrigerate overnight. Serve.

Nutrition:
Calories: 331, Fat: 3g, Sodium: 141mg, Carbohydrates: 59g, Fiber: 8g, Sugars: 26g, Protein: 22g.

103. Steel-Cut Oatmeal with Plums and Pear

Preparation Time: 15 minutes
Cooking Time: 25 minutes
Servings: 4
Ingredients:
- 2 cups of water
- 1 cup nonfat or low-fat milk
- 1 cup steel-cut oats
- 1 cup dried plums, chopped
- 1 medium pear, cored, and skin removed, diced

- 4 tablespoons almonds, roughly chopped

Directions:
1. Mix the water, milk, plus oats in a medium pot and bring to a boil over high heat. Reduce the heat and cover. Simmer for about 10 minutes, stirring occasionally.
2. Add the plums and pear, and cover. Simmer for another 10 minutes. Turn off the heat and let stand within 5 minutes until all the liquid is absorbed. To serve, top each portion with a sprinkling of almonds.

Nutrition:
Calories: 307, Fat: 6g, Sodium: 132mg, Potassium: 640mg, Carbohydrates: 58g, Fiber: 9g, Sugars: 24g, Protein: 9g.

104. French Toast with Applesauce

Preparation Time: 5 minutes
Cooking Time: 5 minutes
Servings: 6
Ingredients:
- ¼ c. unsweetened applesauce
- ½ c. skim milk
- 2 packets Stevia
- 2 eggs
- 6 slices whole-wheat bread
- 1 tsp. ground cinnamon

Directions:
1. Mix well applesauce, sugar, cinnamon, milk, and eggs in a mixing bowl. Soak the bread into the applesauce mixture until wet. On medium fire, heat a large nonstick skillet.
2. Add soaked bread on one side and another on the other side. Cook in a single layer within 2-3 minutes per side on medium-low fire or until lightly browned. Serve and enjoy.

Nutrition:
Calories: 122.6, Fat: 2.6g, Carbs: 18.3g, Protein: 6.5g, Sugars: 14.8g, Sodium: 11mg, Potassium: 123mg.

105. Banana-Peanut Butter and Greens Smoothie

Preparation Time: 5 minutes
Cooking Time: 0 minutes
Servings: 1

Ingredients:
- 1 c. chopped and packed Romaine lettuce
- 1 frozen medium banana
- 1 tbsp. all-natural peanut butter
- 1 c. cold almond milk

Directions:
1. In a heavy-duty blender, add all ingredients. Puree until smooth and creamy. Serve and enjoy.

Nutrition:
Calories: 349.3, Fat: 9.7g, Carbs: 57.4g, Protein: 8.1g, Sugars: 4.3g, Sodium: 18mg, Potassium: 120mg.

106. Baking Powder Biscuits

Preparation Time: 5 minutes
Cooking Time: 5 minutes
Servings: 1
Ingredients:
- 1 egg white
- 1 c. white whole-wheat flour
- 4 tbsps. non-hydrogenated vegetable shortening
- 1 tbsp. sugar
- 2/3 c. low-fat milk
- 1 c. unbleached all-purpose flour
- 4 tsp. sodium-free baking powder

Directions:
1. Heat the oven to 450°F. Put the flour, sugar, plus baking powder into a mixing bowl and mix. Split the shortening into the batter using your fingers until it resembles coarse crumbs. Put the egg white plus milk and stir to combine.
2. Put the dough out onto a lightly floured surface and knead for 1 minute. Roll dough to ¾ inch thickness and cut into 12 rounds. Place rounds on the baking sheet. Bake 10 minutes, then remove the baking sheet and place biscuits on a wire rack to cool.

Nutrition:
Calories: 118, Fat: 4g, Carbs: 16g, Protein: 3g, Sugars: 0.2g, Sodium: 6mg, Potassium: 90mg.

107. Oatmeal Banana Pancakes with Walnuts

Preparation Time: 15 minutes
Cooking Time: 5 minutes
Servings: 8
Ingredients:
- 1 finely diced firm banana
- 1 c. whole wheat pancake mix
- 1/8 c. chopped walnuts
- ¼ c. old-fashioned oats

Directions:
1. Make the pancake mix, as stated in the directions on the package. Add walnuts, oats, and the chopped banana. Coat a griddle with cooking spray. Add about ¼ cup of the pancake batter onto the griddle when hot.
2. Turn pancake over when bubbles form on top. Cook until golden brown. Serve immediately.

Nutrition:
Calories: 155, Fat: 4g, Carbs: 28g, Protein: 7g, Sugars: 2.2g, Sodium: 16mg, Potassium: 100mg.

108. Creamy Oats, Greens & Blueberry Smoothie

Preparation Time: 4 minutes
Cooking Time: 0 minutes
Servings: 1
Ingredients:
- 1 c. cold fat-free milk
- 1 c. salad greens
- ½ c. fresh frozen blueberries
- ½ c. frozen cooked oatmeal
- 1 tbsp. sunflower seeds

Directions:
1. Blend all ingredients using a powerful blender until smooth and creamy. Serve and enjoy.

Nutrition:
Calories: 280, Fat: 6.8g, Carbs: 44.0g, Protein: 14.0g, Sugars: 32g, Sodium: 141mg, Potassium: 110mg.

109. Banana & Cinnamon Oatmeal

Preparation Time: 5 minutes
Cooking Time: 0 minutes
Servings: 6

Ingredients:
- 2 c. quick-cooking oats
- 4 c. Fat-free milk
- 1 tsp. ground cinnamon
- 2 chopped large ripe banana
- 4 tsp. brown sugar
- Extra ground cinnamon

Directions:
1. Place milk in a skillet and bring to boil. Add oats and cook over medium heat until thickened, for two to four minutes.
2. Stir intermittently. Add cinnamon, brown sugar, and banana and stir to combine. If you want, serve with the extra cinnamon and milk. Enjoy!

Nutrition:
Calories: 215, Fat: 2g, Carbs: 42g, Protein: 10g, Sugars: 1g, Sodium: 40mg, Potassium: 112mg.

110. Bagels Made Healthy

Preparation Time: 5 minutes
Cooking Time: 40 minutes
Servings: 8
Ingredients:
- 1 ½ c. warm water
- 1 ¼ c. bread flour
- 2 tbsps. honey
- 2 c. whole wheat flour
- 2 tsp. yeast
- 1 ½ tbsps. olive oil
- 1 tbsp. vinegar

Directions:
1. In a bread machine, mix all the ingredients, and then process in the dough cycle. Once done, create 8 flattened ball-shaped pieces. Create a donut shape by using your thumb to make a hole in the center of each ball.
2. Place the donut-shaped dough on a greased baking sheet and then cover and let rise for about ½ hour. Prepare about 2 inches of water to boil in a large saucepan.
3. In boiling water, drop one at a time the bagels and boil them for 1 minute, then turn them once. Remove them and return them to the baking sheet and bake at 350F0F for about 20 to 25 minutes until golden brown.

Nutrition:
Calories: 228, Fat: 3.7g, Carbs: 41.8g, Protein: 6.9g, Sugars: 0g, Sodium: 15mg, Potassium: 120mg.

111. Cereal with Cranberry-Orange Twist

Preparation Time: 5 minutes
Cooking Time: 0 minutes
Servings: 1
Ingredients:
- ½ c. water
- ½ c. orange juice
- 1/3 c. oat bran
- ¼ c. dried cranberries
- Sugar
- Milk

Directions:
1. In a bowl, combine all ingredients. For about 2 minutes, microwave the bowl; then serve with sugar and milk. Enjoy!

Nutrition:
Calories: 220, Fat: 2.4g, Carbs: 43.5g, Protein: 6.2g, Sugars: 8g, Sodium: 1mg, Potassium: 80mg.

112. No-Cook Overnight Oats

Preparation Time: 5 minutes
Cooking Time: 0 minutes
Servings: 1
Ingredients:
- 1 ½ c. low-fat milk
- 5 whole almond pieces
- 1 tsp. chia seeds
- 2 tbsps. oats
- 1 tsp. sunflower seeds
- 1 tbsp. craisins

Directions:
1. In a jar or mason bottle with a cap, mix all ingredients. Refrigerate overnight. Enjoy for breakfast.

Nutrition:
Calories: 271, Fat: 9.8g, Carbs: 35.4g, Protein: 16.7g, Sugars: 9, Sodium: 103mg, Potassium: 70mg.

113. Avocado Cup with Egg

Preparation Time: 5 minutes
Cooking Time: 0 minutes
Servings: 4
Ingredients:
- 4 tsp. parmesan cheese
- 1 chopped stalk scallion
- 4 dashes pepper
- 4 dashes paprika
- 2 ripe avocados
- 4 medium eggs

Directions:

1. Preheat oven to 375F. Slice avocadoes in half and discard the seed. Slice the rounded portions of the avocado to make it level and sit well on a baking sheet.
2. Place avocadoes on a baking sheet and crack one egg in each hole of the avocado. Season each egg evenly with pepper and paprika. Bake within 25 minutes or until eggs are cooked to your liking. Serve with a sprinkle of parmesan.

Nutrition:
Calories: 206, Fat: 15.4g, Carbs: 11.3g, Protein: 8.5g, Sugars: 0.4g, Sodium: 21mg, Potassium: 130mg.

114. Mediterranean Toast

Preparation Time: 10 minutes
Cooking Time: 0 minutes
Servings: 2
Ingredients:
- 1 ½ tsp. reduced-fat crumbled feta
- 3 sliced Greek olives
- ¼ mashed avocado
- 1 slice good whole wheat bread
- 1 tbsp. roasted red pepper hummus
- 3 sliced cherry tomatoes
- 1 sliced hardboiled egg

Directions:
1. First, toast the bread and top it with ¼ mashed avocado and 1 tablespoon hummus. Add the cherry tomatoes, olives, hardboiled egg, and feta. To taste, season with salt and pepper.

Nutrition:
Calories: 333.7, Fat: 17g, Carbs: 33.3g, Protein: 16.3g, Sugars: 1g, Sodium: 19mg, Potassium: 90mg.

115. Instant Banana Oatmeal

Preparation Time: 1 minute
Cooking Time: 2 minutes
Servings: 1
Ingredients:
- 1 mashed ripe banana
- ½ c. water
- ½ c. quick oats

Directions:

1. Measure the oats and water into a microwave-safe bowl and stir to combine. Place bowl in microwave and heat on high for 2 minutes. Remove the bowl, then stir in the mashed banana and serve.

Nutrition:
Calories: 243, Fat: 3g, Carbs: 50g, Protein: 6g, Sugars: 20g, Sodium: 30mg, Potassium: 145mg.

116. Almond Butter-Banana Smoothie

Preparation Time: 5 minutes
Cooking Time: 0 minutes
Servings: 1
Ingredients:
- 1 tbsp. almond butter
- ½ c. ice cubes
- ½ c. packed spinach
- 1 peeled and a frozen medium banana
- 1 c. Fat-free milk

Directions:
1. Blend all the listed fixing above in a powerful blender until smooth and creamy. Serve and enjoy.

Nutrition:
Calories: 293, Fat: 9.8g, Carbs: 42.5g, Protein: 13.5g, Sugars: 12g, Sodium: 40mg, Potassium: 70mg.

117. Brown Sugar Cinnamon Oatmeal

Preparation Time: 1 minute
Cooking Time: 3 minutes
Servings: 4
Ingredients:
- ½ tsp. ground cinnamon
- 1 ½ tsp. pure vanilla extract
- ¼ c. light brown sugar
- 2 c. low- Fat milk
- 1 1/3 c. quick oats

Directions:
1. Put the milk plus vanilla into a medium saucepan and boil over medium-high heat.
2. Lower the heat to medium once it boils. Mix in oats, brown sugar, plus cinnamon, and cook, stirring 2–3 minutes. Serve immediately.

Nutrition:
Calories: 208, Fat: 3g, Carbs: 38g, Protein: 8g, Sugars: 15g,

Sodium: 33mg, Potassium: 50mg.

118. Buckwheat Pancakes with Vanilla Almond Milk

Preparation Time: 10 minutes
Cooking Time: 10 minutes
Servings: 1
Ingredients:
- ½ c. unsweetened vanilla almond milk
- 2-4 packets of natural sweetener
- 1/8 tsp. salt
- ½ cup buckwheat flour
- ½ tsp. double-acting baking powder

Directions:
1. Prepare a nonstick pancake griddle, grease with the cooking spray and place over medium heat. Whisk the buckwheat flour, salt, baking powder, and stevia in a small bowl and stir in the almond milk after.
2. Onto the pan, scoop a large spoonful of batter. Cook until bubbles no longer pop on the surface and the entire surface looks dry and (2-4 minutes). Flip and cook for another 2-4 minutes. Repeat with all the remaining batter.

Nutrition:
Calories: 240, Fat: 4.5g, Carbs: 2g, Protein: 11g, Sugars: 17g, Sodium: 38mg, Potassium: 80mg.

119. Salmon and Egg Scramble

Preparation Time: 15 minutes
Cooking Time: 4 minutes
Servings: 4
Ingredients:
- 1 teaspoon of olive oil
- 3 organic whole eggs
- 3 tablespoons of water
- 1 minced garlic
- 6 Oz. smoked salmon, sliced
- 2 avocados, sliced
- Black pepper to taste
- 1 green onion, chopped

Directions:
1. Heat olive oil in a large skillet and sauté onion in it. Take a medium bowl and whisk eggs in it; add water and make a scramble with the help of a fork. Add to the skillet the smoked

salmon along with garlic and black pepper.

2. Stir for about 4 minutes until all ingredients get fluffy. At this stage, add the egg mixture. Once the eggs get firm, serve on a plate with a garnish of avocados.

Nutrition:
Calories: 120, Carbs: 3g, Fat: 4g, Protein: 19g, Sodium: 298mg, Potassium: 129mg.

120. Pumpkin Muffins

Preparation Time: 15 minutes
Cooking Time: 20 minutes
Servings: 4
Ingredients:
- 4 cups of almond flour
- 2 cups of pumpkin, cooked and pureed
- 2 large whole organic eggs
- 3 teaspoons of baking powder
- 2 teaspoons of ground cinnamon
- 1/2 cup raw honey
- 4 teaspoons almond butter

Directions:
1. Preheat the oven at 400 degrees F. Line the muffin paper on the muffin tray. Mix almond flour, pumpkin puree, eggs, baking powder, cinnamon, almond butter, and honey in a large bowl.
2. Put the prepared batter into a muffin tray and bake within 20 minutes. Once golden-brown, serve and enjoy.

Nutrition:
Calories: 136, Carbs: 22g, Fat: 5g, Protein: 2g, Sodium: 11mg, Potassium: 699mg.

121. Sweet Berries Pancake

Preparation Time: 15 minutes
Cooking Time: 15 minutes
Servings: 4
Ingredients:
- 4 cups of almond flour
- Pinch of sea salt
- 2 organic eggs
- 4 teaspoons of walnut oil
- 1 cup of strawberries, mashed
- 1 cup of blueberries, mashed
- 1 teaspoon baking powder
- Honey for topping, optional

Directions:

1. Take a bowl and add almond flour, baking powder, and sea salt. Take another bowl and add eggs, walnut oil, strawberries, and blueberries mash. Combine ingredients of both bowls.
2. Heat a bit of walnut oil in a cooking pan and pour the spoonful mixture to make pancakes. Once the bubble comes on the top, flip the pancake to cook from the other side. Once done, serve with the glaze of honey on top.

Nutrition:
Calories: 161, Carbs: 23g, Fat: 6g, Protein: 3g, Cholesterol: 82mg, Sodium: 91mg, Potassium: 252mg.

122. Zucchini Pancakes

Preparation Time: 15 minutes
Cooking Time: 10 minutes
Servings: 4
Ingredients:
- 4 large zucchinis
- 4 green onions, diced
- 1/3 cup of milk
- 1 organic egg
- Sea Salt, just a pinch
- Black pepper, grated
- 2 tablespoons of olive oil

Directions:
1. First, wash the zucchinis and grate them with a cheese grater. Mix the egg and add in the grated zucchinis and milk in a large bowl. Warm oil in a skillet and sauté onions in it.
2. Put the egg batter into the skillet and make pancakes. Once cooked from both sides. Serve by sprinkling salt and pepper on top.

Nutrition:
Calories: 70, Carbs: 8g, Fat: 3g, Protein: 2g, Cholesterol: 43mg, Sodium: 60mg, Potassium: 914mg.

123. Breakfast Banana Split

Preparation Time: 15 minutes
Cooking Time: 0 minutes
Servings: 3
Ingredients:
- 2 bananas, peeled
- 1 cup oats, cooked
- 1/2 cup low-fat strawberry yogurt
- 1/3 teaspoon honey, optional

- 1/2 cup pineapple, chunks

Directions:
1. Peel the bananas and cut lengthwise. Place half of the banana in each separate bowl. Spoon strawberry yogurt on top and pour cooked oats with pineapple chunks on each banana. Serve immediately with a glaze of honey of liked.

Nutrition:
Calories: 145, Carbs: 18g, Fat: 7g, Protein: 3g, Sodium: 2mg, Potassium: 380mg.

124. Easy Veggie Muffins

Preparation Time: 10 minutes
Cooking Time: 40 minutes
Servings: 4
Ingredients:
- 3/4 cup cheddar cheese, shredded
- 1 cup green onion, chopped
- 1 cup tomatoes, chopped
- 1 cup broccoli, chopped
- 2 cups non-fat milk
- 1 cup biscuit mix
- 4 eggs
- Cooking spray
- 1 teaspoon Italian seasoning
- A pinch of black pepper

Directions:
1. Grease a muffin tray with cooking spray and divide broccoli, tomatoes, cheese, and onions in each muffin cup.
2. In a bowl, combine green onions with milk, biscuit mix, eggs, pepper, and Italian seasoning, whisk well and pour into the muffin tray as well.
3. Cook the muffins in the oven at 375 degrees F for 40 minutes, divide them between plates and serve.

Nutrition:
Calories: 80, Carbs: 3g, Fat: 5g, Protein: 7g, Sodium: 25mg, Potassium: 189mg.

125. Carrot Muffins

Preparation Time: 10 minutes
Cooking Time: 30 minutes
Servings: 5
Ingredients:
- 1 and ½ cups whole wheat flour
- ½ cup stevia
- 1 teaspoon baking powder
- ½ teaspoon cinnamon powder

- ½ teaspoon baking soda
- ¼ cup natural apple juice
- ¼ cup olive oil
- 1 egg
- 1 cup fresh cranberries
- 2 carrots, grated
- 2 teaspoons ginger, grated
- ¼ cup pecans, chopped
- Cooking spray

Directions:
1. Mix the flour with the stevia, baking powder, cinnamon and baking soda in a large bowl. Add the apple juice, oil, egg, cranberries, carrots, ginger and walnuts and stir well.
2. Grease a muffin pan with cooking spray. Divide the muffin mixture, place in the oven and bake at 375 degrees F in 30 minutes. Divide muffins between plates and serve for breakfast.

Nutrition:
Calories: 34, Carbs: 6g, Fat: 1g, Protein: 0g, Sodium: 52mg, Potassium: 189mg.

126. Pineapple Oatmeal

Preparation Time: 10 minutes
Cooking Time: 25 minutes
Servings: 4
Ingredients:
- 2 cups old-fashioned oats
- 1 cup walnuts, chopped
- 2 cups pineapple, cubed
- 1 tablespoon ginger, grated
- 2 cups non-fat milk
- 2 eggs
- 2 tablespoons stevia
- 2 teaspoons vanilla extract

Directions:
1. In a bowl, combine the oats with the pineapple, walnuts, and ginger, stir and divide into 4 ramekins. Mix the milk with the eggs, stevia, and vanilla in a bowl and pour over the oats mix. Bake at 400 degrees F within 25 minutes. 4. Serve for breakfast.

Nutrition:
Calories: 200, Carbs: 40g, Fat: 1g, Protein: 3g, Sodium: 275mg, Potassium: 180mg.

127. Spinach Muffins

Preparation Time: 10 minutes
Cooking Time: 30 minutes

Servings: 6
Ingredients:
- 6 eggs
- ½ cup non-fat milk
- 1 cup low-fat cheese, crumbled
- 4 ounces spinach
- ½ cup roasted red pepper, chopped
- 2 ounces prosciutto, chopped
- Cooking spray

Directions:
1. Mix the eggs with the milk, cheese, spinach, red pepper, and prosciutto in a bowl. Grease a muffin tray with cooking spray, divide the muffin mix, introduce in the oven, and bake at 350 degrees F within 30 minutes. Divide between plates and serve for breakfast.

Nutrition:
Calories: 112, Carbs: 19g, Fat: 3g, Protein: 2g, Sodium: 274mg, Potassium: 99mg.

128. Chia Seeds Breakfast Mix

Preparation Time: 8 hours
Cooking Time: 0 minutes
Servings: 4
Ingredients:
- 2 cups old-fashioned oats
- 4 tablespoons chia seeds
- 4 tablespoons coconut sugar
- 3 cups of coconut milk
- 1 teaspoon lemon zest, grated
- 1 cup blueberries

Directions:
1. In a bowl, combine the oats with chia seeds, sugar, milk, lemon zest, and blueberries, stir, divide into cups and keep in the fridge for 8 hours. 2. Serve for breakfast.

Nutrition:
Calories: 69, Carbs: 0g, Fat: 5g, Protein: 3g, Sodium: 0mg, Potassium: 209mg.

129. Breakfast Fruits Bowls

Preparation Time: 10 minutes
Cooking Time: 0 minutes
Servings: 2
Ingredients:
- 1 cup mango, chopped
- 1 banana, sliced
- 1 cup pineapple, chopped
- 1 cup almond milk

Directions:

1. Mix the mango with the banana, pineapple, and almond milk in a bowl, stir, divide into smaller bowls, and serve.

Nutrition:
Calories: 10, Carbs: 0g, Fat: 1g, Protein: 0g, Sodium: 0mg, Potassium: 90mg.

130. Pumpkin Cookies

Preparation Time: 10 minutes
Cooking Time: 25 minutes
Servings: 6
Ingredients:
- 2 cups whole wheat flour
- 1 cup old-fashioned oats
- 1 teaspoon baking soda
- 1 teaspoon pumpkin pie spice
- 15 ounces pumpkin puree
- 1 cup coconut oil, melted
- 1 cup of coconut sugar
- 1 egg
- ½ cup pepitas, roasted
- ½ cup cherries, dried

Directions:
1. Mix the flour the oats, baking soda, pumpkin spice, pumpkin puree, oil, sugar, egg, pepitas, and cherries in a bowl, stir well, shape medium cookies out of this mix, arrange them all on a baking sheet, then bake within 25 minutes at 350 degrees F. Serve the cookies for breakfast.

Nutrition:
Calories: 150, Carbs: 24g, Fat: 8g, Protein: 1g, Sodium: 220mg, Potassium: 100mg.

131. Veggie Scramble

Preparation Time: 10 minutes
Cooking Time: 2 minutes
Servings: 1
Ingredients:
- 1 egg
- 1 tablespoon water
- ¼ cup broccoli, chopped
- ¼ cup mushrooms, chopped
- A pinch of black pepper
- 1 tablespoon low-fat mozzarella, shredded
- 1 tablespoon walnuts, chopped
- Cooking spray

Directions:
1. Grease a ramekin with cooking spray, add the egg, water, pepper, mushrooms, and broccoli, and whisk well. Introduce in the microwave and

cook for 2 minutes. Add mozzarella and walnuts on top and serve for breakfast.

Nutrition:
Calories: 128, Carbs: 24g, Fat: 0g, Protein: 9g, Sodium: 86mg, Potassium: 170mg.

132. Mushrooms and Turkey Breakfast

Preparation Time: 10 minutes
Cooking Time: 1 hour and 5 minutes
Servings: 12
Ingredients:
- 8 ounces whole-wheat bread, cubed
- 12 ounces turkey sausage, chopped
- 2 cups fat-free milk
- 5 ounces low-fat cheddar, shredded
- 3 eggs
- ½ cup green onions, chopped
- 1 cup mushrooms, chopped
- ½ teaspoon sweet paprika
- A pinch of black pepper
- 2 tablespoons low-fat parmesan, grated

Directions:
1. Put the bread cubes on a prepared lined baking sheet, bake at 400 degrees F for 8 minutes. Meanwhile, heat a pan over medium-high flame. Add turkey sausage, stir, and brown for 7 minutes.
2. In a bowl, combine the milk with the cheddar, eggs, parmesan, black pepper, and paprika and whisk well.
3. Add mushrooms, sausage, bread cubes, and green onions.
4. Stir, pour into a baking dish and bake at 350 degrees F within 50 minutes.
5. Slice, divide between plates and serve for breakfast.

Nutrition:
Calories: 88, Carbs: 1g, Fat: 9g, Protein: 1g, Sodium: 74mg, Potassium: 169mg.

133. Mushrooms and Cheese Omelet

Preparation Time: 10 minutes
Cooking Time: 15 minutes
Servings: 4
Ingredients:

- 2 tablespoons olive oil
- A pinch of black pepper
- 3 ounces mushrooms, sliced
- 1 cup baby spinach, chopped
- 3 eggs, whisked
- 2 tablespoons low-fat cheese, grated
- 1 small avocado, peeled, pitted, and cubed
- 1 tablespoons parsley, chopped

Directions:
1. Add mushrooms, stir, cook them for 5 minutes and transfer to a bowl on a heated pan with the oil over medium-high heat.
2. Heat the same pan over medium-high flame. Add eggs and black pepper, spread into the pan, cook within 7 minutes, and transfer to a plate.
3. Spread mushrooms, spinach, avocado, and cheese on half of the omelet. Fold the other half over this mix, sprinkle parsley on top, and serve.

Nutrition:
Calories: 136, Carbs: 5g, Fat: 5g, Protein: 16g, Sodium: 192mg, Potassium: 189mg.

134. Egg White Breakfast Mix

Preparation Time: 10 minutes
Cooking Time: 10 minutes
Servings: 4
Ingredients:
- 1 yellow onion, chopped
- 3 plum tomatoes, chopped
- 10 ounces spinach, chopped
- A pinch of black pepper
- 2 tablespoons water
- 12 egg whites
- Cooking spray

Directions:
1. Mix the egg whites with water and pepper in a bowl. Grease a pan with cooking spray, heat over medium flame. Add ¼ of the egg whites, spread into the pan, and cook for 2 minutes.
2. Spoon ¼ of the spinach, tomatoes, and onion, fold and add to a plate. Serve for breakfast. Enjoy!

Nutrition:
Calories: 31, Carbs: 0g, Fat: 2g, Protein: 3g, Sodium: 55mg, Potassium: 150mg.

135. Pesto Omelet

Preparation Time: 10 minutes
Cooking Time: 6 minutes

Servings: 2
Ingredients:
- 2 teaspoons olive oil
- Handful cherry tomatoes, chopped
- 3 tablespoons pistachio pesto
- A pinch of black pepper
- 4 eggs

Directions:
1. In a bowl, combine the eggs with cherry tomatoes, black pepper, and pistachio pesto and whisk well. Add eggs mix, spread into the pan, cook for 3 minutes, flip, cook for 3 minutes more, divide between 2 plates, and serve on a heated pan with the oil over medium-high heat.

Nutrition:
Calories: 240, Carbs: 23g, Fat: 9g, Protein: 17g, Sodium: 292mg, Potassium: 130mg.

136. Quinoa Bowls

Preparation Time: 10 minutes
Cooking Time: 20 minutes
Servings: 2
Ingredients:
- 1 peach, sliced
- 1/3 cup quinoa, rinsed
- 2/3 cup low-fat milk
- ½ teaspoon vanilla extract
- 2 teaspoons brown sugar
- 12 raspberries
- 14 blueberries

Directions:
1. Mix the quinoa with the milk, sugar, and vanilla in a small pan. Simmer over medium heat, cover the pan, cook for 20 minutes and flip with a fork. Divide this mix into 2 bowls, top each with raspberries and blueberries and serve for breakfast.

Nutrition:
Calories: 170, Carbs: 31g, Fat: 3g, Protein: 6g, Sodium: 120mg, Potassium: 169mg.

137. Strawberry Sandwich

Preparation Time: 10 minutes
Cooking Time: 0 minutes
Servings: 4
Ingredients:
- 8 ounces low-fat cream cheese, soft
- 1 tablespoon stevia
- 1 teaspoon lemon zest, grated
- 4 whole-wheat English muffins, toasted

- 2 cups strawberries, sliced

Directions:

1. In your food processor, combine the cream cheese with the stevia and lemon zest and pulse well. Spread 1 tablespoon of this mix on 1 muffin half and top with some of the sliced strawberries. Repeat with the rest of the muffin halves and serve for breakfast. Enjoy!

Nutrition:

Calories: 150, Carbs: 23g, Fat: 7g, Protein: 2g, Sodium: 70mg, Potassium: 140mg.

138. Apple Quinoa Muffins

Preparation Time: 10 minutes
Cooking Time: 35 minutes
Servings: 4
Ingredients:

- ½ cup natural, unsweetened applesauce
- 1 cup banana, peeled and mashed
- 1 cup quinoa
- 2 and ½ cups old-fashioned oats
- ½ cup almond milk
- 2 tablespoons stevia
- 1 teaspoon vanilla extract
- 1 cup of water
- Cooking spray
- 1 teaspoon cinnamon powder
- 1 apple, cored, peeled, and chopped

Directions:

1. Put the water in a small pan, bring to a simmer over medium heat. Add quinoa, cook within 15 minutes, fluff with a fork, and transfer to a bowl.
2. Add all ingredients, stir, divide into a muffin pan greased with cooking spray, place in the oven and bake for 20 minutes at 375 degrees F. Serve for breakfast.

Nutrition:

Calories: 241, Carbs: 31g, Fat: 11g, Protein: 5g, Sodium: 251mg, Potassium: 100mg.

139. Very Berry Muesli

Preparation Time: 15 minutes
Cooking Time: 0 minutes
Servings: 2
Ingredients:

- 1 c. oats
- 1 c. fruit flavored yogurt
- ½ c. milk

- 1/8 tsp. salt
- ½ c dried raisins
- ½ c. chopped apple
- ½ c. frozen blueberries
- ¼ c. chopped walnuts

Directions:

1. Combine yogurt, salt, and oats in a medium bowl. Mix well, and then cover it tightly. Fridge for at least 6 hours. Add your raisins and apples the gently fold. Top with walnuts and serve. Enjoy!

Nutrition:

Calories: 195, Protein: 6g, Carbs: 31g, Fat: 4g, Sodium: 0mg, Potassium: 50mg.

140. Veggie Quiche Muffins

Preparation Time: 15 minutes
Cooking Time: 40 minutes
Servings: 12
Ingredients:

- 3/4 c. shredded cheddar
- 1 c. chopped green onion
- 1 c. chopped broccoli
- 1 c. diced tomatoes
- 2 c. milk
- 4 eggs
- 1 c. pancake mix
- 1 tsp. oregano
- 1/2 tsp. salt
- 1/2 tsp. pepper

Directions:

1. Preheat your oven to 375F, and lightly grease a 12-cup muffin tin with oil. Sprinkle your tomatoes, broccoli, onions, and cheddar into your muffin cups.
2. Combine your remaining ingredients in a medium bowl. Whisk to combine, then pour evenly on top of your veggies.
3. Set to bake in your preheated oven for about 40 minutes or until golden brown. Allow to cool slightly (about 5 minutes), then serve. Enjoy!

Nutrition:

Calories: 58.5, Protein: 5.1g, Carbs: 2.9g, Fat: 3.2g, Sodium: 340mg, Potassium: 80mg.

141. Turkey Sausage and Mushroom Strata

Preparation Time: 15 minutes
Cooking Time: 8 minutes
Servings: 12

Ingredients:

- 8 oz. cubed Ciabatta bread
- 12 oz. chopped turkey sausage
- 2 c. milk
- 4 oz. shredded cheddar
- 3 large eggs
- 12 oz. egg substitute
- ½ c. chopped green onion
- 1 c. diced mushroom
- ½ tsp. paprika
- ½ tsp. pepper
- 2 tbsps. grated Parmesan cheese

Directions:

1. Set the oven to preheat to 400F. Lay your bread cubes flat on a baking tray and set it to toast for about 8 minutes. Meanwhile, add a skillet over medium heat with sausage and cook while stirring, until fully brown and crumbled.
2. Mix salt, pepper, paprika, parmesan cheese, egg substitute, eggs, cheddar cheese, and milk in a large bowl. Add in your remaining ingredients and toss well to incorporate.
3. Transfer mixture to a large baking dish (preferably a 9x13-inch), then tightly cover and allow to rest in the refrigerator overnight. Set your oven to preheat to 350F, remove the cover from your casserole, and set to bake until golden brown and cooked through. Slice and serve.

Nutrition:

Calories: 288.2, Protein: 24.3g, Carbs: 18.2g, Fat: 12.4g, Sodium: 355mg, Potassium: 100mg.

142. Bacon Bits

Preparation Time: 15 minutes
Cooking Time: 60 minutes
Servings: 4
Ingredients:

- 1 c. millet
- 5 c. water
- 1 c. diced sweet potato
- 1 tsp. ground cinnamon
- 2 tbsps. brown sugar
- 1 medium diced apple
- 1/4 c. honey

Directions:

1. In a deep pot, add your sugar, sweet potato, cinnamon, water, and millet. Stir to combine, then boil on high heat. After that, simmer on low.
2. Cook like this for about an hour until your water is fully

absorbed and the millet is cooked. Stir in your remaining ingredients and serve.

Nutrition:
Calories: 136, Protein: 3.1g, Carbs: 28.5g, Fat: 1.0g, Sodium: 120mg, Potassium: 130mg

143. Steel Cut Oat Blueberry Pancakes

Preparation Time: 15 minutes
Cooking Time: 15 minutes
Servings: 4
Ingredients:
- 11/2 c. water
- 1/2 c. steel-cut oats
- 1/8 tsp. salt
- 1 c. whole wheat flour
- 1/2 tsp. baking powder
- 1/2 tsp. baking soda
- 1 egg
- 1 c. milk
- 1/2 c. Greek yogurt
- 1 c. frozen blueberries
- 3/4 c. Agave nectar

Directions:
1. Combine your oats, salt, and water in a medium saucepan, stir, and allow to come to a boil over high heat. Adjust the heat to low, and allow to simmer for about 10 minutes, or until oats get tender. Set aside.
2. Combine all your remaining ingredients, except agave nectar, in a medium bowl, then fold in oats. Preheat your skillet and lightly grease it. Cook ¼ cup of milk batter at a time for about 3 minutes per side. Garnish with Agave nectar.

Nutrition:
Calories: 257, Protein: 14g, Carbs: 46g, Fat: 7g, Sodium: 123mg, Potassium: 120mg.

144. Spinach, Mushroom, and Feta Cheese Scramble

Preparation Time: 15 minutes
Cooking Time: 4 minutes
Servings: 1
Ingredients:
- Olive oil cooking spray
- ½ c. sliced mushroom
- 1 c. chopped spinach

- 3 eggs
- 2 tbsps. feta cheese
- Pepper

Directions:
1. Set a lightly greased, medium skillet over medium heat. Add spinach and mushrooms and cook until spinach wilts.
2. Combine egg whites, cheese, pepper, and whole egg in a medium bowl, whisk to combine. Pour into your skillet and cook, while stirring, until set (about 4 minutes). Serve.

Nutrition:
Calories: 236.5, Protein: 22.2g, Carbs: 12.9g, Fat: 11.4g, Sodium: 405mg, Potassium: 110mg.

145. Red Velvet Pancakes with Cream Cheese Topping

Preparation Time: 15 minutes
Cooking Time: 10 minutes
Servings: 2
Ingredients:
Cream Cheese Topping:
- 2 oz. cream cheese
- 3 tbsps. yogurt
- 3 tbsps. honey
- 1 tbsp. milk

Pancakes:
- 1/2 c. whole wheat flour
- 1/2 c. all-purpose flour
- 2 1/4tsp. baking powder
- 1/2 tsp. unsweetened cocoa powder
- 1/4 tsp. salt
- 1/4 c. sugar
- 1 large egg
- 1 c. + 2 tbsps. milk
- 1 tsp. vanilla
- 1 tsp. red paste food coloring

Directions:
1. Combine all your topping ingredients in a medium bowl and set aside. Add all your pancake ingredients to a large bowl and fold until combined. Set a greased skillet over medium heat to get hot.
2. Add ¼ cup of pancake batter onto the hot skillet and cook until bubbles begin to form on the top. Flip and cook until set. Repeat until your batter is done well. Add your toppings and serve.

Nutrition:

Calories: 231, Protein: 7g, Carbs: 43g, Fat: 4g, Sodium: 0mg, Potassium: 70mg.

146. Peanut Butter & Banana Breakfast Smoothie

Preparation Time: 15 minutes
Cooking Time: 0 minutes
Servings: 1
Ingredients:
- 1 c. non-fat milk
- 1 tbsp. peanut butter
- 1 banana
- 1/2 tsp. vanilla

Directions:
1. Place non-fat milk, peanut butter, and banana in a blender. Blend until smooth.

Nutrition:
Calories: 295, Protein: 133g, Carbs: 42g, Fat: 8.4g, Sodium: 100mg, Potassium: 140mg.

147. No-Bake Breakfast Granola Bars

Preparation Time: 15 minutes
Cooking Time: 0 minutes
Servings: 18
Ingredients:
- 2 c. old fashioned oatmeal
- 1/2 c. raisins
- 1/2 c. brown sugar
- 2 1/2 c. corn rice cereal
- 1/2 c. syrup
- 1/2 c. peanut butter
- 1/2 tsp. vanilla

Directions:
1. In a suitable size mixing bowl, mix using a wooden spoon, rice cereal, oatmeal, and raisins. In a saucepan, combine corn syrup and brown sugar. On a medium-high flame, continuously stir the mixture and bring to a boil.
2. On boiling, take away from heat. In a saucepan, stir vanilla and peanut into the sugar mixture. Stir until very smooth.
3. Spoon peanut butter mixture on the cereal and raisins into the mixing bowl and combine — shape mixture into a 9 x 13 baking tin. Allow to cool properly, then cut into bars (18 pcs).

Nutrition:

Calories: 152, Protein: 4g, Carbs: 26g, Fat: 4.3g, Sodium: 160mg, Potassium: 130mg.

148. Mushroom Shallot Frittata

Preparation Time: 15 minutes
Cooking Time: 25 minutes
Servings: 4
Ingredients:
- 1 tsp. butter
- 4 chopped shallots
- ½ lb. chopped mushrooms
- 2 tsp. chopped parsley
- 1 tsp. dried thyme
- Black pepper
- 3 medium Eggs
- 5 large egg whites
- 1 tbsp. milk
- ¼ c. grated parmesan cheese

Directions:
1. Preheat oven to 350F. In a suitable size oven-proof skillet, heat butter over medium flame. Add shallots and sauté for about 5 minutes, or until golden brown. Add to pot, thyme, parsley, chopped mushroom, and black pepper to taste.
2. Whisk milk, egg whites, parmesan, and eggs into a bowl. Pour the mixture into the skillet, ensuring the mushroom is covered completely. Transfer the skillet to the oven as soon as the edges begin to set.
3. Bake until frittata is cooked (15-20 mins). Should be served warm, cut into equal wedges (4 pcs).

Nutrition:
Calories: 346, Protein: 19.1g, Carbs: 48.3g, Fat: 12g, Sodium: 218mg, Potassium: 112mg.

149. Jack-o-Lantern Pancakes

Preparation Time: 15 minutes
Cooking Time: 5 minutes
Servings: 8
Ingredients:
- 1 Egg
- 1/2 c. canned pumpkin
- 1 3/4 c. low-fat milk
- 2 tbsps. vegetable oil
- 2 c. flour
- 2 tbsps. brown sugar
- 1 tbsp. baking powder
- 1 tsp. pumpkin pie spice

- 1 tsp. salt

Directions:
1. In a mixing bowl, mix milk, pumpkin, eggs, and oil. Add dry ingredients to the egg mixture. Stir gently. Coat skillet lightly with cooking spray and heat on medium.
2. When the skillet is hot, spoon (using a dessert spoon) batter onto the skillet. When bubbles start bursting, flip pancakes over and cook until it's a nice golden-brown color.

Nutrition:
Calories: 313, Protein: 15g, Carbs: 28g, Fat: 16g, Sodium: 1mg, Potassium: 120mg.

150. Fruit Pizza

Preparation Time: 15 minutes
Cooking Time: 0 minutes
Servings: 2
Ingredients:
- 1 English muffin
- 2 tbsps. fat-free cream cheese
- 2 tbsps. sliced strawberries
- 2 tbsps. blueberries
- 2 tbsps. crushed pineapple

Directions:
1. Cut English muffin in half and toast halves until slightly browned. Coat both halves with cream cheese. Arrange fruits atop cream cheese on muffin halves. Serve soon after preparation. Any leftovers refrigerate within 2 hours.

Nutrition:
Calories: 119, Protein: 6g, Carbs: 23g, Fat: 1g, Sodium: 288mg, Potassium: 100mg.

151. Flax Banana Yogurt Muffins

Preparation Time: 15 minutes
Cooking Time: 20 minutes
Servings: 12
Ingredients:
- 1 c. whole wheat flour
- 1 c. old-fashioned rolled oats
- 1 tsp. baking soda
- 2 tbsps. ground flaxseed
- 3 large ripe bananas
- 1/2 c. Greek yogurt
- 1/4 c. unsweetened applesauce
- 1/4 c. brown sugar
- 2 tsp. vanilla extract

Directions:
1. Set the oven to 355F and preheat. Prepare muffin tin, or you can use cooking spray or

cupcake liners. Combine dry ingredients in a mixing bowl.
2. In a separate bowl, mix yogurt, banana, sugar, vanilla, and applesauce. Combine both mixtures and mix. Do not over mix. The batter should not be smooth but lumpy. Bake for 20 minutes, or when inserted, toothpick comes out clean.

Nutrition:
Calories: 136, Protein: 4g, Carbs: 30g, Fat: 2g, Sodium: 242mg, Potassium: 60mg.

152. Apple Oats

Preparation Time: 5 minutes
Cooking Time: 5 minutes
Servings: 2
Ingredients:
- 1/2 cup oats
- 1 cup of water
- 1 apple, chopped
- 1 teaspoon olive oil
- 1/2 teaspoon vanilla extract

Directions:
1. Pour olive oil in the saucepan and add oats. Cook them for 2 minutes, stir constantly.
2. After this, add water and mix up.
3. Close the lid and cook oats on low heat for 5 minutes.
4. After this, add chopped apples and vanilla extract. Stir the meal.

Nutrition:
Calories: 159, Protein: 3g, Carbohydrates: 29.4g, Fat: 3.9g, Fiber: 4.8g, Cholesterol: 0mg, Sodium: 6mg, Potassium: 196mg.

153. Buckwheat Crepes

Preparation Time: 8 minutes
Cooking Time: 15 minutes
Servings: 6
Ingredients:
- 1 cup buckwheat flour
- 1/3 cup whole grain flour
- 1 egg, beaten
- 1 cup skim milk
- 1 teaspoon olive oil
- 1/2 teaspoon ground cinnamon

Directions:
1. In the mixing bowl, mix all ingredients and whisk until you get a smooth batter.
2. Heat the non-stick skillet on high flame for 3 minutes.

3. With the help of the ladle, pour the small amount of batter into the skillet and flatten it in the shape of the crepe.
4. Cook it for 1 minute and flip on another side. Cook it for 30 seconds more.
5. Repeat the same steps with the remaining batter.

Nutrition:
Calories: 122, Protein: 5.7g, Carbohydrates: 211g, Fat: 2.2g, Fiber: 2g, Cholesterol: 28mg, Sodium: 34mg, Potassium: 216mg.

154. Whole Grain Pancakes

Preparation Time: 10 minutes
Cooking Time: 5 minutes
Servings: 4
Ingredients:
- 1/2 teaspoon baking powder
- 1/4 cup skim milk
- 1 cup whole-grain wheat flour
- 2 teaspoons liquid honey
- 1 teaspoon olive oil

Directions:
1. Mix baking powder and flour in the bowl.
2. Add skim milk and olive oil. Whisk the mixture well.
3. Preheat the non-stick skillet and pour the small amount of dough inside in the shape of the pancake. Cook it for 2 minutes from each side or until the pancake is golden brown.
4. Top the cooked pancakes with liquid honey.

Nutrition:
Calories: 129, Protein: 4.6g, Carbohydrates: 25.7g, Fat: 1.7g, Fiber: 3.7g, Cholesterol: 0mg, Sodium: 10mg, Potassium: 211mg.

155. Granola Parfait

Preparation Time: 10 minutes
Cooking Time: 0 minutes
Servings: 2
Ingredients:
- ½ cup low-fat yogurt
- 4 tablespoons granola

Directions:
1. Put ½ tablespoon of granola in every glass.
2. Then add 2 tablespoons of low-fat yogurt.
3. Repeat the steps till you use all ingredients.

4. Store the parfait in the fridge for up to 2 hours.

Nutrition:
Calories: 79, Protein: 8g, Carbohydrates: 20.6g, Fat: 8.1g, Fiber: 2.8g, Cholesterol: 4mg, Sodium: 51mg.

156. Curry Tofu Scramble

Preparation Time: 10 minutes
Cooking Time: 5 minutes
Servings: 3
Ingredients:
- 12 oz. tofu, crumbled
- 1 teaspoon curry powder
- 1/4 cup skim milk
- 1 teaspoon olive oil
- 1/4 teaspoon chili flakes

Directions:
1. Heat olive oil in the skillet.
2. Add crumbled tofu and chili flakes.
3. In the bowl, mix the curry powder and skim milk.
4. Pour the liquid over the crumbled tofu and stir well.
5. Cook the scrambled tofu for 3 minutes on medium-high heat.

Nutrition:
Calories: 102, Protein: 10g, Carbohydrates: 3.3g, Fat: 6.4g, Fiber: 1.2g, Cholesterol: 0mg, Sodium: 25mg, Potassium: 210mg.

157. Scallions Omelet

Preparation Time: 10 minutes
Cooking Time: 10 minutes
Servings: 2
Ingredients:
- 1 oz. scallions, chopped
- 2 eggs, beaten
- 1 tablespoon low-fat sour cream
- 1/4 teaspoon ground black pepper
- 1 teaspoon olive oil

Directions:
1. Heat olive oil in the skillet.
2. Meanwhile, in the mixing bowl, mix all remaining ingredients.
3. Pour the egg mixture into the hot skillet, flatten well and cook for 7 minutes over medium-low heat.
4. The omelet is cooked when it is set.

Nutrition:
Calories: 101, Protein: 6g, Carbohydrates: 1.8g, Fat: 8g, Fiber: 0.4g, Cholesterol: 166mg,

Sodium: 67mg, Potassium: 110mg.

158. Breakfast Almond Smoothie

Preparation Time: 5 minutes
Cooking Time: 2 minutes
Servings: 3
Ingredients:
- 1/2 cup almonds, chopped
- 1 cup low-fat milk
- 1 banana, peeled, chopped

Directions:
1. Put all ingredients in the blender and blend until smooth.
2. Pour the smoothie into the serving glasses.

Nutrition:
Calories: 161, Protein: 6.5g, Carbohydrates: 16.4g, Fat: 8.8g, Fiber: 3g, Cholesterol: 4mg, Sodium: 36mg, Potassium: 379mg.

159. Fruits and Rice Pudding

Preparation Time: 10 minutes
Cooking Time: 10 minutes
Servings: 3
Ingredients:
- 1/2 cup long-grain rice
- 1 1/2 cup low-fat milk
- 1 teaspoon vanilla extract
- 2 oz. apricots, chopped

Directions:
1. Pour milk and add rice to the saucepan.
2. Close the lid and cook the rice on medium-high heat for 10 minutes.
3. Then add vanilla extract and stir the rice well.
4. Transfer the pudding to the bowls and top with apricots.

Nutrition:
Calories: 171, Protein: 6.4g, Carbohydrates: 32.9g, Fat: 0.3g, Fiber: 0.8g, Cholesterol: 2mg, Sodium: 67mg, Potassium: 276mg.

160. Asparagus Omelet

Preparation Time: 5 minutes
Cooking Time: 10 minutes
Servings: 2
Ingredients:
- 3 oz. asparagus, boiled, chopped

- 1/4 teaspoon ground paprika
- 1/2 teaspoon ground cumin
- 3 eggs, beaten
- 2 tablespoons low-fat milk
- 1 teaspoon avocado oil

Directions:
1. Heat avocado oil in the skillet.
2. Meanwhile, mix ground paprika, ground cumin, eggs and milk.
3. Pour the liquid into the hot skillet and cook it for 2 minutes.
4. Then add chopped asparagus and close the lid.
5. Cook the omelet for 5 minutes on low heat.

Nutrition:
Calories: 115, Protein: 9.9g, Carbohydrates: 3.4g, Fat: 7.2g, Fiber: 1.2g, Cholesterol: 246mg, Sodium: 101mg, Potassium: 220mg.

161. Bean Frittata

Preparation Time: 5 minutes
Cooking Time: 12 minutes
Servings: 4
Ingredients:
- 4 eggs, beaten
- 1/2 cup red kidney beans, canned
- 1/2 onion, diced
- 1 tablespoon margarine
- 1 teaspoon dried dill

Directions:
1. Toss the margarine in the skillet. Add onion and sauté it for 4 minutes or until it is soft.
2. Then add red kidney beans and dried dill. Mix the mixture up.
3. Pour the eggs over it and close the lid.
4. Cook the frittata on medium-low heat for 7 minutes or until it is set or bake it in the oven at 390F for 5 minutes.

Nutrition:
Calories: 172, Protein: 11g, Carbohydrates: 15.9g, Fat: 7.5g, Fiber: 3.8g, Cholesterol: 164mg, Sodium: 99mg, Potassium: 401mg.

162. Peach Pancakes

Preparation Time: 10 minutes
Cooking Time: 10 minutes
Servings: 6
Ingredients:
- 1 cup whole-wheat flour
- 1 egg, beaten
- 1 teaspoon vanilla extract
- 2 peaches, chopped

- 1 tablespoon margarine
- 1/2 teaspoon baking powder
- 1 teaspoon apple cider vinegar
- 1/4 cup skim milk

Directions:
1. Make the pancake batter: in the mixing bowl, mix eggs, whole-wheat flour, vanilla extract, baking powder, apple cider vinegar, and skim milk.
2. Then melt the margarine in the skillet.
3. Pour the prepared batter into the skillet with the help of the ladle and flatten in the shape of the pancake.
4. Cook the pancakes for 2 minutes from each side over medium-low heat.
5. Top the cooked pancakes with peaches.

Nutrition:
Calories: 129, Protein: 3.9g, Carbohydrates: 21.5g, Fat: 3g, Fiber: 1.3g, Cholesterol: 27mg, Sodium: 39mg, Potassium: 188mg.

163. Breakfast Splits

Preparation Time: 15 minutes
Cooking Time: 0 minutes
Servings: 2
Ingredients:
- 2 bananas, peeled
- 4 tablespoons granola
- 2 tablespoons low-fat yogurt
- 1/2 teaspoon ground cinnamon
- 1 strawberry, chopped

Directions:
1. In the mixing bowl, mix yogurt with ground cinnamon and strawberries.
2. Then make the lengthwise cuts in bananas and fill them with the yogurt mass.
3. Top the fruits with granola.

Nutrition:
Calories: 154, Protein: 6.8g, Carbohydrates: 45.2g, Fat: 8g, Fiber: 6.3g, Cholesterol: 1mg, Sodium: 20mg, Potassium: 635mg.

164. Banana Pancakes

Preparation Time: 10 minutes
Cooking Time: 15 minutes
Servings: 5
Ingredients:
- 2 bananas, mashed
- 1/2 cup 1% milk

- 1 1/2 cup whole-grain flour
- 1 teaspoon liquid honey
- 1 teaspoon vanilla extract
- 1 teaspoon baking powder
- 1 tablespoon lemon juice
- 1 tablespoon olive oil

Directions:
1. Mix mashed bananas and milk.
2. Then add flour, liquid honey, vanilla extract, baking powder, and lemon juice.
3. Whisk the mixture until you get a smooth batter.
4. After this, heat olive oil in the skillet.
5. When the oil is hot, pour the pancake mixture into the skillet and flatten it in the shape of pancakes.
6. Cook them for 1 minute and then flip on another side. Cook the pancakes for 1 minute more.

Nutrition:
Calories: 207, Protein: 6.3g, Carbohydrates: 39.9g, Fat: 3.9g, Fiber: 5.7g, Cholesterol: 1mg, Sodium: 15mg, Potassium: 458mg.

165. Aromatic Breakfast Granola

Preparation Time: 10 minutes
Cooking Time: 25 minutes
Servings: 2
Ingredients:
- 2 tablespoons avocado oil
- 1 tablespoon liquid honey
- 1/4 teaspoon ground cinnamon
- 1/4 cup almonds, chopped
- 1 tablespoon chia seeds
- 1 teaspoon sesame seeds
- 2 tablespoons cut oats
- Cooking spray

Directions:
1. Heat avocado oil and liquid honey until you get a homogenous mixture.
2. Then add ground cinnamon, almonds, chia seeds, sesame seeds, and cut oats.
3. Stir until homogenous.
4. Grease the baking tray with cooking spray and place the almond mixture inside.
5. Flatten it in the shape of a square.
6. Bake the granola at 345F for 20 minutes.
7. Cut it into servings.

Nutrition:

Calories: 203, Protein: 5.7g, Carbohydrates: 22.3g, Fat: 11.4g, Fiber: 5.9g, Cholesterol: 0mg, Sodium: 2mg, Potassium: 211mg.

166. Morning Sweet Potatoes

Preparation Time: 5 minutes
Cooking Time: 20 minutes
Servings: 2
Ingredients:
- 2 sweet potatoes
- 1 tablespoon chives, chopped
- 2 teaspoons margarine
- 1/4 teaspoon chili flakes

Directions:
1. Preheat the oven to 400F.
2. Put the sweet potatoes in the oven and cook them for 20 minutes or until the vegetables are soft.
3. Then cut the sweet potato into halves and top with margarine, chives, and chili flakes. Wait till margarine starts to melt.

Nutrition:
Calories: 35, Protein: 0.1g, Carbohydrates: 0.4g, Fat: 3.8g, Fiber: 0.1g, Cholesterol: 0mg, Sodium: 45mg, Potassium: 15mg.

167. Egg Toasts

Preparation Time: 5 minutes
Cooking Time: 5 minutes
Servings: 3
Ingredients:
- 3 eggs
- 3 whole-grain bread slices
- 1 teaspoon olive oil
- 1/4 teaspoon minced garlic
- 1/4 teaspoon ground black pepper

Directions:
1. Heat olive oil in the skillet.
2. Crack the eggs inside and cook them for 4 minutes.
3. Meanwhile, rub the bread slices with minced garlic.
4. Top the bread with cooked eggs and sprinkle with ground black pepper.

Nutrition:
Calories: 157, Protein: 8.6g, Carbohydrates: 13.5g, Fat: 7.4g, Fiber: 2.1g, Cholesterol: 164mg, Sodium: 182mg, Potassium: 62mg.

168. Sweet Yogurt with Figs

Preparation Time: 5 minutes
Cooking Time: 0 minutes
Servings: 1
Ingredients:
- 1/3 cup low-fat yogurt
- 1 teaspoon almond flakes
- 1 fresh fig, chopped
- 1 teaspoon liquid honey
- 1/4 teaspoon sesame seeds

Directions:
1. Mix yogurt and honey and pour the mixture into the serving glass.
2. Top it with chopped fig, almond flakes, and sesame seeds.

Nutrition:
Calories: 178, Protein: 6.2g, Carbohydrates: 24.4g, Fat: 6.8g, Fiber: 3.1g, Cholesterol: 5mg, Sodium: 44mg, Potassium: 283mg.

169. Vanilla Toasts

Preparation Time: 10 minutes
Cooking Time: 5 minutes
Servings: 3
Ingredients:
- 3 whole-grain bread slices
- 1 teaspoon vanilla extract
- 1 egg, beaten
- 2 tablespoons low-fat sour cream
- 1 tablespoon margarine

Directions:
1. Melt the butter in the skillet.
2. Meanwhile, in the bowl, mix vanilla extract, eggs, and low-fat sour cream.
3. Dip the bread slices in the egg mixture well.
4. Then transfer them in the melted margarine and roast for 2 minutes from each side.

Nutrition:
Calories: 166, Protein: 5.1g, Carbohydrates: 18.7g, Fat: 7.9g, Fiber: 2g, Cholesterol: 58mg, Sodium: 229mg, Potassium: 39mg.

170. Raspberry Yogurt

Preparation Time: 5 minutes
Cooking Time: 0 minutes
Servings: 2
Ingredients:
- 1/2 cup low-fat yogurt
- 1/2 cup raspberries

- 1 teaspoon almond flakes

Directions:
1. Mix yogurt and raspberries and transfer them to the serving glasses.
2. Top yogurt with almond flakes.

Nutrition:
Calories: 77, Protein: 3.9g, Carbohydrates: 8.6g, Fat: 3.4g, Fiber: 2.6g, Cholesterol: 4mg, Sodium: 32mg, Potassium: 192mg.

171. Salsa Eggs

Preparation Time: 10 minutes
Cooking Time: 10 minutes
Servings: 4
Ingredients:
- 2 tomatoes, chopped
- 1 chili pepper, chopped
- 2 cucumbers, chopped
- 1 red onion, chopped
- 2 tablespoons parsley, chopped
- 1 tablespoon olive oil
- 1 tablespoon lemon juice
- 4 eggs
- 1 cup water for cooking eggs

Directions:
1. Put eggs in the water and boil them for 7 minutes. Cool the cooked eggs in the cold water and peel.
2. After this, make salsa salad: Mix tomatoes, chili pepper, cucumbers, red onion, parsley, olive oil, and lemon juice.
3. Cut the eggs into the halves and sprinkle generously with cooked salsa salad.

Nutrition:
Calories: 140, Protein: 7.5g, Carbohydrates: 11.1g, Fat: 8.3g, Fiber: 2.2g, Cholesterol: 164mg, Sodium: 71mg, Potassium: 484mg.

172. Fruit Scones

Preparation Time: 10 minutes
Cooking Time: 12 minutes
Servings: 8
Ingredients:
- 2 cups whole-grain wheat flour
- ½ teaspoon baking powder
- ¼ cup cranberries, dried
- ¼ cup chia seeds
- ¼ cup apricots, chopped
- ¼ cup almonds, chopped
- 1 tablespoon liquid honey
- 1 egg, whisked

Directions:
1. In the bowl, mix all the ingredients and knead the dough.

2. Cut the dough into 16 pieces (scones)
3. Bake them at 350 degrees F for 12 minutes in the lined baking paper tray.
4. Cool the scones well.

Nutrition:
Calories: 156, Protein: 6.1g, Carbohydrates: 27.1g, Fat: 3.7g, Fiber: 5.5g, Cholesterol: 20mg, Sodium: 10mg, Potassium: 216mg.

173. Berry Pancakes

Preparation Time: 10 minutes
Cooking Time: 8 minutes
Servings: 12
Ingredients:
- 2 eggs, whisked
- 4 tablespoons almond milk
- 1 cup low-fat yogurt
- 3 tablespoons margarine, melted
- ½ teaspoon vanilla extract
- 1 cup almond flour
- 1 cup strawberries

Directions:
1. Pour the margarine into the skillet.
2. Mix all remaining ingredients and blend with the help of the mixer.
3. Then pour the dough into the hot skillet in the shape of the pancakes and cook for 1.5 minutes from each side.

Nutrition:
Calories: 80, Protein: 2.8g, Carbohydrates: 3.3g, Fat: 6.2g, Fiber: 0.6g, Cholesterol: 29mg, Sodium: 60mg, Potassium: 91mg.

174. Western Omelet Quiche

Preparation Time: 10 minutes
Cooking Time: 30 minutes
Servings: 4-6
Ingredients:
- 6 beaten eggs
- 1/8 teaspoon of mineral salt and black pepper
- ¾ cup diced peppers
- ¾ spring onions, sliced
- ¾ cup shredded cheese
- ½ cup half and half
- 8 oz., chopped Canadian bacon
- ¼ cup shredded cheddar cheese to garnish

Directions:

1. Add two cups of water to the bottom of the Instant Pot and then add the trivet.
2. Spray a soufflé dish with butter or cooking spray, and then in a mixing bowl, add the eggs, salt, milk, and pepper together.
3. Add the rest of the ingredients to the dish and mix it well.
4. Put it in a soufflé dish, and from there, add to the Instant Pot, cooking on high pressure for 30 minutes of cook time.
5. Open up the lid and sprinkle the top of it with more cheese.

Nutrition: Calories: 365, Fat: 15g, Carbs: 6g, Net Carbs: 4g, Protein: 24g, Fiber: 2g, Sodium: 45mg, Potassium: 92mg.

175. Ginger French toast

Preparation Time: 10 minutes
Cooking Time: 5 minutes
Servings: 2
Ingredients:
- 4 whole-wheat bread slices
- ½ cup low-fat milk
- 2 eggs, whisked
- 1 teaspoon ground ginger
- Cooking spray

Directions:
1. Grease the skillet with cooking spray.
2. In the mixing bowl, mix milk and eggs.
3. Then add ginger and dip the bread in the liquid.
4. Roast the bread in the preheated skillet for 2 minutes from each side.

Nutrition:
Calories: 229, Protein: 15.6g, Carbohydrates: 29.4g, Fat: 8g, Fiber: 4g, Cholesterol: 167mg, Sodium: 388mg, Potassium: 150mg.

176. Fruit Muffins

Preparation Time: 35 minutes
Cooking Time: 10 minutes
Servings: 6
Ingredients:
- 1 cup apple, grated
- 1 cup quinoa
- 2 cups oatmeal
- ½ cup of coconut milk
- 1 tablespoon liquid honey
- 1 teaspoon vanilla extract
- 1 tablespoon olive oil
- 1 cup of water
- 1 teaspoon ground nutmeg

Directions:

1. Mix water and quinoa and the mixture for 15 minutes, fluff with a fork and transfer to a bowl.
2. Add all remaining ingredients and mix well.
3. Transfer the batter to the muffin molds and bake them at 375F for 20 minutes.

Nutrition:
Calories: 308, Protein: 8.2g, Carbohydrates: 46g, Fat: 10.8g, Fiber: 6.2g, Cholesterol: 0mg, Sodium: 7mg, Potassium: 355mg.

177. Omelet with Peppers

Preparation Time: 10 minutes
Cooking Time: 15 minutes
Servings: 4
Ingredients:
- 4 eggs, beaten
- 1 tablespoon margarine
- 1 cup bell peppers, chopped
- 2 oz. scallions, chopped

Directions:
1. Toss the margarine in the skillet and melt it.
2. In the mixing bowl, mix eggs and bell peppers. Add scallions.
3. Pour the egg mixture into the hot skillet and roast the omelet for 12 minutes.

Nutrition:
Calories: 102, Protein: 6.1g, Carbohydrates: 3.7g, Fat: 7.3g, Fiber: 0.8g, Cholesterol: 164mg, Sodium: 98mg, Potassium: 156mg.

178. Quinoa Hashes

Preparation Time: 10 minutes
Cooking Time: 25 minutes
Servings: 2
Ingredients:
- 3 oz. quinoa
- 6 oz. water
- 2 potatoes, grated
- 1 egg, beaten
- 1 tablespoon avocado oil
- 1 teaspoon chives, chopped

Directions:
1. Cook quinoa in water for 15 minutes.
2. Heat avocado oil in the skillet.
3. Then mix all remaining ingredients in the bowl. Add quinoa and mix well.
4. Add quinoa hash browns, cook for 5 minutes on each side.

Nutrition:
Calories: 344, Protein: 12.5g, Carbohydrates: 61.3g, Fat: 5.9g, Fiber: 8.4g, Cholesterol: 82mg, Sodium: 49mg, Potassium: 1160mg.

179. Artichoke Eggs

Preparation Time: 5 minutes
Cooking Time: 20 minutes
Servings: 4
Ingredients:
- 5 eggs, beaten
- 2 oz. low-fat feta, chopped
- 1 yellow onion, chopped
- 1 tablespoon canola oil
- 1 tablespoon cilantro, chopped
- 1 cup artichoke hearts, canned, chopped

Directions:
1. Grease 4 ramekins with oil.
2. Mix all remaining ingredients and divide the mixture between prepared ramekins.
3. Bake the meal at 380F for 20 minutes.

Nutrition:
Calories: 177, Protein: 10.6g, Carbohydrates: 7.4g, Fat: 12.2g, Fiber: 2.5g, Cholesterol: 217mg, Sodium: 259mg, Potassium: 235mg.

180. Quinoa Cakes

Preparation Time: 25 minutes
Cooking Time: 10 minutes

Servings: 4
Ingredients:
- 7 oz. quinoa
- 1 cup cauliflower, shredded
- 1 cup of water
- ½ cup vegan parmesan, grated
- 1 egg, beaten
- 1 tablespoon olive oil
- ½ teaspoon ground black pepper

Directions:
1. Mix the quinoa with the cauliflower, water, and ground black pepper, stir, bring to a simmer over medium heat and cook for 15 minutes.
2. Cool the mixture and add parmesan and the eggs; stir well. Shape medium cakes out of this mix.
3. Heat a pan with the oil over medium-high heat and add the quinoa cakes. Cook them for 4-5 minutes per side.

Nutrition:
Calories: 280, Protein: 14.9g, Carbohydrates: 36.4g, Fat: 7.6g, Fiber: 4.2g, Cholesterol: 41mg, Sodium: 222mg, Potassium: 374mg.

181. Bean Casserole

Preparation Time: 10 minutes
Cooking Time: 30 minutes
Servings: 8
Ingredients:
- 5 eggs, beaten

- ½ cup bell pepper, chopped
- 1 cup red kidney beans, cooked
- ½ cup white onions, chopped
- 1 cup low-fat mozzarella cheese, shredded

Directions:
1. Spread the beans over the casserole mold. Add onions and bell pepper.
2. Add the eggs mixed with the cheese.
3. Bake the casserole at 380F for 30 minutes.

Nutrition:
Calories: 142, Protein: 12.8g, Carbohydrates: 16g, Fat: 3g, Fiber: 4.3g, Cholesterol: 105mg, Sodium: 162mg, Potassium: 374mg.

182. Grape Yogurt

Preparation Time: 10 minutes
Cooking Time: 0 minutes
Servings: 3
Ingredients:
- 1 ½ cup low-fat yogurt
- ½ cup grapes, chopped
- 1 oz. walnuts, chopped

Directions:
1. Mix all ingredients and transfer them to the serving glasses.

Nutrition:
Calories: 156, Protein: 9.4g, Carbohydrates: 12.2g, Fat: 7.1g, Fiber: 0.8g, Cholesterol: 7mg, Sodium: 86mg, Potassium: 365mg.

Chapter 7. Snacks

183. Herb-Marinated Feta and Artichokes

Preparation Time: 10 minutes, plus 4 hours inactive time
Cooking Time: 10 minutes
Servings: 2
Ingredients:

- 4 ounces traditional Greek feta, cut into ½-inch cubes
- 4 ounces drained artichoke hearts, quartered lengthwise
- 1/3 cup extra-virgin olive oil
- Zest and juice of 1 lemon
- 2 tablespoons roughly chopped fresh rosemary
- 2 tablespoons roughly chopped fresh parsley
- ½ teaspoon black peppercorns

Directions:

1. In a glass bowl, combine the feta and artichoke hearts. Add the olive oil, lemon zest and juice, rosemary, parsley, and peppercorns. Toss gently to coat, being sure not to crumble the feta.
2. Cool for 4 hours, or up to 4 days. Take out of the refrigerator 30 minutes before serving.

Nutrition:
Calories: 235, Fat: 23g, Carbohydrates: 1g, Protein: 4g, Sodium: 43mg, Potassium: 123mg.

184. Yellowfin Croquettes

Preparation Time: 40 minutes, plus hours to overnight to chill
Cooking Time: 25 minutes
Servings: 36
Ingredients:

- 6 tablespoons extra-virgin olive oil, plus 1 to 2 cups
- 5 tablespoons almond flour, plus 1 cup, divided
- 1¼ cups heavy cream
- 1 (4-ounce) can olive oil-packed yellowfin tuna
- 1 tablespoon chopped red onion
- 2 teaspoons minced capers
- ½ teaspoon dried dill
- ¼ teaspoon freshly ground black pepper
- 2 large eggs
- 1 cup panko breadcrumbs (or a gluten-free version)

Directions:

1. In a large skillet, heat 6 tablespoons of olive oil over medium-low fire. Add 5 tablespoons almond flour and cook, stirring constantly, until a smooth paste forms and the flour browns slightly, 2 to 3 minutes.
2. Select the heat to medium-high and gradually mix in the heavy cream, whisking constantly until completely smooth and thickened, another 4 to 5 minutes. Remove and add in the tuna, red onion, capers, dill, and pepper.
3. Transfer the mixture to an 8-inch square baking dish well coated with olive oil and set aside at room temperature. Wrap and cool for 4 hours or up to overnight. To form the croquettes, set out three bowls. In one, beat together the eggs. In another, add the remaining almond flour. In the third, add the panko. Line a baking sheet with parchment paper.
4. Scoop about one tablespoon of cold prepared dough into the flour mixture and roll to coat. Shake off excess and, using your hands, roll into an oval.
5. Dip the croquette into the beaten egg, then lightly coat in panko. Set on a lined baking sheet and repeat with the remaining dough.
6. In a small saucepan, heat the remaining 1 to 2 cups of olive oil over medium-high heat.
7. Once the oil is heated, fry the croquettes 3 or 4 at a time, depending on the size of your pan, removing with a slotted spoon when golden brown. You will need to adjust the temperature of the oil occasionally to prevent burning. If the croquettes get dark brown very quickly, lower the temperature.

Nutrition:
Calories: 245, Fat: 22g, Carbohydrates: 1g, Protein: 6g, Sodium: 63mg, Potassium: 123mg.

185. All-Spiced Olives

Preparation Time: 4 hours and 10 minutes
Cooking Time: 0 minutes
Servings: 2
Ingredients:

- 2 cups mixed green olives with pits
- ¼ cup red wine vinegar
- ¼ cup extra-virgin olive oil
- 4 garlic cloves, finely minced
- Zest and juice of 1 large orange
- 1 teaspoon red pepper flakes
- 2 bay leaves
- ½ teaspoon ground cumin
- ½ teaspoon ground allspice

Directions:

1. Incorporate the olives, vinegar, oil, garlic, orange zest and juice, red pepper flakes, bay leaves, cumin, and allspice and mix well. Seal and chill for 4 hours or up to a week to allow the olives to marinate, tossing again before serving.

Nutrition:
Calories: 133, Fat: 14g, Carbohydrates: 2g, Protein: 1g, Sodium: 53mg, Potassium: 133mg.

186. Pitted Olives and Anchovies

Preparation Time: 1 hour and 10 minutes
Cooking Time: 0 minutes
Servings: 2
Ingredients:

- 2 cups pitted Kalamata olives or other black olives
- 2 anchovy fillets, chopped
- 2 teaspoons chopped capers
- 1 garlic clove, finely minced
- 1 cooked egg yolk
- 1 teaspoon Dijon mustard
- ¼ cup extra-virgin olive oil
- Seedy Crackers, Versatile Sandwich Round, or vegetables, for serving (optional)

Directions:

1. Wash the olives in cold water and strain well. In a food processor, blender or large pitcher (if using an immersion blender), place the drained

olives, anchovies, capers, garlic, egg yolk and Dijon. Process until a thick paste forms. While processing, gradually add the olive oil.

2. Transfer to a small bowl, cover and refrigerate at least 1 hour for flavors to develop. Serve with crackers, on a versatile sandwich or with your favorite crunchy vegetables.

Nutrition:
Calories: 179, Fat: 19g, Carbohydrates: 2g, Protein: 2g, Sodium: 43mg, Potassium: 113mg.

187. Medi Deviled Eggs

Preparation Time: 45 minutes
Cooking Time: 15 minutes
Servings: 4
Ingredients:
- 4 large hardboiled eggs
- 2 tablespoons Roasted Garlic Aioli
- ½ cup finely crumbled feta cheese
- 8 pitted Kalamata olives, finely chopped
- 2 tablespoons chopped sun-dried tomatoes
- 1 tablespoon minced red onion
- ½ teaspoon dried dill
- ¼ teaspoon freshly ground black pepper

Directions:
1. Chop the hardboiled eggs half lengthwise, remove the yolks, and place the yolks in a medium bowl. Reserve the egg white halves and set them aside. Smash the yolks well with a fork. Add the aioli, feta, olives, sun-dried tomatoes, onion, dill, and pepper and stir to combine until smooth and creamy.
2. Spoon the filling into each egg white half and chill for 30 minutes, or up to 24 hours, covered.

Nutrition:
Calories: 147, Fat: 11g, Carbohydrates: 6g, Protein: 9g, Sodium: 43mg, Potassium: 123mg.

188. Cheese Crackers

Preparation Time: 1 hour and 15 minutes
Cooking Time: 15 minutes

Servings: 20
Ingredients:
- 4 tablespoons butter at room temperature
- 1 cup finely shredded Manchego cheese
- 1 cup almond flour
- 1 teaspoon salt, divided
- ¼ teaspoon freshly ground black pepper
- 1 large egg

Directions:
1. With an electric mixer, beat the butter and grated cheese until well combined and smooth. Stir in the almond flour with ½ teaspoon salt and pepper. Gradually incorporate the almond flour mixture into the cheese, mixing constantly until the dough comes together to form a ball.
2. Place on a piece of parchment or plastic wrap and roll into a cylindrical log about 1½ inches thick. Seal well and freeze for at least 1 hour. Preheat oven to 350°F. Place parchment paper or silicone baking mats on 2 baking sheets.
3. To make the egg wash, scourge together the egg and remaining ½ teaspoon salt. Slice the refrigerated dough into small rounds, about ¼ inch thick, and place on the lined baking sheets.
4. Egg wash the tops of the crackers and bake until the crackers are golden and crispy. Put on a wire rack to cool.
5. Serve warm or, once fully cooled, store in an airtight container in the refrigerator for up to 1 week.

Nutrition:
Calories: 243, Fat: 23g, Carbohydrates: 1g, Protein: 8g, Sodium: 63mg, Potassium: 123mg.

189. Cheesy Caprese Stack

Preparation Time: 5 minutes
Cooking Time: 0 minutes
Servings: 4
Ingredients:
- 1 large organic tomato, preferably heirloom
- ½ teaspoon salt
- ¼ teaspoon freshly ground black pepper
- 1 (4-ounce) ball burrata cheese
- 8 fresh basil leaves, thinly sliced

- 2 tablespoons extra-virgin olive oil
- 1 tablespoon red wine or balsamic vinegar

Directions:
1. Cut the tomato into 4 thick slices, removing the hard center core and sprinkle with salt and pepper. Place the tomatoes, seasoned side up, on a plate. On another rimmed plate, cut the burrata into 4 thick slices and place a slice on top of each tomato slice. Top each with a quarter of the basil and pour the reserved burrata cream onto the rimmed plate on top.
2. Dash with olive oil and vinegar and serve with a fork and knife.

Nutrition:
Calories: 153, Fat: 13g, Carbohydrates: 1g, Protein: 7g, Sodium: 63mg, Potassium: 123mg.

190. Zucchini-Cheese Fritters with Aioli

Preparation Time: 10 minutes, plus 20 minutes rest time
Cooking Time: 25 minutes
Servings: 4
Ingredients:
- 1 large or 2 small/medium zucchini
- 1 teaspoon salt, divided
- ½ cup whole-milk ricotta cheese
- 2 scallions
- 1 large egg
- 2 garlic cloves, finely minced
- 2 tablespoons chopped fresh mint (optional)
- 2 teaspoons grated lemon zest
- ¼ teaspoon freshly ground black pepper
- ½ cup almond flour
- 1 teaspoon baking powder
- 8 tablespoons extra-virgin olive oil
- 8 tablespoons Roasted Garlic Aioli or avocado oil mayonnaise

Directions:
1. Put the shredded zucchini in a colander or on several layers of paper towels. Sprinkle with ½ teaspoon salt and let sit for 10 minutes.
2. Using another layer of paper towel, press down on the zucchini to release any excess moisture and pat dry. Incorporate the drained zucchini, ricotta, scallions, egg,

garlic, mint (if using), lemon zest, remaining ½ teaspoon salt, and pepper.
3. Scourge together the almond flour and baking powder. Fold in the flour mixture into the zucchini mixture and let rest for 10 minutes. In a large skillet, working in four batches, fry the fritters.
4. For each batch of four, heat 2 tablespoons of olive oil over medium-high heat. Add 1 heaping tablespoon of zucchini batter per fritter, pressing down with the back of a spoon to form 2- to 3-inch fritters. Cover and let fry 2 minutes before flipping. Fry another 2 to 3 minutes, covered, or until crispy and golden and cooked through. You may need to reduce heat to medium to prevent burning. Remove from the pan and keep warm.
5. Repeat for the remaining three batches, using 2 tablespoons of olive oil for each batch. Serve fritters warm with aioli.

Nutrition:
Calories: 448, Fat: 42g, Carbohydrates: 2g, Protein: 8g, Sodium: 53mg, Potassium: 123mg.

191. Cucumbers Filled with Salmon

Preparation Time: 10 minutes
Cooking Time: 0 minutes
Servings: 4
Ingredients:
- 2 large cucumbers, peeled
- 1 (4-ounce) can red salmon
- 1 medium very ripe avocado
- 1 tablespoon extra-virgin olive oil
- Zest and juice of 1 lime
- 3 tablespoons chopped fresh cilantro
- ½ teaspoon salt
- ¼ teaspoon freshly ground black pepper

Directions:
1. Cut the cucumber into 1-inch-thick wedges and, using a spoon, scrape the seeds from the center of each wedge and stand it upright on a plate. In a medium bowl, combine the salmon, avocado, olive oil, lime zest and juice, cilantro, salt and pepper and mix until creamy.

2. Scoop the salmon mixture into the center of each cucumber segment and serve chilled.

Nutrition:
Calories: 159, Fat: 11g, Carbohydrates: 3g, Protein: 9g, Sodium: 65mg, Potassium: 123mg.

192. Smoked Mackerel Pâté

Preparation Time: 10 minutes
Cooking Time: 0 minutes
Servings: 4
Ingredients:
- 4 ounces olive oil-packed wild-caught mackerel
- 2 ounces goat cheese
- Zest and juice of 1 lemon
- 2 tablespoons chopped fresh parsley
- 2 tablespoons chopped fresh arugula
- 1 tablespoon extra-virgin olive oil
- 2 teaspoons chopped capers
- 1 to 2 teaspoons fresh horseradish (optional)
- Crackers, cucumber rounds, endive spears, or celery for serving (optional)

Directions:
1. In a food processor, blender, or large bowl with an immersion blender, combine the mackerel, goat cheese, lemon zest and juice, parsley, arugula, olive oil, capers, and horseradish (if using). Process or blend until smooth and creamy.
2. Serve with crackers, cucumber rounds, endive spears, or celery. Seal covered in the refrigerator for up to 1 week.

Nutrition:
Calories: 118, Fat: 8g, Carbohydrates: 6g, Protein: 9g, Sodium: 43mg, Potassium: 123mg.

193. Medi Fat Bombs

Preparation Time: 4 hours and 15 minutes
Cooking Time: 0 minutes
Servings: 6
Ingredients:
- 1 cup crumbled goat cheese
- 4 tablespoons jarred pesto
- 12 pitted Kalamata olives, finely chopped

- ½ cup finely chopped walnuts
- 1 tablespoon chopped fresh rosemary

Directions:
1. In a medium bowl, scourge the goat cheese, pesto, and olives and mix well using a fork. Freeze for 4 hours to toughen.
2. With your hands, create the mixture into 6 balls, about ¾-inch diameter. The mixture will be sticky.
3. In a small bowl, place the walnuts and rosemary and roll the goat cheese balls in the nut mixture to coat. Store the fat bombs in the refrigerator for up to 1 week or in the freezer for up to 1 month.

Nutrition:
Calories: 166, Fat: 15g, Carbohydrates: 1g, Protein: 5g, Sodium: 55mg, Potassium: 123mg.

194. Avocado Cold Soup

Preparation Time: 15 minutes
Cooking Time: 10 minutes
Servings: 4
Ingredients:
- 2 cups chopped tomatoes
- 2 large ripe avocados, halved and pitted
- 1 large cucumber, peeled and seeded
- 1 medium bell pepper (red, orange or yellow), chopped
- 1 cup plain whole-milk Greek yogurt
- ¼ cup extra-virgin olive oil
- ¼ cup chopped fresh cilantro
- ¼ cup chopped scallions, green part only
- 2 tablespoons red wine vinegar
- Juice of 2 limes or 1 lemon
- ½ to 1 teaspoon salt
- ¼ teaspoon freshly ground black pepper

Directions:
1. Using an immersion blender, combine the tomatoes, avocados, cucumber, bell pepper, yogurt, olive oil, cilantro, scallions, vinegar, and lime juice. Blend until smooth.
2. Season and blend to combine the flavors. Serve cold.

Nutrition:
Calories: 392, Fat: 32g, Carbohydrates: 9g, Protein: 6g, Sodium: 53mg, Potassium: 133mg.

195. Crab Cake Lettuce Cups

Preparation Time: 35 minutes
Cooking Time: 20 minutes
Servings: 4
Ingredients:
- 1-pound jumbo lump crab
- 1 large egg
- 6 tablespoons Roasted Garlic Aioli
- 2 tablespoons Dijon mustard
- ½ cup almond flour
- ¼ cup minced red onion
- 2 teaspoons smoked paprika
- 1 teaspoon celery salt
- 1 teaspoon garlic powder
- 1 teaspoon dried dill (optional)
- ½ teaspoon freshly ground black pepper
- ¼ cup extra-virgin olive oil
- 4 large Bibb lettuce leaves, thick spine removed

Directions:
1. Put the crabmeat in a large bowl and pick out any visible shells, then break apart the meat with a fork. In a small bowl, scourge together the egg, 2 tablespoons aioli, and Dijon mustard. Add to the crabmeat and blend with a fork. Add the almond flour, red onion, paprika, celery salt, garlic powder, dill (if using), and pepper and combine well. Allow rest at room temperature for 10 to 15 minutes.
2. Form into 8 small cakes, about 2 inches in diameter. Cook the olive oil over medium-high heat. Fry the cakes until browned, 2 to 3 minutes per side. Wrap, decrease the heat to low and cook for another 6 to 8 minutes, or until set in the center. Remove from the skillet.
3. To serve, wrap 2 small crab cakes in each lettuce leaf and top with 1 tablespoon aioli.

Nutrition:
Calories: 344, Fat: 24g, Carbohydrates: 2g, Protein: 24g, Sodium: 45mg, Potassium: 123mg.

196. Orange-Tarragon Chicken Salad Wrap

Preparation Time: 15 minutes
Cooking Time: 0 minutes
Servings: 4
Ingredients:
- ½ cup plain whole-milk Greek yogurt
- 2 tablespoons Dijon mustard
- 2 tablespoons extra-virgin olive oil
- 2 tablespoons fresh tarragon
- ½ teaspoon salt
- ¼ teaspoon freshly ground black pepper
- 2 cups cooked shredded chicken
- ½ cup slivered almonds
- 4 to 8 large Bibb lettuce leaves, tough stem removed
- 2 small ripe avocados, peeled and thinly sliced
- Zest of 1 clementine, or ½ small orange (about 1 tablespoon)

Directions:
1. In a medium bowl, mix the yogurt, mustard, olive oil, tarragon, orange zest, salt, and pepper and whisk until creamy. Add the shredded chicken and almonds and stir to coat.
2. To assemble the wraps, place about ½ cup chicken salad mixture in the center of each lettuce leaf and top with sliced avocados.

Nutrition:
Calories: 440, Fat: 32g, Carbohydrates: 8g, Protein: 26g, Sodium: 63mg, Potassium: 123mg.

197. Feta and Quinoa Stuffed Mushrooms

Preparation Time: 5 minutes
Cooking Time: 8 minutes
Servings: 6
Ingredients:
- 2 tablespoons finely diced red bell pepper
- 1 garlic clove, minced
- ¼ cup cooked quinoa
- 1/8 teaspoon salt
- ¼ teaspoon dried oregano
- 24 button mushrooms, stemmed
- 2 ounces crumbled feta
- 3 tablespoons whole wheat bread crumbs
- Olive oil cooking spray

Directions:
1. Preheat the Air Fryer to 360°F. In a small bowl, mix the red bell pepper, garlic, quinoa, salt and oregano. Spoon the quinoa filling into the mushrooms until full. Add a small piece of feta cheese to the top of each mushroom. Sprinkle a pinch of bread crumbs over the feta on each mushroom.
2. Put the basket of the Air Fryer with olive oil cooking spray, then gently place the mushrooms into the basket, making sure that they don't touch each other.
3. Lay the basket into the Air Fryer and bake for 8 minutes. Remove from the Air Fryer and serve.

Nutrition:
Calories: 97, Fat: 4g, Carbohydrates: 11g, Protein: 7g, Sodium: 53mg, Potassium: 123mg.

198. Five-Ingredient Falafel with Garlic-Yogurt Sauce

Preparation Time: 5 minutes
Cooking Time: 15 minutes
Servings: 4
Ingredients:
For the Falafel
- 1 (15-ounce) can chickpeas, drained and rinsed
- ½ cup fresh parsley
- 2 garlic cloves, minced
- ½ tablespoon ground cumin
- 1 tablespoon whole wheat flour
- Salt

For the Garlic-Yogurt Sauce
- 1 cup nonfat plain Greek yogurt
- 1 garlic clove, minced
- 1 tablespoon chopped fresh dill
- 2 tablespoons lemon juice

Directions:
To Make the Falafel
1. Preheat the Air Fryer to 360°F. Put the chickpeas into a food processor. Pulse until mostly chopped, then add the parsley, garlic, and cumin and pulse for another minute, until the ingredients turn into a dough.
2. Add the flour. Pulse a couple more times until combined. The dough will have texture, but the chickpeas should be crushed into small pieces. With clean hands, make 8 balls of the same size and flatten them a bit so they are like half-thick discs.
3. Put the basket of the Air Fryer with olive oil cooking spray, then place the falafel patties in

the basket in a single layer, making sure they don't touch each other. Fry in the Air Fryer for 15 minutes.

To Make the Garlic-Yogurt Sauce
4. Mix together the yogurt, garlic, dill and lemon juice. Once the falafel is cooked and nicely browned on all sides, remove from the Air Fryer and season with salt. Serve it hot with the dipping sauce.
Nutrition:
Calories: 151, Fat: 2g, Carbohydrates: 10g, Protein: 12g, Sodium: 53mg, Potassium: 133mg.

199. Lemon Shrimp with Garlic Olive Oil

Preparation Time: 5 minutes
Cooking Time: 6 minutes
Servings: 4
Ingredients:
- 1-pound medium shrimp, cleaned and deveined
- ¼ cup plus 2 tablespoons olive oil, divided
- Juice of ½ lemon
- 3 garlic cloves, minced and divided
- ½ teaspoon salt
- ¼ teaspoon red pepper flakes
- Lemon wedges, for serving (optional)
- Marinara sauce, for dipping (optional)
Directions:
1. Preheat the Air Fryer to 380°F. Toss in the shrimp with 2 tablespoons of olive oil, lemon juice, 1/3 of minced garlic, salt, and red pepper flakes and coat well.
2. In a small ramekin, combine the remaining ¼ cup of olive oil and the remaining minced garlic. Tear off a 12-by-12-inch sheet of aluminum foil. Place the shrimp into the center of the foil, then fold the sides up and crimp the edges so that it forms an aluminum foil bowl that is open on top. Place this packet into the Air Fryer basket.
3. Roast the shrimp for 4 minutes, open the Air Fryer and place the ramekin with oil and garlic in the basket beside the shrimp packet. Cook for 2 more

minutes. Transfer the shrimp on a serving plate or platter with the ramekin of garlic olive oil on the side for dipping. You may also serve with lemon wedges and marinara sauce if desired.
Nutrition:
Calories: 264, Fat: 21g, Carbohydrates: 10g, Protein: 16g, Sodium: 63mg, Potassium: 123mg.

200. Crispy Green Bean Fries with Lemon-Yogurt Sauce

Preparation Time: 5 minutes
Cooking Time: 5 minutes
Servings: 4
Ingredients:
For the Green Beans
- 1 egg
- 2 tablespoons water
- 1 tablespoon whole wheat flour
- ¼ teaspoon paprika
- ½ teaspoon garlic powder
- ½ teaspoon salt
- ¼ cup whole wheat bread crumbs
- ½ pound whole green beans

For the Lemon-Yogurt Sauce
- ½ cup nonfat plain Greek yogurt
- 1 tablespoon lemon juice
- ¼ teaspoon salt
- 1/8 teaspoon cayenne pepper
Directions:
To Make the Green Beans
1. Preheat the Air Fryer to 380°F.
2. In a medium shallow bowl, combine the egg and water until frothy. In a separate medium shallow bowl, whisk together the flour, paprika, garlic powder, and salt, then mix in the bread crumbs.
3. Spread the bottom of the Air Fryer with cooking spray. Dip each green bean into the egg mixture, then into the bread crumb mixture, coating the outside with the crumbs. Put the green beans in a single layer in the bottom of the Air Fryer basket.
4. Fry in the Air Fryer for 5 minutes, or until the breading is golden brown.

To Make the Lemon-Yogurt Sauce

5. Incorporate the yogurt, lemon juice, salt, and cayenne. Serve the green bean fries alongside the lemon-yogurt sauce as a snack or appetizer.
Nutrition:
Calories: 88, Fat: 2g, Carbohydrates: 10g, Protein: 7g, Sodium: 63mg, Potassium: 123mg.

201. Homemade Sea Salt Pita Chips

Preparation Time: 2 minutes
Cooking Time: 8 minutes
Servings: 2
Ingredients:
- 2 whole wheat pitas
- 1 tablespoon olive oil
- ½ teaspoon kosher salt
Directions:
1. Preheat the Air Fryer to 360°F. Cut each pita into 8 wedges. In a medium bowl, mix the pita wedges, olive oil, and salt until the wedges are coated and the olive oil and salt are evenly distributed.
2. Place the pita wedges into the Air Fryer basket in an even layer and fry for 6 to 8 minutes.
3. Season with additional salt, if desired. Serve alone or with a favorite dip.
Nutrition:
Calories: 230, Fat: 8g, Carbohydrates: 11g, Protein: 6g, Sodium: 53mg, Potassium: 123mg.

202. Baked Spanakopita Dip

Preparation Time: 10 minutes
Cooking Time: 15 minutes
Servings: 2
Ingredients:
- Olive oil cooking spray
- 3 tablespoons olive oil, divided
- 2 tablespoons minced white onion
- 2 garlic cloves, minced
- 4 cups fresh spinach
- 4 ounces cream cheese, softened
- 4 ounces feta cheese, divided
- Zest of 1 lemon
- ¼ teaspoon ground nutmeg
- 1 teaspoon dried dill
- ½ teaspoon salt

- Pita chips, carrot sticks, or sliced bread for serving (optional)

Directions:
1. Preheat the Air Fryer to 360°F. Coat the inside of a 6-inch ramekin or baking dish with olive oil cooking spray.
2. Using a skillet over medium heat, cook 1 tablespoon of the olive oil. Add the onion, then cook for 1 minute. Add in the garlic and cook, stirring for 1 minute more.
3. Lower heat and combine the spinach and water. Cook until the spinach has wilted. Remove the skillet from the heat. In a medium bowl, scourge the cream cheese, 2 ounces of the feta, and the rest of olive oil, lemon zest, nutmeg, dill, and salt. Mix until just combined.
4. Add the vegetables to the cheese base and stir until combined. Pour the dip mixture into the prepared ramekin and top with the remaining 2 ounces of feta cheese.
5. Place the dip into the Air Fryer basket and cook for 10 minutes, or until heated through and bubbling. Serve with pita chips, carrot sticks, or sliced bread.

Nutrition:
Calories: 550, Fat: 52g, Carbohydrates: 21g, Protein: 14g, Sodium: 63mg, Potassium: 123mg.

203. Roasted Pearl Onion Dip

Preparation Time: 5 minutes
Cooking Time: 12 minutes plus 1 hour to chill
Servings: 4
Ingredients:
- 2 cups peeled pearl onions
- 3 garlic cloves
- 3 tablespoons olive oil, divided
- ½ teaspoon salt
- 1 cup nonfat plain Greek yogurt
- 1 tablespoon lemon juice
- ¼ teaspoon black pepper
- 1/8 teaspoon red pepper flakes
- Pita chips, vegetables, or toasted bread for serving (optional)

Directions:
1. Preheat the Air Fryer to 360°F. In a large bowl, combine the pearl onions and garlic with 2 tablespoons of olive oil until the onions are well coated.

2. Pour the garlic and onion mixture into the basket of the Air Fryer and roast for 12 minutes. Place garlic and onion in a food processor. Pulse the vegetables several times until the onions are minced but still have some chunks.
3. Toss in the garlic and onions and the remaining 1 tablespoon of olive oil, along with the salt, yogurt, lemon juice, black pepper, and red pepper flakes. Chill for 1 hour before serving with pita chips, vegetables, or toasted bread.

Nutrition:
Calories: 150, Fat: 10g, Carbohydrates: 6g, Protein: 7g, Sodium: 63mg, Potassium: 123mg.

204. Red Pepper Tapenade

Preparation Time: 5 minutes
Cooking Time: 5 minutes
Servings: 4
Ingredients:
- 1 large red bell pepper
- 2 tablespoons plus 1 teaspoon olive oil
- ½ cup Kalamata olives, pitted and roughly chopped
- 1 garlic clove, minced
- ½ teaspoon dried oregano
- 1 tablespoon lemon juice

Directions:
1. Preheat the Air Fryer to 380°F. Brush the outside of a whole red bell pepper with 1 teaspoon of olive oil and place inside the Air Fryer basket. Roast for 5 minutes. Meanwhile, in a medium bowl incorporate the remaining 2 tablespoons of olive oil with the olives, garlic, oregano and lemon juice.
2. Remove the red bell pepper from the Air Fryer, then gently cut out the stem and remove the seeds. Chop the roasted bell pepper into small pieces.
3. Add the red pepper to the olive mixture and stir all together until combined. Serve with pita chips, crackers, or crusty bread.

Nutrition:
Calories: 104, Fat: 10g, Carbohydrates: 9g, Protein: 1g, Sodium: 63mg, Potassium: 123mg.

205. Greek Potato Skins with Olives and Feta

Preparation Time: 5 minutes
Cooking Time: 45 minutes
Servings: 4
Ingredients:
- 2 russet potatoes
- 3 tablespoons olive oil
- 1 teaspoon kosher salt, divided
- ¼ teaspoon black pepper
- 2 tablespoons fresh cilantro
- ¼ cup Kalamata olives, diced
- ¼ cup crumbled feta
- Chopped fresh parsley for garnish (optional)

Directions:
1. Preheat the Air Fryer to 380°F. Using a fork, poke 2 to 3 holes in the potatoes, then coat each with about ½ tablespoon olive oil and ½ teaspoon salt.
2. Put the potatoes into the Air Fryer basket and bake for 30 minutes. Remove the potatoes from the Air Fryer, and slice them in half. Scrape out the flesh of the potatoes using a spoon, leaving a ½-inch layer of potato inside the skins, and set the skins aside.
3. In a medium bowl, combine the scooped potato middles with the remaining 2 tablespoons of olive oil, ½ teaspoon of salt, black pepper, and cilantro. Mix until well combined. Divide the potato filling into the now-empty potato skins, spreading it evenly over them. Top each potato with a tablespoon of each of the olives and feta.
4. Place the loaded potato skins back into the Air Fryer and bake for 15 minutes. Serve with additional chopped cilantro or parsley and a drizzle of olive oil, if desired.

Nutrition:
Calories: 270, Sodium: 63mg, Potassium: 123mg, Fat: 13g, Carbohydrates: 34g, Protein: 5g.

206. Artichoke and Olive Pita Flatbread

Preparation Time: 5 minutes
Cooking Time: 10 minutes
Servings: 4
Ingredients:
- 2 whole wheat pitas
- 2 tablespoons olive oil, divided

- 2 garlic cloves, minced
- ¼ teaspoon salt
- ½ cup canned artichoke hearts, sliced
- ¼ cup Kalamata olives
- ¼ cup shredded Parmesan
- ¼ cup crumbled feta
- Chopped fresh parsley for garnish (optional)

Directions:
1. Preheat the Air Fryer to 380°F. Brush each pita with 1 tablespoon olive oil, then sprinkle the minced garlic and salt over the top.
2. Distribute the artichoke hearts, olives, and cheeses evenly between the two pitas, and place both into the Air Fryer to bake for 10 minutes. Remove the pitas and cut them into 4 pieces each before serving. Sprinkle parsley over the top, if desired.

Nutrition:
Calories: 243, Fat: 15g, Carbohydrates: 10g, Sodium: 43mg, Potassium: 123mg, Protein: 7g.

207. Mini Crab Cakes

Preparation Time: 10 minutes
Cooking Time: 10 minutes
Servings: 6
Ingredients:
- 8 ounces lump crab meat
- 2 tablespoons diced red bell pepper
- 1 scallion, white parts and green parts, diced
- 1 garlic clove, minced
- 1 tablespoon capers, minced
- 1 tablespoon nonfat plain Greek yogurt
- 1 egg, beaten
- ¼ cup whole wheat bread crumbs
- ¼ teaspoon salt
- 1 tablespoon olive oil
- 1 lemon, cut into wedges

Directions:
1. Preheat the Air Fryer to 360°F. In a medium bowl, mix the crab, bell pepper, scallion, garlic, and capers until combined. Add the yogurt and egg. Stir until incorporated. Mix in the bread crumbs and salt.
2. Portion this mixture into 6 equal parts and pat out into patties. Place the crab cakes inside the Air Fryer basket on a single layer, separately. Grease the

tops of each patty with a bit of olive oil. Bake for 10 minutes.
3. Pull out the crab cakes from the Air Fryer and serve with lemon wedges on the side.

Nutrition:
Calories: 87, Fat: 4g, Sodium: 45mg, Potassium: 53mg, Carbohydrates: 6g, Protein: 9g.

208. Zucchini Feta Roulades

Preparation Time: 10 minutes
Cooking Time: 10 minutes
Servings: 6
Ingredients:
- ½ cup feta
- 1 garlic clove, minced
- 2 tablespoons fresh basil, minced
- 1 tablespoon capers, minced
- 1/8 teaspoon salt
- 1/8 teaspoon red pepper flakes
- 1 tablespoon lemon juice
- 2 medium zucchinis
- 12 toothpicks

Directions:
1. Preheat the Air Fryer to 360°F. (If using a grill attachment, make sure it is inside the Air Fryer during preheating.) In a small bowl, mix the feta, garlic, basil, capers, salt, red pepper flakes, and lemon juice.
2. Slice the zucchini into 1/8-inch strips lengthwise. (Each zucchini should yield around 6 strips.) Spread 1 tablespoon of the cheese filling onto each slice of zucchini, then roll it up and locked it with a toothpick through the middle.
3. Place zucchini rolls in the basket of the Air Fryer in a single layer. Bake or grill in the Air Fryer for 10 minutes. Remove the zucchini roulades from the Air Fryer and gently remove the toothpicks before serving.

Nutrition:
Calories: 46, Fat: 3g, Carbohydrates: 6g, Protein: 3g, Sodium: 52mg, Potassium: 123mg.

209. Garlic-Roasted Tomatoes and Olives

Preparation Time: 5 minutes
Cooking Time: 20 minutes

Servings: 6
Ingredients:
- 2 cups cherry tomatoes
- 4 garlic cloves, roughly chopped
- ½ red onion, roughly chopped
- 1 cup black olives
- 1 cup green olives
- 1 tablespoon fresh basil, minced
- 1 tablespoon fresh oregano, minced
- 2 tablespoons olive oil
- ¼ to ½ teaspoon salt

Directions:
1. Preheat the Air Fryer to 380°F. In a large bowl, incorporate all the ingredients and toss them together so that the tomatoes and olives are coated well with the olive oil and herbs.
2. Pour the mixture into the Air Fryer basket, and roast for 10 minutes. Stir the mixture well, then continue roasting for an additional 10 minutes. Remove from the Air Fryer, transfer to a serving bowl, and enjoy.

Nutrition:
Calories: 109, Fat: 10g, Carbohydrates: 5g, Protein: 1g, Sodium: 63mg, Potassium: 123mg.

210. Goat Cheese and Garlic Crostini

Preparation Time: 3 minutes
Cooking Time: 5 minutes
Servings: 4
Ingredients:
- 1 whole wheat baguette
- ¼ cup olive oil
- 2 garlic cloves, minced
- 4 ounces goat cheese
- 2 tablespoons fresh basil, minced

Directions:
1. Preheat the Air Fryer to 380°F. Cut the baguette into ½-inch-thick slices. In a small bowl, incorporate the olive oil and garlic, then brush it over one side of each slice of bread.
2. Place the olive-oil-coated bread in a single layer in the Air Fryer basket and bake for 5 minutes. In the meantime, combine the goat cheese and basil. Remove the toast from the Air Fryer, then spread a thin layer of the goat cheese mixture over each piece and serve.

Nutrition:

Calories: 365, Fat: 21g, Sodium: 43mg, Potassium: 123mg, Carbohydrates: 10g, Protein: 12g.

211. Rosemary-Roasted Red Potatoes

Preparation Time: 5 minutes
Cooking Time: 20 minutes
Servings: 6
Ingredients:

- 1-pound red potatoes, quartered
- ¼ cup olive oil
- ½ teaspoon kosher salt
- ¼ teaspoon black pepper
- 1 garlic clove, minced
- 4 rosemary sprigs

Directions:

1. Preheat the Air Fryer to 360°F.
2. In a large bowl, toss potatoes with olive oil, salt, pepper and garlic until well coated. Fill the Air Fryer basket with the potatoes and top with the rosemary sprigs.
3. Roast for 10 minutes, then stir or toss the potatoes and roast for 10 minutes more. Remove the rosemary sprigs and serve the potatoes. Season well.

Nutrition:
Calories: 133, Fat: 9g, Sodium: 53mg, Potassium: 143mg, Carbohydrates: 5g, Protein: 1g.

212. Guaca Egg Scramble

Preparation Time: 8 minutes
Cooking Time: 15 minutes
Servings: 4
Ingredients:

- 4 eggs, beaten
- 1 white onion, diced
- 1 tablespoon avocado oil
- 1 avocado, finely chopped
- ½ teaspoon chili flakes
- 1 oz Cheddar cheese, shredded
- ½ teaspoon salt
- 1 tablespoon fresh parsley

Directions:

1. Pour the avocado oil into the pan and bring to a boil. Then add the diced onion and roast until lightly browned. Meanwhile, mix the chili flakes, beaten eggs and salt.
2. Spoon the egg mixture over the cooked onion and cook the mixture for 1 minute over medium heat. Then, scramble the eggs well with the help of a fork or spatula. Cook the eggs until they are solid but soft.
3. Then, add the chopped avocado and grated cheese. Stir the scrambled eggs well and transfer them to serving plates. Sprinkle the food with fresh parsley.

Nutrition:
Calories: 236, Fat: 20g, Carbohydrates: 4g, Protein: 8.6g, Sodium: 63mg, Potassium: 123mg.

213. Morning Tostadas

Preparation Time: 15 minutes
Cooking Time: 6 minutes
Servings: 6
Ingredients:

- ½ white onion, diced
- 1 tomato, chopped
- 1 cucumber, chopped
- 1 tablespoon fresh cilantro, chopped
- ½ jalapeno pepper, chopped
- 1 tablespoon lime juice
- 6 corn tortillas
- 1 tablespoon canola oil
- 2 oz Cheddar cheese, shredded
- ½ cup white beans, canned, drained
- 6 eggs
- ½ teaspoon butter
- ½ teaspoon Sea salt

Directions:

1. Make Pico de Gallo: in the salad bowl, combine diced white onion, tomato, cucumber, fresh cilantro, and jalapeno pepper. Then add lime juice and a ½ tablespoon of canola oil. Mix the mixture well. Pico de Gallo is cooked.
2. After this, preheat the oven to 390F. Line the tray with baking paper. Arrange the corn tortillas on the baking paper and brush with remaining canola oil from both sides. Bake the tortillas until they start to be crunchy. Chill the cooked crunchy tortillas well. Meanwhile, toss the butter in the skillet.
3. Crack the eggs into the melted butter and sprinkle with sea salt. Fry the eggs until the whites turn white (cooked). Approximately 3-5 minutes over medium heat. Then mash the beans to a puree texture. Spread the mashed beans on the corn tortillas.
4. Add fried eggs. Then top the eggs with Pico de Gallo and shredded Cheddar cheese.

Nutrition:
Calories: 246, Fat: 11g, Carbohydrates: 4.7g, Protein: 13.7g, Sodium: 63mg, Potassium: 123mg.

214. Cheese Omelet

Preparation Time: 5 minutes
Cooking Time: 10 minutes
Servings: 2
Ingredients:

- 1 tablespoon cream cheese
- 2 eggs, beaten
- ¼ teaspoon paprika
- ½ teaspoon dried oregano
- ¼ teaspoon dried dill
- 1 oz Parmesan, grated
- 1 teaspoon coconut oil

Directions:

1. Mix the cream cheese with the eggs, dried oregano and dill. Pour the coconut oil into the skillet and heat it until it coats the entire skillet.
2. Next, fill the pan with the egg mixture and flatten it. Add the grated Parmesan and close the lid. Cook the omelet for 10 minutes over low heat. Then transfer the cooked omelet onto the serving plate and sprinkle with paprika.

Nutrition:
Calories: 148, Fat: 11.5g, Carbohydrates: 0.3g, Protein: 10.6g, Sodium: 33mg, Potassium: 123mg.

215. Fruity Pizza

Preparation Time: 10 minutes
Cooking Time: 0 minutes
Servings: 2
Ingredients:

- 9 oz watermelon slice
- 1 tablespoon Pomegranate sauce
- 2 oz Feta cheese, crumbled
- 1 tablespoon fresh cilantro, chopped

Directions:

1. Place the watermelon slice on the plate and sprinkle with crumbled Feta cheese. Add fresh cilantro. After this, sprinkle the pizza with Pomegranate juice generously. Cut the pizza into servings.

Nutrition:
Calories: 143, Fat: 6.2g, Carbohydrates: 0.6g, Protein: 5.1g, Sodium: 63mg, Potassium: 123mg.

216. Herb and Ham Muffins

Preparation Time: 10 minutes
Cooking Time: 15 minutes
Servings: 4
Ingredients:
- 3 oz ham, chopped
- 4 eggs, beaten
- 2 tablespoons coconut flour
- ½ teaspoon dried oregano
- ¼ teaspoon dried cilantro
- Cooking spray

Directions:
1. Grease muffin tins with cooking spray from the inside. In the bowl, mix the beaten eggs, coconut flour, dried oregano, coriander and ham. When the liquid is homogeneous, pour it into the prepared muffin tins.
2. Bake the muffins for 15 minutes at 360F. Cool the baked food well and only after that remove it from the molds.

Nutrition:
Calories: 128, Fat: 7.2g, Carbohydrates: 2.9g, Protein: 10.1g, Sodium: 63mg, Potassium: 123mg.

217. Morning Sprouts Pizza

Preparation Time: 15 minutes
Cooking Time: 20 minutes
Servings: 6
Ingredients:
- ½ cup wheat flour, whole grain
- 2 tablespoons butter, softened
- ¼ teaspoon baking powder
- ¾ teaspoon salt
- 5 oz chicken fillet, boiled
- 2 oz Cheddar cheese, shredded
- 1 teaspoon tomato sauce
- 1 oz bean sprouts

Directions:
1. Make the pizza crust: Mix wheat flour, butter, baking powder, and salt. Knead the soft and non-sticky dough. Add more wheat flour if needed. Leave the dough for 10 minutes to chill. Then place the dough on the baking paper. Cover it with the second baking paper sheet.

2. Roll up the dough with the help of the rolling pin to get the round pizza crust. After this, remove the upper baking paper sheet. Transfer the pizza crust to the tray.
3. Spread the crust with tomato sauce. Then shred the chicken fillet and arrange it over the pizza crust. Add shredded Cheddar cheese. Bake pizza for 20 minutes at 355F. Then top the cooked pizza with bean sprouts and slice into the servings.

Nutrition:
Calories: 157, Fat: 8.8g, Carbohydrates: 0.3g, Protein: 10.5g, Sodium: 63mg, Potassium: 123mg.

218. Quinoa with Banana and Cinnamon

Preparation Time: 10 minutes
Cooking Time: 12 minutes
Servings: 4
Ingredients:
- 1 cup quinoa
- 2 cup milk
- 1 teaspoon vanilla extract
- 1 teaspoon honey
- 2 bananas, sliced
- ¼ teaspoon ground cinnamon

Directions:
1. Pour the milk into the saucepan and add the quinoa. Close the lid and cook over medium heat for 12 minutes or until the quinoa absorbs all the liquid. Then chill the quinoa for 10-15 minutes and place in the serving mason jars.
2. Add honey, vanilla extract, and ground cinnamon. Stir well. Top quinoa with banana and stir before serving.

Nutrition:
Calories: 279, Fat: 5.3g, Carbohydrates: 4.6g, Protein: 10.7g, Sodium: 63mg, Potassium: 123mg.

219. Egg Casserole

Preparation Time: 10 minutes
Cooking Time: 28 minutes
Servings: 4
Ingredients:
- 2 eggs, beaten
- 1 red bell pepper, chopped

- 1 chili pepper, chopped
- ½ red onion, diced
- 1 teaspoon canola oil
- ½ teaspoon salt
- 1 teaspoon paprika
- 1 tablespoon fresh cilantro, chopped
- 1 garlic clove, diced
- 1 teaspoon butter, softened
- ¼ teaspoon chili flakes

Directions:
1. Brush the casserole mold with canola oil and pour beaten eggs inside. After this, toss the butter in the skillet and melt it over medium heat. Add chili pepper and red bell pepper.
2. Next, add red onion and cook the vegetables for 7-8 minutes over medium heat. Stir them from time to time. Transfer the vegetables to the casserole mold.
3. Add salt, paprika, cilantro, diced garlic, and chili flakes. Stir mildly with the help of a spatula to get a homogenous mixture. Bake the casserole for 20 minutes at 355F in the oven. Then chill the meal well and cut it into servings. Transfer the casserole to the serving plates with the help of the spatula.

Nutrition:
Calories: 68, Fat: 4.5g, Carbohydrates: 1g, Protein: 3.4g, Sodium: 63mg, Potassium: 123mg.

220. Cheese-Cauliflower Fritters

Preparation Time: 10 minutes
Cooking Time: 10 minutes
Servings: 2
Ingredients:
- 1 cup cauliflower, shredded
- 1 egg, beaten
- 1 tablespoon wheat flour, whole grain
- 1 oz Parmesan, grated
- ½ teaspoon ground black pepper
- 1 tablespoon canola oil

Directions:
1. In the mixing bowl, combine shredded cauliflower and egg. Add wheat flour, grated Parmesan, and ground black pepper. Stir the mixture with the help of the fork until it is homogenous and smooth.
2. Pour the canola oil into the pan and bring it to a boil. Make the

fritters with the cauliflower mixture with the help of your fingertips or use a spoon and transfer them into the hot oil. Grill the fritters for 4 minutes on each side over medium-low heat.

Nutrition:

Calories: 167, Fat: 12.3g, Carbohydrates: 1.5g, Protein: 8.8g, Sodium: 53mg, Potassium: 123mg.

221. Creamy Oatmeal Figs

Preparation Time: 10 minutes
Cooking Time: 20 minutes
Servings: 5
Ingredients:

- 2 cups oatmeal
- 1 ½ cup milk
- 1 tablespoon butter
- 3 figs, chopped
- 1 tablespoon honey

Directions:

1. Pour milk into the saucepan. Add oatmeal and close the lid. Cook the oatmeal for 15 minutes over medium-low heat. Then add chopped figs and honey.
2. Add butter and mix the oatmeal well. Cook it for 5 minutes more. Close the lid and let the cooked breakfast rest for 10 minutes before serving.

Nutrition:

Calories: 222, Fat: 6g, Carbohydrates: 4.4g, Protein: 7.1g, Sodium: 63mg, Potassium: 123mg.

222. Baked Cinnamon Oatmeal

Preparation Time: 10 minutes
Cooking Time: 25 minutes
Servings: 4
Ingredients:

- 1 cup oatmeal
- 1/3 cup milk
- 1 pear, chopped
- 1 teaspoon vanilla extract
- 1 tablespoon Splenda
- 1 teaspoon butter
- ½ teaspoon ground cinnamon
- 1 egg, beaten

Directions:

1. In the large bowl, mix the oat flour, milk, egg, vanilla extract, Splenda and ground cinnamon. Melt the butter and add it to the oat mixture. Then add the chopped pear and stir well.
2. Spoon the oat mixture into the pan and gently flatten. Cover with the foil and secure the edges. Bake the oatmeal for 25 minutes at 350F.

Nutrition:

Calories: 151, Fat: 3.9g, Carbohydrates: 3.3g, Protein: 4.9g, Sodium: 63mg, Potassium: 123mg.

223. Chia and Nut Porridge

Preparation Time: 10 minutes
Cooking Time: 30 minutes
Servings: 4
Ingredients:

- 3 cups organic almond milk
- 1/3 cup chia seeds, dried
- 1 teaspoon vanilla extract
- 1 tablespoon honey
- ¼ teaspoon ground cardamom

Directions:

1. Pour the almond milk into the saucepan and bring to a boil. Then cool the almond milk to room temperature (or appx. for 10-15 minutes). Add vanilla extract, honey, and ground cardamom. Stir well. After this, add chia seeds and stir again. Close the lid and let chia seeds soak the liquid for 20-25 minutes.
2. Transfer the cooked porridge into the serving ramekins.

Nutrition:

Calories: 150, Fat: 7.3g, Carbohydrates: 6.1g, Protein: 3.7g, Sodium: 63mg, Potassium: 123mg.

224. Chocolate Oatmeal

Preparation Time: 10 minutes
Cooking Time: 15 minutes
Servings: 2
Ingredients:

- 1 ½ cup oatmeal
- 1 tablespoon cocoa powder
- ½ cup heavy cream
- ¼ cup of water
- 1 teaspoon vanilla extract
- 1 tablespoon butter
- 2 tablespoons Splenda

Directions:

1. Mix oatmeal with cocoa powder and Splenda. Transfer the mixture to the saucepan. Add vanilla extract, water, and heavy cream. Stir it gently with the help of the spatula.
2. Close the lid and cook it for 10-15 minutes over medium-low heat. Remove the cooked cocoa oatmeal from the heat and add butter. Stir it well.

Nutrition:

Calories: 230, Fat: 10.6g, Carbohydrates: 3.5g, Protein: 4.6g, Sodium: 63mg, Potassium: 123mg.

225. Cinnamon Roll Oats

Preparation Time: 7 minutes
Cooking Time: 10 minutes
Servings: 4
Ingredients:

- ½ cup rolled oats
- 1 cup milk
- 1 teaspoon vanilla extract
- 1 teaspoon ground cinnamon
- 2 teaspoon honey
- 2 tablespoons Plain yogurt
- 1 teaspoon butter

Directions:

1. Put the milk in the saucepan and bring to a boil. Add the oat flakes and stir well. Close the lid and cook the oatmeal for 5 minutes over medium heat. The cooked oatmeal will absorb all the milk.
2. Next, add the butter and stir the oatmeal well. In a separate bowl, whisk the plain yogurt with the honey, cinnamon and vanilla extract. Spoon the cooked oatmeal into the serving bowls. Top the oats with the yogurt mixture in the shape of the wheel.

Nutrition:

Calories: 243, Fat: 20.2g, Carbohydrates: 1g, Protein: 13.3g, Sodium: 63mg, Potassium: 123mg.

226. Pumpkin Oatmeal with Spices

Preparation Time: 10 minutes
Cooking Time: 13 minutes
Servings: 6
Ingredients:

- 2 cups oatmeal
- 1 cup of coconut milk
- 1 cup milk
- 1 teaspoon Pumpkin pie spices

- 2 tablespoons pumpkin puree
- 1 tablespoon honey
- ½ teaspoon butter

Directions:

1. Pour coconut milk and milk into the saucepan. Add butter and bring the liquid to a boil. Add oatmeal, stir well with the help of a spoon and close the lid.

2. Simmer the oatmeal for 7 minutes over medium heat. Meanwhile, Mix honey, pumpkin pie spices, and pumpkin puree. When the oatmeal is cooked, add pumpkin puree mixture and stir well. Transfer the cooked breakfast to the serving plates.

Nutrition:

Calories: 232, Fat: 12.5g, Carbohydrates: 3.8g, Protein: 5.9g, Sodium: 53mg, Potassium: 123mg.

Chapter 8. Mains

227. Zucchini Zoodles with Chicken and Basil

Preparation Time: 10 minutes
Cooking Time: 10 minutes
Servings: 3
Ingredients:

- 2 chicken fillets, cubed
- 2 tablespoons ghee
- 1 pound tomatoes, diced
- ½ cup basil, chopped
- ¼ cup almond milk
- 1 garlic clove, peeled, minced
- 1 zucchini, shredded

Directions:

1. Sauté cubed chicken in ghee until no longer pink.
2. Add tomatoes and season with sunflower seeds.
3. Simmer and reduce the liquid.
4. Prepare your zucchini Zoodles by shredding zucchini in a food processor.
5. Add basil, garlic, coconut almond milk to the chicken and cook for a few minutes.
6. Add half of the zucchini Zoodles to a bowl and top with creamy tomato basil chicken.
7. Enjoy!

Nutrition:

Calories: 156, Protein: 9.4g, Carbohydrates: 12.2g, Fat: 7.1g, Fiber: 0.8g, Cholesterol: 7mg, Sodium: 86mg, Potassium: 365mg.

228. Parmesan Baked Chicken

Preparation Time: 5 minutes
Cooking Time: 20 minutes
Servings: 2
Ingredients:

- 2 tablespoons ghee
- 2 boneless chicken breasts, skinless
- Pink sunflower seeds
- Freshly ground black pepper
- ½ cup mayonnaise, low fat
- ¼ cup parmesan cheese, grated
- 1 tablespoon dried Italian seasoning, low fat, low sodium
- ¼ cup crushed pork rinds

Directions:

1. Preheat your oven to 425 degrees F.
2. Take a large baking dish and coat with ghee.
3. Pat chicken breasts dry and wrap with a towel.
4. Season with sunflower seeds and pepper.
5. Place in baking dish.
6. Take a small bowl and add mayonnaise, parmesan cheese, Italian seasoning.
7. Slather mayo mix evenly over chicken breast.
8. Sprinkle crushed pork rinds on top.
9. Bake for 20 minutes until topping is browned.
10. Serve and enjoy!

Nutrition:

Calories: 156, Protein: 9.4g, Carbohydrates: 12.2g, Fat: 7.1g, Fiber: 0.8g, Cholesterol: 7mg, Sodium: 86mg, Potassium: 365mg.

229. Crazy Japanese Potato and Beef Croquettes

Preparation Time: 10 minutes
Cooking Time: 20 minutes
Servings: 10
Ingredients:

- 3 medium russet potatoes, peeled and chopped
- 1 tablespoon almond butter
- 1 tablespoon vegetable oil
- 3 onions, diced
- ¾ pound ground beef
- 4 teaspoons light coconut aminos
- All-purpose flour for coating
- 2 eggs, beaten
- Panko bread crumbs for coating
- ½ cup oil, frying

Directions:

1. Take a saucepan and place it over medium-high heat; add potatoes and sunflower seeds water, boil for 16 minutes.
2. Remove water and put potatoes in another bowl. Add almond butter and mash the potatoes.
3. Take a frying pan and place it over medium heat. Add 1 tablespoon oil and let it heat. Add onions and stir fry until tender.
4. Add coconut aminos to beef to onions.
5. Keep frying until beef is browned.
6. Mix the beef with the potatoes evenly.
7. Take another frying pan and place it over medium heat; add half a cup of oil.
8. Form croquettes using the mashed potato mixture and coat them with flour, then eggs and finally breadcrumbs.
9. Fry patties until golden on all sides.
10. Enjoy!

Nutrition:

Calories: 156, Protein: 9.4g, Carbohydrates: 12.2g, Fat: 7.1g, Fiber: 0.8g, Cholesterol: 7mg, Sodium: 86mg, Potassium: 365mg.

230. Golden Eggplant Fries

Preparation Time: 10 minutes
Cooking Time: 15 minutes
Servings: 8
Ingredients:

- 2 eggs
- 2 cups almond flour
- 2 tablespoons coconut oil, spray
- 2 eggplants, peeled and cut thinly
- Sunflower seeds and pepper

Directions:

1. Preheat your oven to 400 degrees F.
2. Take a bowl and mix with sunflower seeds and black pepper.
3. Take another bowl and beat eggs until frothy.
4. Dip the eggplant pieces into the eggs.
5. Then coat them with the flour mixture.
6. Add another layer of flour and egg.
7. Then, take a baking sheet and grease with coconut oil on top.
8. Bake for about 15 minutes.
9. Serve and enjoy!

Nutrition:

Calories: 156, Protein: 9.4g, Carbohydrates: 12.2g, Fat: 7.1g, Fiber: 0.8g, Cholesterol: 7mg, Sodium: 86mg, Potassium: 365mg.

231. Very Wild Mushroom Pilaf

Preparation Time: 10 minutes
Cooking Time: 3 hours
Servings: 4
Ingredients:
- 1 cup wild rice
- 2 garlic cloves, minced
- 6 green onions, chopped
- 2 tablespoons olive oil
- ½ pound baby Bella mushrooms
- 2 cups water

Directions:
1. Add rice, garlic, onion, oil, mushrooms and water to your Slow Cooker.
2. Stir well until mixed.
3. Place lid and cook on LOW for 3 hours.
4. Stir pilaf and divide between serving platters.
5. Enjoy!

Nutrition:
Calories: 156, Protein: 9.4g, Carbohydrates: 12.2g, Fat: 7.1g, Fiber: 0.8g, Cholesterol: 7mg, Sodium: 86mg, Potassium: 365mg.

232. Sporty Baby Carrots

Preparation Time: 5 minutes
Cooking Time: 5 minutes
Servings: 4
Ingredients:
- 1 pound baby carrots
- 1 cup water
- 1 tablespoon clarified ghee
- 1 tablespoon chopped up fresh mint leaves
- Sea flavored vinegar as needed

Directions:
1. Place a steamer rack on top of your pot and add the carrots.
2. Add water.
3. Lock the lid and cook at HIGH pressure for 2 minutes.
4. Do a quick release.
5. Pass the carrots through a strainer and drain them.
6. Wipe the insert clean.
7. Return the insert to the pot and set the pot to Sauté mode.
8. Add clarified butter and allow it to melt.

9. Add mint and sauté for 30 seconds.
10. Add carrots to the insert and sauté well.
11. Remove them and sprinkle with a bit of flavored vinegar on top. Enjoy

Nutrition:
Calories: 156, Protein: 9.4g, Carbohydrates: 12.2g, Fat: 7.1g, Fiber: 0.8g, Cholesterol: 7mg, Sodium: 86mg, Potassium: 365mg.

233. Garden Salad

Preparation Time: 5 minutes
Cooking Time: 20 minutes
Servings: 6
Ingredients:
- 1 pound raw peanuts in the shell
- 1 bay leaf
- 2 medium-sized chopped up tomatoes
- ½ cup diced up green pepper
- ½ cup diced up sweet onion
- ¼ cup finely diced hot pepper
- ¼ cup diced up celery
- 2 tablespoons olive oil
- ¾ teaspoon flavored vinegar
- ¼ teaspoon freshly ground black pepper

Directions:
1. Boil your peanuts for 1 minute and rinse them.
2. The skin will be soft; so, discard the skin.
3. Add 2 cups of water to the Instant Pot.
4. Add bay leaf and peanuts.
5. Lock the lid and cook on HIGH pressure for 20 minutes.
6. Drain the water.
7. Take a large bowl and add the peanuts, diced vegetables.
8. Whisk in olive oil, lemon juice, pepper in another bowl.
9. Pour the mixture over the salad and mix. Enjoy!

Nutrition:
Calories: 156, Protein: 9.4g, Carbohydrates: 12.2g, Fat: 7.1g, Fiber: 0.8g, Cholesterol: 7mg, Sodium: 86mg, Potassium: 200mg.

234. Baked Smoky Broccoli and Garlic

Preparation Time: 5 minutes
Cooking Time: 20 minutes
Servings: 6
Ingredients:

- Cooking spray
- 1 tablespoon extra-virgin olive oil
- 3 cloves garlic, minced
- 1/2 teaspoon sea salt
- 1/4 teaspoon ground black pepper
- ½ tsp. cumin
- ½ tsp. annatto seeds
- 3 1/2 cups sliced broccoli
- 1 lime, cut into wedges
- 1 tablespoon chopped fresh cilantro

Directions:
1. Preheat your oven to 450 degrees F.
2. Line a baking sheet with foil and grease with olive oil.
3. Mix the olive oil, garlic, cumin, annatto seeds, salt, and pepper in a bowl.
4. Add in the cauliflower, carrots, and broccoli.
5. Combine until well coated.
6. Spread them out in a single layer on the baking sheet.
7. Add the lime wedges.
8. Roast in the oven until vegetables become caramelized, for about 25 minutes.
9. Take out the lime wedges and top with the cilantro.

Nutrition:
Calories: 156, Protein: 9.4g, Carbohydrates: 12.2g, Fat: 7.1g, Fiber: 0.8g, Cholesterol: 7mg, Sodium: 86mg, Potassium: 0mg.

235. Roasted Cauliflower and Lima Beans

Preparation Time: 5 minutes
Cooking Time: 20 minutes
Servings: 6
Ingredients:
- Cooking spray
- 1 tablespoon melted vegan butter/margarine
- 9 cloves garlic, minced
- 1/2 teaspoon sea salt
- 1/4 teaspoon ground black pepper
- 1 1/2 cups sliced cauliflower
- 3 1/2 cups cherry tomatoes
- 1 (15 ounce) can lima beans, drained
- 1 lemon, cut into wedges

Directions:
1. Preheat your oven to 450 degrees F.

2. Line a baking sheet with foil and grease with melted vegan butter or margarine.
3. Mix the olive oil, garlic, salt, and pepper in a bowl.
4. Add in the cauliflower, tomatoes, and lima beans
5. Combine until well coated.
6. Spread them out in a single layer on the baking sheet.
7. Add the lemon wedges.
8. Roast in the oven until vegetables become caramelized, for about 25 minutes.
9. Take out the lemon wedges.

Nutrition:
Calories: 156, Protein: 9.4g, Carbohydrates: 12.2g, Fat: 7.1g, Fiber: 0.8g, Cholesterol: 7mg, Sodium: 86mg, Potassium: 160mg.

236. Thai Roasted Spicy Black Beans and Choy Sum

Preparation Time: 5 minutes
Cooking Time: 20 minutes
Servings: 6
Ingredients:
- Cooking spray
- 1 tablespoon sesame oil
- 3 cloves garlic, minced
- 1/2 teaspoon sea salt
- 1 tbsp. Thai chili paste
- 1/4 teaspoon ground black pepper
- 3 1/2 cups Choy Sum, coarsely chopped
- 2 1/2 cups cherry tomatoes
- 1 (15 ounce) can black beans, drained
- 1 lime, cut into wedges
- 1 tablespoon chopped fresh cilantro

Directions:
1. Preheat your oven to 450 degrees F.
2. Line a baking sheet with foil and grease with sesame oil. Mix the olive oil, garlic, salt, Thai chili paste, and pepper in a bowl.
3. Add in the Choy sum, tomatoes, and black beans. Combine until well coated.
4. Spread them out in a single layer on the baking sheet.
5. Add the lime wedges.
6. Roast in the oven until vegetables become caramelized, for about 25 minutes.
7. Take out the lime wedges and top with the cilantro.

Nutrition:
Calories: 156, Protein: 9.4g, Carbohydrates: 12.2g, Fat: 7.1g, Fiber: 0.8g, Cholesterol: 7mg, Sodium: 86mg, Potassium: 150mg.

237. Simple Roasted Broccoli and Cauliflower

Preparation Time: 5 minutes
Cooking Time: 20 minutes
Servings: 6
Ingredients:
- Cooking spray
- 1 tablespoon extra-virgin olive oil
- 3 cloves garlic, minced
- 1/2 teaspoon sea salt
- 1/4 teaspoon ground black pepper
- 3 1/2 cups broccoli florets
- 2 1/2 cups cauliflower florets
- 1 tablespoon chopped fresh thyme

Directions:
1. Preheat your oven to 450 degrees F.
2. Line a baking sheet with foil and grease with olive oil.
3. Mix the olive oil, garlic, salt, and pepper in a bowl.
4. Add in the cauliflower and tomatoes. Combine until well coated.
5. Spread them out in a single layer on the baking sheet.
6. Roast in the oven until vegetables become caramelized, for about 25 minutes.
7. Top with the thyme.

Nutrition:
Calories: 156, Protein: 9.4g, Carbohydrates: 12.2g, Fat: 7.1g, Fiber: 0.8g, Cholesterol: 7mg, Sodium: 86mg, Potassium: 80mg.

238. Roasted Napa Cabbage and Turnips Extra

Preparation Time: 5 minutes
Cooking Time: 20 minutes
Servings: 6
Ingredients:
- Cooking spray
- 1 tablespoon extra-virgin olive oil
- 1/2 teaspoon sea salt
- 1/4 teaspoon ground black pepper
- 1/2 medium Napa cabbage, sliced thinly
- 1 medium turnip, sliced thinly

Directions:
1. Preheat your oven to 450 degrees F.
2. Line a baking sheet with foil and grease with olive oil.
3. Mix the extra ingredients thoroughly. Add in the main ingredients
4. Combine until well coated. Spread them out in a single layer on the baking sheet.
5. Roast in the oven until vegetables become caramelized, for about 25 minutes.

Nutrition:
Calories: 156, Protein: 9.4g, Carbohydrates: 12.2g, Fat: 7.1g, Fiber: 0.8g, Cholesterol: 7mg, Sodium: 86mg, Potassium: 90mg.

239. Simple Roasted Kale Artichoke Heart and Choy Sum Extra

Preparation Time: 5 minutes
Cooking Time: 20 minutes
Servings: 6
Ingredients:
- Cooking spray
- 1 tablespoon extra-virgin olive oil
- 1/2 teaspoon sea salt
- 1/4 teaspoon ground black pepper
- 1 bunch of kale, rinsed and drained
- 1 cup canned artichoke hearts
- 1/2 medium Chinese flowery cabbage (Choy sum), coarsely chopped

Directions:
1. Preheat your oven to 450 degrees F.
2. Line a baking sheet with foil and grease with olive oil. Mix the extra ingredients thoroughly. Add in the main ingredients
3. Combine until well coated. Spread them out in a single layer on the baking sheet.
4. Roast in the oven until vegetables become caramelized, for about 25 minutes.

Nutrition:

Calories: 156, Protein: 9.4g, Carbohydrates: 12.2g, Fat: 7.1g, Fiber: 0.8g, Cholesterol: 7mg, Sodium: 86mg, Potassium: 45mg.

240. Roasted Kale and Bok Choy Extra

Preparation Time: 5 minutes
Cooking Time: 20 minutes
Servings: 6
Ingredients:

- Cooking spray
- 1 tablespoon extra-virgin olive oil
- 1/2 teaspoon sea salt
- 1/4 teaspoon ground black pepper
- 1 bunch of kale, rinsed and drained
- 1 bunch of bok Choy, rinsed, drained and coarsely chopped

Directions:

1. Preheat your oven to 450 degrees F. Line a baking sheet with foil and grease with olive oil.
2. Mix the extra ingredients thoroughly. Add in the main ingredients
3. Combine until well coated. Spread them out in a single layer on the baking sheet.
4. Roast in the oven until vegetables become caramelized, for about 25 minutes.

Nutrition:
Calories: 156, Protein: 9.4g, Carbohydrates: 12.2g, Fat: 7.1g, Fiber: 0.8g, Cholesterol: 7mg, Sodium: 86mg, Potassium: 30mg.

241. Roasted Soy Beans and Winter Squash

Preparation Time: 5 minutes
Cooking Time: 20 minutes
Servings: 6
Ingredients:

- 2 (15 ounce) cans soy beans, rinsed and drained
- 1/2 winter squash - peeled, seeded, and cut into 1-inch pieces
- 1 red onion, diced 1 sweet potato, peeled and cut into 1-inch cubes
- 2 large carrots, cut into 1-inch pieces

- 3 medium potatoes, cut into 1-inch pieces
- 4 tablespoons extra virgin oil

Seasoning

- 1 teaspoon salt
- 1/2 teaspoon ground black pepper
- 1 teaspoon onion powder
- 1 teaspoon dried basil
- 1 teaspoon Italian seasoning

Garnishing

- 2 green onions, chopped (optional)

Directions:

1. Preheat your oven to 350 degrees F. Grease your baking pan.
2. Combine the beans, squash, onion, sweet potato, carrots, and russet potatoes on the prepared sheet pan. Drizzle with the oil and toss to coat.
3. Combine the seasoning ingredients in a bowl. Sprinkle them over the vegetables on the pan and toss to coat with seasonings. Bake in the oven for 25 minutes.
4. Stir frequently until vegetables are soft and lightly browned and beans are crisp, for about 20 to 25 minutes more. Season with more salt and black pepper to taste, top with the green onion before serving.

Nutrition:
Calories: 156, Protein: 9.4g, Carbohydrates: 12.2g, Fat: 7.1g, Fiber: 0.8g, Cholesterol: 7mg, Sodium: 86mg, Potassium: 79mg.

242. Roasted Button Mushrooms and Squash

Preparation Time: 5 minutes
Cooking Time: 20 minutes
Servings: 6
Ingredients:

- 2 (15 ounce) cans button mushrooms, rinsed and drained
- 1/2 summer squash - peeled, seeded, and cut into 1-inch pieces
- 1 red onion, diced
- 2 large turnips, cut into 1-inch pieces
- 2 large parsnips, cut into 1-inch pieces

- 1 medium potatoes, cut into 1-inch pieces
- 3 tablespoons butter Seasoning ingredients
- 1 teaspoon salt
- 1/2 teaspoon ground black pepper
- 1 teaspoon onion powder
- 2 teaspoon garlic powder
- 1 teaspoon Herbs de Provence

Garnishing

- 2 sprigs of thyme, chopped (optional)

Directions:

1. Preheat your oven to 350 degrees F. Grease your baking pan.
2. Combine the main ingredients on the prepared sheet pan. Drizzle with the melted butter or margarine and toss to coat.
3. Combine the seasoning ingredients in a bowl. Sprinkle them over the vegetables on the pan and toss to coat with seasonings.
4. Bake in the oven for 25 minutes. Stir frequently until vegetables are soft and lightly browned and chickpeas are crisp, for about 20 to 25 minutes more.
5. Season with more salt and black pepper to taste, top with thyme before serving.

Nutrition:
Calories: 156, Protein: 9.4g, Carbohydrates: 12.2g, Fat: 7.1g, Fiber: 0.8g, Cholesterol: 7mg, Sodium: 86mg, Potassium: 78mg.

243. Roasted Tomatoes Rutabaga and Kohlrabi Main

Preparation Time: 5 minutes
Cooking Time: 20 minutes
Servings: 6
Ingredients:

- 3 large tomatoes, cut into 1-inch pieces
- 3 red onions, diced
- 1 rutabaga, peeled and cut into 1-inch cubes
- 2 large carrots, cut into 1-inch pieces
- 3 medium kohlrabi, cut into 1-inch pieces
- 3 tablespoons extra virgin olive oil

Seasoning
- 1 teaspoon salt
- 1/2 teaspoon ground black pepper
- 1 teaspoon onion powder
- 2 teaspoon garlic powder
- 1 teaspoon Spanish paprika
- 1 teaspoon cumin

Garnishing
- 2 sprigs parsley, chopped (optional)

Directions:
1. Preheat your oven to 350 degrees F. Grease your baking pan.
2. Combine the main ingredients on the prepared sheet pan. Drizzle with the oil and toss to coat.
3. Combine the seasoning ingredients in a bowl. Sprinkle them over the vegetables on the pan and toss to coat with seasonings.
4. Bake in the oven for 25 minutes. Stir frequently until vegetables are soft, for about 20 to 25 minutes more. Season with more salt and black pepper to taste, top with the parsley before serving.

Nutrition:
Calories: 156, Protein: 9.4g, Carbohydrates: 12.2g, Fat: 7.1g, Fiber: 0.8g, Cholesterol: 7mg, Sodium: 86mg, Potassium: 98mg.

244. Roasted Brussels Sprouts and Broccoli

Preparation Time: 5 minutes
Cooking Time: 20 minutes
Servings: 6
Ingredients:
- 1 large broccoli, sliced
- 1 cup bean sprouts
- 1 red onion, diced
- 3 large kohlrabi, cut into 1-inch pieces
- 2 large carrots, cut into 1-inch pieces
- 3 medium potatoes, cut into 1-inch pieces
- 3 tablespoons extra virgin olive oil

Seasoning
- 1 teaspoon salt

- 1/2 teaspoon ground black pepper
- 1 teaspoon onion powder
- 2 teaspoon garlic powder
- 1 teaspoon ground fennel seeds
- 1 teaspoon dried rubbed sage

Garnishing
- 2 green onions, chopped (optional)

Directions:
1. Preheat your oven to 350 degrees F. Grease your baking pan.
2. Combine the main ingredients on the prepared sheet pan. Drizzle with the oil and toss to coat.
3. Combine the seasoning ingredients in a bowl. Sprinkle them over the vegetables on the pan and toss to coat with seasonings.
4. Bake in the oven for 25 minutes. Stir frequently until vegetables are soft and lightly browned and chickpeas are crisp, for about 20 to 25 minutes more.
5. Season with more salt and black pepper to taste, top with the green onion before serving.

Nutrition:
Calories: 156, Protein: 9.4g, Carbohydrates: 12.2g, Fat: 7.1g, Fiber: 0.8g, Cholesterol: 7mg, Sodium: 86mg, Potassium: 67mg.

245. Roasted Broccoli Sweet Potatoes & Bean Sprouts

Preparation Time: 5 minutes
Cooking Time: 20 minutes
Servings: 6
Ingredients:
- 1 large broccoli, sliced
- 1 cup bean sprouts
- 1 yellow onion, diced
- 1 sweet potato, peeled and cut into 1-inch cubes
- 2 large carrots, cut into 1-inch pieces
- 3 medium potatoes, cut into 1-inch pieces
- 3 tablespoons canola oil

Seasoning
- 1 teaspoon salt
- 1/2 teaspoon ground black pepper
- 1 teaspoon onion powder

- 2 teaspoon garlic powder
- ½ cup grated gouda cheese
- ¼ cup parmesan cheese

Garnishing
- 2 green onions, chopped (optional)

Directions:
1. Preheat your oven to 350 degrees F. Grease your baking pan.
2. Combine the main ingredients on the prepared sheet pan. Drizzle with the oil and toss to coat.
3. Combine the seasoning ingredients in a bowl. Sprinkle them over the vegetables on the pan and toss to coat with seasonings.
4. Bake in the oven for 25 minutes. Stir frequently until vegetables are soft and lightly browned and chickpeas are crisp, for about 20 to 25 minutes more.
5. Season with more salt and black pepper to taste, top with the green onion before serving.

Nutrition:
Calories: 156, Protein: 9.4g, Carbohydrates: 12.2g, Fat: 7.1g, Fiber: 0.8g, Cholesterol: 7mg, Sodium: 86mg, Potassium: 78mg.

246. Roasted Sweet Potato and Red Beets

Preparation Time: 5 minutes
Cooking Time: 20 minutes
Servings: 6
Ingredients:
- 1 ½ cups Brussels sprouts, trimmed
- 1 cup large sweet potato chunks
- 1 cup large carrot chunks
- 1 ½ cup broccoli florets
- 1 cup cubed red beets
- 1/2 cup yellow onion chunks
- 2 tablespoons sesame seed oil
- salt and ground black pepper to taste

Directions:
1. Preheat your oven to 425 degrees F (220 degrees C). Set the rack to the second-lowest level in the oven.
2. Pour some lightly salted water into a bowl. Submerge the Brussels sprouts in salted water for 15 minutes and drain.
3. Place the rest of the ingredients together in a bowl. Spread the

vegetables in a single layer onto a baking pan.

4. Roast in the oven until the vegetables start to brown and cook through, for about 45 minutes.

Nutrition:

Calories: 156, Protein: 9.4g, Carbohydrates: 12.2g, Fat: 7.1g, Fiber: 0.8g, Cholesterol: 7mg, Sodium: 86mg, Potassium: 78mg.

247. Sichuan Style Baked Chioggia Beets and Broccoli Florets

Preparation Time: 5 minutes
Cooking Time: 20 minutes
Servings: 6
Ingredients:

- 1 ½ cups Brussels sprouts, trimmed
- 1 cup broccoli florets
- 1 cup Chioggia beets, cut into chunks
- 1 ½ cup cauliflower florets
- 1 cup button mushrooms, sliced
- 1/2 cup red onion chunks
- 2 tablespoons sesame oil
- ½ tsp. Sichuan peppercorns
- salt ground black pepper to taste

Directions:

1. Preheat your oven to 425 degrees F (220 degrees C). Set the rack to the second-lowest level in the oven.
2. Pour some lightly salted water into a bowl. Submerge the Brussels sprouts in salted water for 15 minutes and drain.
3. Place the rest of the ingredients together in a bowl. Spread the vegetables in a single layer onto a baking pan.
4. Roast in the oven until the vegetables start to brown and cook through, for about 45 minutes.

Nutrition:

Calories: 156, Protein: 9.4g, Carbohydrates: 12.2g, Fat: 7.1g, Fiber: 0.8g, Cholesterol: 7mg, Sodium: 86mg, Potassium: 60mg.

248. Baked Enoki and Mini Cabbage

Preparation Time: 5 minutes

Cooking Time: 20 minutes
Servings: 6
Ingredients:

- 1 ½ cups mini cabbage, trimmed
- 1 cup broccoli florets
- 1 cup enoki mushrooms, sliced
- 1 ½ cup cauliflower florets
- 1 cup oyster mushrooms
- 1/2 cup red onion chunks
- 2 tablespoons olive oil
- salt and ground black pepper to taste

Directions:

1. Preheat your oven to 425 degrees F (220 degrees C). Set the rack to the second-lowest level in the oven.
2. Pour some lightly salted water into a bowl. Submerge the Brussels sprouts in salted water for 15 minutes and drain.
3. Place the rest of the ingredients together in a bowl. Spread the vegetables in a single layer onto a baking pan.
4. Roast in the oven until the vegetables start to brown and cook through, for about 45 minutes.

Nutrition:

Calories: 156, Protein: 9.4g, Carbohydrates: 12.2g, Fat: 7.1g, Fiber: 0.8g, Cholesterol: 7mg, Sodium: 86mg, Potassium: 89mg.

249. Roasted Triple Mushrooms

Preparation Time: 5 minutes
Cooking Time: 20 minutes
Servings: 6
Ingredients:

- 2 cups spinach, rinsed
- 1 cup oyster mushrooms
- 1 cup button mushrooms, sliced
- 1 ½ cup enoki mushrooms
- 1/2 cup red onion chunks
- 2 tablespoons extra-virgin olive oil
- salt and ground black pepper to taste
- 1/4 cup Ricotta cheese

Directions:

1. Preheat your oven to 425 degrees F (220 degrees C). Set the rack to the second-lowest level in the oven.
2. Pour some lightly salted water into a bowl. Submerge the spinach in salted water for 15 minutes and drain.

3. Place the rest of the ingredients together in a bowl. Spread the vegetables in a single layer onto a baking pan.
4. Roast in the oven until the vegetables start to brown and cook through, for about 45 minutes.

Nutrition:

Calories: 156, Protein: 9.4g, Carbohydrates: 12.2g, Fat: 7.1g, Fiber: 0.8g, Cholesterol: 7mg, Sodium: 86mg, Potassium: 45mg.

250. Roasted Mini Cabbage and Sweet Potato

Preparation Time: 5 minutes
Cooking Time: 20 minutes
Servings: 6
Ingredients:

- 1 ½ cups mini cabbage, trimmed
- 1 cup large potato chunks
- 1 cup large rainbow carrot chunks
- 1 ½ cup potato chunks
- 1 cup parsnips
- 1/2 cup red onion chunks
- 2 tablespoons extra-virgin olive oil
- Sea salt
- Rainbow peppercorns to taste
- 1/4 cup cottage cheese

Directions:

1. Preheat your oven to 425 degrees F (220 degrees C). Set the rack to the second-lowest level in the oven.
2. Pour some lightly salted water into a bowl. Submerge the mini cabbage in salted water for 15 minutes and drain.
3. Place the rest of the ingredients together in a bowl. Spread the vegetables in a single layer onto a baking pan.
4. Roast in the oven until the vegetables start to brown and cook through, for about 45 minutes.

Nutrition:

Calories: 156, Protein: 9.4g, Carbohydrates: 12.2g, Fat: 7.1g, Fiber: 0.8g, Cholesterol: 7mg, Sodium: 86mg, Potassium: 89mg.

251. Tofu & Green Bean Stir-Fry

Preparation Time: 15 minutes
Cooking Time: 20 minutes
Servings: 4
Ingredients:
- 1 (14-ounce) package extra-firm tofu
- 2 tablespoons canola oil
- 1-pound green beans, chopped
- 2 carrots, peeled and thinly sliced
- ½ cup Stir-Fry Sauce or store-bought lower-sodium stir-fry sauce
- 2 cups Fluffy Brown Rice
- 2 scallions, thinly sliced
- 2 tablespoons sesame seeds

Directions:
1. Place the tofu on the dish lined with a dish towel, place another dish towel over the tofu and place a heavy pot on top, changing the towels each time they get soaked. Let stand for 15 minutes to remove moisture. Cut the tofu into 1-inch cubes.
2. Heat the canola oil in a large wok or skillet to medium-high heat. Add the tofu cubes and cook, flipping every 1 to 2 minutes, so all sides become browned. Remove from the skillet and place the green beans and carrots in the hot oil. Stir-fry for 4 to 5 minutes, occasionally tossing, until crisp and slightly tender.
3. While the vegetables are cooking, prepare the Stir-Fry Sauce (if using homemade). Place the tofu back in the skillet. Put the sauce over the tofu and vegetables and let simmer for 2 to 3 minutes. Serve over rice, then top with scallions and sesame seeds.

Nutrition:
Calories: 380, Fat: 15g, Sodium: 440mg, Potassium: 454mg, Carbohydrates: 45g, Protein: 16g.

252. Peanut Vegetable Pad Thai

Preparation Time: 15 minutes
Cooking Time: 20 minutes
Servings: 6
Ingredients:
- 8 ounces brown rice noodles
- 1/3 cup natural peanut butter
- 3 tablespoons unsalted vegetable broth
- 1 tablespoon low-sodium soy sauce
- 2 tablespoons of rice wine vinegar
- 1 tablespoon honey
- 2 teaspoons sesame oil
- 1 teaspoon sriracha (optional)
- 1 tablespoon canola oil
- 1 red bell pepper, thinly sliced
- 1 zucchini, cut into matchsticks
- 2 large carrots, cut into matchsticks
- 3 large eggs, beaten
- ¾ teaspoon kosher or sea salt
- ½ cup unsalted peanuts, chopped
- ½ cup cilantro leaves, chopped

Directions:
1. Boil a large pot of water. Cook the rice noodles as stated in package directions. Mix the peanut butter, vegetable broth, soy sauce, rice wine vinegar, honey, sesame oil, and sriracha in a bowl. Set aside.
2. Heat canola oil over medium heat in a large nonstick skillet. Add the red bell pepper, zucchini, and carrots, and sauté for 2 to 3 minutes, until slightly soft. Stir in the eggs and fold with a spatula until scrambled. Add the cooked rice noodles, sauce, and salt. Toss to combine. Spoon into bowls and evenly top with the peanuts and cilantro.

Nutrition:
Calories: 393, Fat: 19g, Sodium: 561mg, Carbohydrates: 45g, Protein: 13g, Potassium: 344mg.

253. Spicy Tofu Burrito Bowls with Cilantro Avocado Sauce

Preparation Time: 15 minutes
Cooking Time: 15 minutes
Servings: 4
Ingredients:
For the sauce:
- ¼ cup plain nonfat Greek yogurt
- ½ cup fresh cilantro leaves
- ½ ripe avocado, peeled
- Zest and juice of 1 lime
- 2 garlic cloves, peeled
- ¼ teaspoon kosher or sea salt
- 2 tablespoons water

For the burrito bowls:
- 1 (14-ounce) package extra-firm tofu
- 1 tablespoon canola oil
- 1 yellow or orange bell pepper, diced
- 2 tablespoons Taco Seasoning
- ¼ teaspoon kosher or sea salt
- 2 cups Fluffy Brown Rice
- 1 (15-ounce) can black beans, drained

Directions:
1. Place all the sauce ingredients in the bowl of a food processor or blender and purée until smooth. Taste and adjust the seasoning, if necessary. Refrigerate until ready for use.
2. Put the tofu on your plate lined with a kitchen towel. Put another kitchen towel over the tofu and place a heavy pot on top, changing towels if they become soaked. Let it stand within 15 minutes to remove the moisture. Cut the tofu into 1-inch cubes.
3. Heat canola oil in a large skillet over medium flame. Add the tofu and bell pepper and sauté, breaking up the tofu into smaller pieces for 4 to 5 minutes. Stir in the taco seasoning, salt, and ¼ cup of water. Evenly divide the rice and black beans among 4 bowls. Top with the tofu/bell pepper mixture and top with the cilantro avocado sauce.

Nutrition:
Calories: 383, Fat: 13g, Sodium: 438mg, Carbohydrates: 48g, Protein: 21g, Potassium: 234mg.

254. Sweet Potato Cakes with Classic Guacamole

Preparation Time: 15 minutes
Cooking Time: 20 minutes
Servings: 4
Ingredients:
For the guacamole:
- 2 ripe avocados, peeled and pitted
- ½ jalapeño, seeded and finely minced
- ¼ red onion, peeled and finely diced
- ¼ cup fresh cilantro leaves, chopped
- Zest and juice of 1 lime
- ¼ teaspoon kosher or sea salt

For the cakes:
- 3 sweet potatoes, cooked and peeled
- ½ cup cooked black beans
- 1 large egg
- ½ cup panko bread crumbs
- 1 teaspoon ground cumin
- 1 teaspoon chili powder
- ½ teaspoon kosher or sea salt
- ¼ teaspoon ground black pepper
- 2 tablespoons canola oil

Directions:
1. Mash the avocado, then stir in the jalapeño, red onion, cilantro, lime zest and juice, and salt in a bowl. Taste and adjust the seasoning, if necessary.
2. Put the cooked sweet potatoes plus black beans in a bowl and mash until a paste forms. Stir in the egg, bread crumbs, cumin, chili powder, salt, and black pepper until combined.
3. Heat canola oil in a large skillet at medium heat. Form the sweet potato mixture into 4 patties, place them in the hot skillet, and cook within 3 to 4 minutes per side until browned and crispy. Serve the sweet potato cakes with guacamole on top.

Nutrition:
Calories: 369, Fat: 22g, Sodium: 521mg, Carbohydrates: 38g, Protein: 8g, Potassium: 155mg.

255. Chickpea Cauliflower Tikka Masala

Preparation Time: 15 minutes
Cooking Time: 40 minutes
Servings: 6
Ingredients:
- 2 tablespoons olive oil
- 1 yellow onion, peeled and diced
- 4 garlic cloves, peeled and minced
- 1-inch piece fresh ginger, peeled and minced
- 2 tablespoons Garam Masala
- 1 teaspoon kosher or sea salt
- ½ teaspoon ground black pepper
- ¼ teaspoon ground cayenne pepper
- ½ small head cauliflower, small florets
- 2 (15-ounce) cans no-salt-added chickpeas, rinsed and drained
- 1 (15-ounce) can no-salt-added petite diced tomatoes, drained

- 1½ cups unsalted vegetable broth
- ½ (15-ounce) can coconut milk
- Zest and juice of 1 lime
- ½ cup fresh cilantro leaves, chopped, divided
- 1½ cups cooked Fluffy Brown Rice, divided

Directions:
1. Heat olive oil over medium heat, then put the onion and sauté within 4 to 5 minutes in a large Dutch oven or stockpot. Stir in the garlic, ginger, garam masala, salt, black pepper, and cayenne pepper and toast for 30 to 60 seconds until fragrant.
2. Stir in the cauliflower florets, chickpeas, diced tomatoes, and vegetable broth and increase to medium-high. Simmer within 15 minutes until the cauliflower is fork-tender.
3. Remove, stir in the coconut milk, lime juice, lime zest, and half of the cilantro. Taste and adjust the seasoning, if necessary. Serve over the rice and the remaining chopped cilantro.

Nutrition:
Calories: 323, Fat: 12g, Sodium: 444mg, Carbohydrates: 44g, Protein: 11g, Potassium: 134mg.

256. Eggplant Parmesan Stacks

Preparation Time: 15 minutes
Cooking Time: 20 minutes
Servings: 4
Ingredients:
- 1 large eggplant, cut into thick slices
- 2 tablespoons olive oil, divided
- ¼ teaspoon kosher or sea salt
- ¼ teaspoon ground black pepper
- 1 cup panko bread crumbs
- ¼ cup freshly grated Parmesan cheese
- 5 to 6 garlic cloves, minced
- ½ pound fresh mozzarella, sliced
- 1½ cups lower-sodium marinara
- ½ cup fresh basil leaves, torn

Directions:
1. Preheat the oven to 425°F. Coat the eggplant slices in 1 tablespoon olive oil and sprinkle with salt and black pepper. Put on a large baking sheet, then

roast for 10 to 12 minutes, until soft with crispy edges. Remove the eggplants and put the oven on low heat.
2. In a bowl, stir the remaining tablespoon of olive oil, bread crumbs, Parmesan cheese, and garlic. Remove the cooled eggplant from the baking sheet and clean it.
3. Create layers on the same baking sheet by stacking a roasted eggplant slice with a slice of mozzarella, a tablespoon of marinara, and a tablespoon of the bread crumb mixture, repeating with 2 layers of each ingredient. Cook under the broiler within 3 to 4 minutes until the cheese is melted and bubbly.

Nutrition:
Calories: 377, Fat: 22g, Sodium: 509mg, Carbohydrates: 29g, Protein: 16g, Potassium: 84mg.

257. Roasted Vegetable Enchiladas

Preparation Time: 15 minutes
Cooking Time: 45 minutes
Servings: 8
Ingredients:
- 2 zucchinis, diced
- 1 red bell pepper, seeded and sliced
- 1 red onion, peeled and sliced
- 2 ears corn
- 2 tablespoons canola oil
- 1 can no-salt-added black beans, drained
- 1½ tablespoons chili powder
- 2 teaspoon ground cumin
- 1/8 teaspoon kosher or sea salt
- ½ teaspoon ground black pepper
- 8 (8-inch) whole-wheat tortillas
- 1 cup Enchilada Sauce or store-bought enchilada sauce
- ½ cup shredded Mexican-style cheese
- ½ cup plain nonfat Greek yogurt
- ½ cup cilantro leaves, chopped

Directions:
1. Preheat oven to 400°F. Place the zucchini, red bell pepper, and red onion on a baking sheet. Place the ears of corn separately on the same baking sheet. Drizzle all with the canola oil and toss to coat. Roast for 10 to 12 minutes until the vegetables

are tender. Remove and reduce the temperature to 375°F.
2. Cut the corn from the cob. Transfer the corn kernels, zucchini, red bell pepper, and onion to a bowl and stir in the black beans, chili powder, cumin, salt, and black pepper until combined.
3. Grease a 9-inch by 13-inch baking dish with cooking spray. Line up the tortillas in the greased baking dish. Evenly spread the vegetable and bean filling on each tortilla. Pour half of the enchilada sauce and sprinkle half of the shredded cheese over the filling.
4. Roll each tortilla into an enchilada shape and place them seam side down. Pour the remaining enchilada sauce and sprinkle the remaining cheese over the enchiladas. Bake for 25 minutes until the cheese is melted and bubbly. Serve the enchiladas with Greek yogurt and chopped cilantro.

Nutrition:
Calories: 335, Fat: 15g, Sodium: 557mg, Carbohydrates: 42g, Protein: 13g, Potassium: 289mg.

258. Lentil Avocado Tacos

Preparation Time: 15 minutes
Cooking Time: 35 minutes
Servings: 6
Ingredients:
- 1 tablespoon canola oil
- ½ yellow onion, peeled and diced
- 2-3 garlic cloves, minced
- 1½ cups dried lentils
- ½ teaspoon kosher or sea salt
- 3 to 3½ cups unsalted vegetable or chicken stock
- 2½ tablespoons Taco Seasoning or store-bought low-sodium taco seasoning
- 16 (6-inch) corn tortillas, toasted
- 2 ripe avocados, peeled and sliced

Directions:
1. Heat the canola oil in a large skillet or Dutch oven over medium heat. Cook the onion within 4 to 5 minutes, until soft. Mix in the garlic and cook within 30 seconds until fragrant. Then add the lentils, salt, and stock. Bring to a simmer for 25 to 35 minutes,

adding additional stock if needed.
2. When there's only a small amount of liquid left in the pan, and the lentils are al dente, stir in the taco seasoning and let simmer for 1 to 2 minutes. Taste and adjust the seasoning, if necessary. Spoon the lentil mixture into tortillas and serve with the avocado slices.

Nutrition:
Calories: 400, Fat: 14g, Sodium: 336mg, Carbohydrates: 64g, Fiber: 15g, Protein: 16g, Potassium: 215mg.

259. Pasta with Basil Pesto

Preparation Time: 15 minutes
Cooking Time: 25 minutes
Servings: 6
Ingredients:
- 12 ounces orecchiette pasta
- 2 tablespoons olive oil
- 1-pint cherry tomatoes, quartered
- ½ cup Basil Pesto or store-bought pesto
- ¼ cup Kalamata olives, sliced
- 1 tablespoon dried oregano leaves
- ¼ teaspoon kosher or sea salt
- ½ teaspoon freshly cracked black pepper
- ¼ teaspoon crushed red pepper flakes
- 2 tablespoons freshly grated Parmesan cheese

Directions:
1. Boil a large pot of water. Cook the orecchiette, drain and transfer the pasta to a large nonstick skillet.
2. Put the skillet over medium-low heat, then heat the olive oil. Stir in the cherry tomatoes, pesto, olives, oregano, salt, black pepper, and crushed red pepper flakes. Cook within 8 to 10 minutes, until heated throughout. Serve the pasta with the freshly grated Parmesan cheese.

Nutrition:
Calories: 332, Fat: 13g, Sodium: 389mg, Carbohydrates: 44g, Protein: 9g, Potassium: 434mg.

260. Italian Stuffed Portobello Mushroom Burgers

Preparation Time: 15 minutes
Cooking Time: 25 minutes
Servings: 4
Ingredients:
- 1 tablespoon olive oil
- 4 large portobello mushrooms, washed and dried
- ½ yellow onion, peeled and diced
- 4 garlic cloves, peeled and minced
- 1 can cannellini beans, drained
- ½ cup fresh basil leaves, torn
- ½ cup panko bread crumbs
- 1/8 teaspoon kosher or sea salt
- ¼ teaspoon ground black pepper
- 1 cup lower-sodium marinara, divided
- ½ cup shredded mozzarella cheese
- 4 whole-wheat buns, toasted
- 1 cup fresh arugula

Directions:
1. Heat the olive oil in a large skillet over medium-high heat. Brown the mushrooms for 4 to 5 minutes per side, until slightly soft. Place them on a baking sheet. Preheat the oven to low heat.
2. Put the onion in the skillet and cook for 4 to 5 minutes, until slightly soft. Mix in the garlic and then cook for 30 to 60 seconds. Transfer the onions plus the garlic to a bowl. Add the cannellini beans and mash with the back of a fork to form a thick paste. Stir in the basil, breadcrumbs, salt and black pepper and half of the marinara. Cook for 5 minutes.
3. Remove the bean mixture from the heat and divide among the mushrooms. Pour the remaining marinara over the stuffed mushrooms and top each with the mozzarella cheese. Grill in 3 to 4 minutes, until the cheese is melted and bubbly. Transfer the burgers to the toasted whole-wheat buns and top with the arugula.

Nutrition:
Calories: 407, Fat: 9g, Sodium: 575mg, Carbohydrates: 63g, Protein: 25g, Potassium: 87mg.

261. Gnocchi with Tomato Basil Sauce

Preparation Time: 15 minutes
Cooking Time: 25 minutes
Servings: 6
Ingredients:

- 2 tablespoons olive oil
- ½ yellow onion, peeled and diced
- 3 cloves garlic, peeled and minced
- 1 (32-ounce) can no-salt-added crushed San Marzano tomatoes
- ¼ cup fresh basil leaves
- 2 teaspoons Italian seasoning
- ½ teaspoon kosher or sea salt
- 1 teaspoon granulated sugar
- ½ teaspoon ground black pepper
- 1/8 teaspoon crushed red pepper flakes
- 1 tablespoon heavy cream (optional)
- 12 ounces gnocchi
- ¼ cup freshly grated Parmesan cheese

Directions:

1. Heat the olive oil in a Dutch oven or stockpot over medium flame. Add the onion and sauté for 5 to 6 minutes, until soft. Stir in the garlic and stir until fragrant, 30 to 60 seconds. Then stir in the tomatoes, basil, Italian seasoning, salt, sugar, black pepper, and crushed red pepper flakes.
2. Bring to a simmer for 15 minutes. Stir in the heavy cream, if desired. For a smooth, puréed sauce, use an immersion blender or transfer sauce to a blender and purée until smooth. Taste and adjust the seasoning, if necessary.
3. While the sauce simmers, cook the gnocchi according to the package instructions, remove with a slotted spoon, and transfer to 6 bowls. Pour the sauce over the gnocchi and top with the Parmesan cheese.

Nutrition:

Calories: 287, Fat: 7g, Sodium: 527mg, Carbohydrates: 41g, Protein: 10g.

262. Creamy Pumpkin Pasta

Preparation Time: 15 minutes
Cooking Time: 30 minutes
Servings: 6
Ingredients:

- 1-pound whole-grain linguine
- 1 tablespoon olive oil
- 3 garlic cloves, peeled and minced
- 2 tablespoons chopped fresh sage
- 1½ cups pumpkin purée
- 1 cup unsalted vegetable stock
- ½ cup low-fat evaporated milk
- ¾ teaspoon kosher or sea salt
- ½ teaspoon ground black pepper
- ½ teaspoon ground nutmeg
- ¼ teaspoon ground cayenne pepper
- ½ cup freshly grated Parmesan cheese, divided

Directions:

1. Cook the whole-grain linguine in a large pot of boiled water. Reserve ½ cup of pasta water and drain the rest. Set the pasta aside.
2. Heat olive oil over medium heat in a large skillet. Add the garlic and sage and sauté for 1 to 2 minutes, until soft and fragrant. Whisk in the pumpkin purée, stock, milk, and reserved pasta water and simmer for 4 to 5 minutes, until thickened.
3. Whisk in the salt, black pepper, nutmeg, cayenne pepper and half of the Parmesan cheese. Stir in the cooked whole-grain linguine. Evenly divide the pasta among 6 bowls and top with the remaining Parmesan cheese.

Nutrition:

Calories: 381, Fat: 8g, Sodium: 175mg, Carbohydrates: 63g, Protein: 15g, Potassium: 128mg.

263. Mexican-Style Potato Casserole

Preparation Time: 15 minutes
Cooking Time: 60 minutes
Servings: 8
Ingredients:

- Cooking spray
- 2 tablespoons canola oil
- ½ yellow onion, peeled and diced
- 4 garlic cloves, peeled and minced
- 2 tablespoons all-purpose flour
- 1¼ cups milk
- 1 tablespoon chili powder
- ½ tablespoon ground cumin
- 1 teaspoon kosher salt or sea salt
- ½ teaspoon ground black pepper
- ¼ teaspoon ground cayenne pepper
- 1½ cups shredded Mexican-style cheese, divided
- 1 (4-ounce) can green chilies, drained
- 1½ pounds baby Yukon Gold or red potatoes, thinly sliced
- 1 red bell pepper, thinly sliced

Directions:

1. Preheat the oven to 400°F. Grease a 9-by-13-inch baking dish with cooking spray. In a large saucepan, warm canola oil on medium heat. Add the onion and sauté for 4 to 5 minutes, until soft. Mix in the garlic, then cook until fragrant, 30 to 60 seconds.
2. Mix in the flour, then put in the milk while whisking. Slow simmer for about 5 minutes until thickened. Whisk in the chili powder, cumin, salt, black pepper, and cayenne pepper.
3. Remove from the heat and whisk in half of the shredded cheese and the green chilies. Taste and adjust the seasoning, if necessary. Line up one-third of the sliced potatoes and sliced bell pepper in the baking dish and top with a quarter of the remaining shredded cheese.
4. Repeat with 2 more layers. Pour the cheese sauce over the top and sprinkle with the remaining shredded cheese. Cover it with aluminum foil and bake within 45 to 50 minutes until the potatoes are tender.
5. Remove the foil and bake again within 5 to 10 minutes, until the topping is slightly browned. Let cool within 20 minutes before slicing into 8 pieces. Serve.

Nutrition:

Calories: 195, Fat: 10g, Sodium: 487mg, Carbohydrates: 19g, Protein: 8g, Potassium: 67mg.

264. Black Bean Stew with Cornbread

Preparation Time: 15 minutes
Cooking Time: 55 minutes

Servings: 6
Ingredients:
For the black bean stew:
- 2 tablespoons canola oil
- 1 yellow onion, peeled and diced
- 4 garlic cloves, peeled and minced
- 1 tablespoon chili powder
- 1 tablespoon ground cumin
- ¼ teaspoon kosher or sea salt
- ½ teaspoon ground black pepper
- 2 cans no-salt-added black beans, drained
- 1 (10-ounce) can fire-roasted diced tomatoes
- ½ cup fresh cilantro leaves, chopped

For the cornbread topping:
- 1¼ cups cornmeal
- ½ cup all-purpose flour
- ½ teaspoon baking powder
- ¼ teaspoon baking soda
- 1/8 teaspoon kosher or sea salt
- 1 cup low-fat buttermilk
- 2 tablespoons honey
- 1 large egg

Directions:
1. Heat canola oil over medium heat in a large Dutch oven or stockpot. Add the onion and sauté for 4 to 6 minutes until the onion is soft. Stir in the garlic, chili powder, cumin, salt, and black pepper.
2. Cook within 1 to 2 minutes, until fragrant. Add the black beans and diced tomatoes. Bring to a simmer and cook for 15 minutes. Remove, then stir in the fresh cilantro. Taste and adjust the seasoning, if necessary.
3. Preheat the oven to 375°F. While the stew simmers, prepare the cornbread topping. Mix the cornmeal, baking soda, flour, baking powder, plus salt in a bowl. In a measuring cup, whisk the buttermilk, honey, and egg until combined. Put the batter into the dry fixing until just combined.
4. In oven-safe bowls or dishes, spoon out the black bean soup. Distribute dollops of the cornbread batter on top and then spread it out evenly with a spatula. Bake within 30 minutes until the cornbread is just set.

Nutrition:
Calories: 359, Fat: 7g, Sodium: 409mg, Carbohydrates: 61g, Protein: 14g, Potassium: 23mg.

265. Mushroom Florentine

Preparation Time: 15 minutes
Cooking Time: 20 minutes
Servings: 4
Ingredients:
- 5 oz. whole-grain pasta
- ¼ cup low-sodium vegetable broth
- 1 cup mushrooms, sliced
- ¼ cup of soy milk
- 1 teaspoon olive oil
- ½ teaspoon Italian seasonings

Directions:
1. Cook the pasta according to the direction of the manufacturer. Then pour olive oil into the saucepan and heat it. Add mushrooms and Italian seasonings. Stir the mushrooms well and cook for 10 minutes.
2. Then add soy milk and vegetable broth. Add cooked pasta and combine the mixture well. Cook it for 5 minutes on low heat.

Nutrition:
Calories: 287, Protein: 12.4g, Carbohydrates: 50.4g, Fat: 4.2g, Sodium: 26mg, Potassium: 98mg.

266. Hassel Back Eggplant

Preparation Time: 15 minutes
Cooking Time: 25 minutes
Servings: 2
Ingredients:
- 2 eggplants, trimmed
- 2 tomatoes, sliced
- 1 tablespoon low-fat yogurt
- 1 teaspoon curry powder
- 1 teaspoon olive oil

Directions:
1. Make the cuts in the eggplants in the shape of the Hassel back. Then rub the vegetables with curry powder and fill with sliced tomatoes. Sprinkle the eggplants with olive oil and yogurt and wrap them in the foil (each Hassel back eggplant wrap separately). Bake the vegetables at 375F for 25 minutes.

Nutrition:
Calories: 188, Protein: 7g, Carbohydrates: 38.1g, Fat: 3g, Sodium: 23mg, Potassium: 66mg.

267. Vegetarian Kebabs

Preparation Time: 15 minutes
Cooking Time: 6 minutes
Servings: 4
Ingredients:
- 2 tablespoons balsamic vinegar
- 1 tablespoon olive oil
- 1 teaspoon dried parsley
- 2 tablespoons water
- 2 sweet peppers
- 2 red onions, peeled
- 2 zucchinis, trimmed

Directions:
1. Cut the sweet peppers and onions into medium size squares. Then slice the zucchini. String all vegetables into the skewers. After this, in the shallow bowl, Mix olive oil, dried parsley, water, and balsamic vinegar.
2. Sprinkle the vegetable skewers with olive oil mixture and transfer them to the preheated oven at 390F. Cook the kebabs during 3 minutes per side or until the vegetables are light brown.

Nutrition:
Calories: 88, Protein: 2.4g, Carbohydrates: 13g, Fat: 3.9g, Sodium: 14mg, Potassium: 35mg.

268. White Beans Stew

Preparation Time: 15 minutes
Cooking Time: 55 minutes
Servings: 4
Ingredients:
- 1 cup white beans, soaked
- 1 cup low-sodium vegetable broth
- 1 cup zucchini, chopped
- 1 teaspoon tomato paste
- 1 tablespoon avocado oil
- 4 cups of water
- ½ teaspoon peppercorns
- ½ teaspoon ground black pepper
- ¼ teaspoon ground nutmeg

Directions:
1. Heat avocado oil in the saucepan, add zucchinis and roast them for 5 minutes. After this, add white beans, vegetable broth, tomato paste, water, peppercorns, ground black pepper, and ground nutmeg. Simmer the stew during 50 minutes on low heat.

Nutrition:
Calories: 184, Protein: 12.3g, Carbohydrates: 32.6g, Fat: 1g, Sodium: 55mg, Potassium: 75mg.

269. Vegetarian Lasagna

Preparation Time: 15 minutes
Cooking Time: 30 minutes
Servings: 6
Ingredients:
- 1 cup carrot, diced
- ½ cup bell pepper, diced
- 1 cup spinach, chopped
- 1 tablespoon olive oil
- 1 teaspoon chili powder
- 1 cup tomatoes, chopped
- 4 oz. low-fat cottage cheese
- 1 eggplant, sliced
- 1 cup low-sodium vegetable broth

Directions:
1. Put carrot, bell pepper, and spinach in the saucepan. Add olive oil and chili powder and stir the vegetables well. Cook them for 5 minutes.
2. Make the sliced eggplant layer in the casserole mold and top it with the vegetable mixture. Add tomatoes, vegetable stock, and cottage cheese. Bake the lasagna for 30 minutes at 375F.

Nutrition:
Calories: 77, Protein: 4.1g, Carbohydrates: 9.7g, Fat: 3g, Sodium: 124mg, Potassium: 90mg.

270. Pan-Fried Salmon with Salad

Preparation Time: 15 minutes
Cooking Time: 20 minutes
Servings: 4
Ingredients:
- Pinch of salt and pepper
- 1 tablespoon extra-virgin olive oil
- 2 tablespoon unsalted butter
- ½ teaspoon fresh dill
- 1 tablespoon fresh lemon juice
- 100g salad leaves, or bag of mixed leaves

Salad Dressing:
- 3 tablespoons olive oil
- 2 tablespoons balsamic vinaigrette
- 1/2 teaspoon maple syrup (honey)

Directions:
1. Pat-dry the salmon fillets with a paper towel and season with a pinch of salt and pepper. In a skillet, heat the oil over medium-high flame and add fillets. Cook each side within 5 to 7 minutes until golden brown.
2. Dissolve butter, dill, and lemon juice in a small saucepan. Put the butter mixture onto the cooked salmon. Lastly, combine all the salad dressing ingredients and drizzle to mixed salad leaves in a large bowl. Toss to coat. Serve with fresh salads on the side. Enjoy!

Nutrition:
Calories: 307, Fat: 22g, Protein: 34.6g, Sodium: 80mg, Carbohydrates: 1.7g, Potassium: 165mg.

271. Veggie Variety

Preparation Time: 15 minutes
Cooking Time: 15 minutes
Servings: 2
Ingredients:
- ½ onion, diced
- 1 teaspoon vegetable oil (corn or sunflower oil)
- 200 g Tofu/ bean curd
- 4 cherry tomatoes, halved
- 30ml vegetable milk (soy or oat milk)
- ½ tsp. curry powder
- 0.25 tsp. paprika
- Pinch of Salt & Pepper
- 2 slices of Vegan protein bread/ Whole grain bread
- Chives for garnish

Directions:
1. Dice the onion and fry in a frying pan with the oil. Break the tofu by hand into small pieces and put them in the pan. Sauté 7-8 minutes. Season with curry, paprika, salt, and pepper, cherry tomatoes and milk. Cook it all over for a few minutes. Serve with bread as desired and sprinkle with chopped chives.

Nutrition:
Calories: 216, Fat: 8.4g, Protein: 14.1g, Sodium: 140mg, Carbohydrates: 24.8g, Potassium: 213mg.

272. Vegetable Pasta

Preparation Time: 15 minutes
Cooking Time: 15 minutes
Servings: 4
Ingredients:
- 1 kg of thin zucchini
- 20 g of fresh ginger
- 350Fg smoked tofu
- 1 lime
- 2 cloves of garlic
- 2 tbsp. sunflower oil
- 2 tablespoons of sesame seeds
- Pinch of salt and pepper
- 4 tablespoons fried onions

Directions:
1. Wash and clean the zucchini and, using a julienne cutter, cut the pulp around the kernel into long thin strips (noodles). Peel and finely chop the ginger. Crumble tofu. Halve lime and squeeze juice. Peel and chop garlic.
2. Heat 1 tablespoon of oil in a large pan and fry the tofu for about 5 minutes. After about 3 minutes, add ginger, garlic, and sesame. Season with soy sauce. Remove from the pan and keep warm.
3. Wipe out the pan, then warm 2 tablespoons of oil in it. Stir fry zucchini strips for about 4 minutes while turning. Season with salt, pepper, and lime juice. Arrange pasta and tofu. Sprinkle with fried onions.

Nutrition:
Calories: 262, Fat: 17.7g, Protein: 15.4g, Sodium: 62mg, Carbohydrates: 17.1g, Potassium: 198mg.

273. Vegetable Noodles with Bolognese

Preparation Time: 15 minutes
Cooking Time: 15 minutes
Servings: 4
Ingredients:
- 4 large zucchinis (e.g., green and yellow)
- 600g of carrots
- 1 onion
- 1 tbsp. olive oil
- 250g of beef steak
- Pinch of salt and pepper
- 2 tablespoons tomato paste
- 1 tbsp. flour
- 1 teaspoon vegetable broth (instant)

- 40g pecorino or parmesan
- Basil

Directions:

1. Clean and peel zucchini and carrots and wash. Using a sharp, long knife, cut first into thin slices, then into long, fine strips. Clean or peel the soup greens, wash and cut into tiny cubes. Peel the onion and chop finely. Heat the Bolognese oil in a large pan. Fry hack in it crumbly. Season with salt and pepper.
2. Briefly sauté the prepared vegetable and onion cubes. Stir in tomato paste. Dust the flour, sweat briefly. Pour in 400 ml of water and stir in the vegetable stock. Boil everything, simmer for 7-8 minutes.
3. Meanwhile, cook the vegetable strips in plenty of salted water for 3-5 minutes. Drain, collecting some cooking water. Add the vegetable strips to the pan and mix well. If the sauce is not liquid enough, stir in some vegetable cooking water and season everything again.
4. Slice the cheese into fine shavings. Wash the basil, shake dry, peel off the leaves, and cut roughly. Arrange vegetable noodles, sprinkle with parmesan and basil

Nutrition:
Calories: 269, Fat: 9.7g, Protein: 25.6g, Sodium: 253mg, Carbohydrates: 21.7g, Potassium: 186mg.

274. Harissa Bolognese with Vegetable Noodles

Preparation Time: 15 minutes
Cooking Time: 30 minutes
Servings: 4
Ingredients:

- 2 onions
- 1 clove of garlic
- 3-4 tbsp. oil
- 400g ground beef
- Pinch salt, pepper, cinnamon
- 1 tsp. Harissa (Arabic seasoning paste, tube)
- 1 tablespoon tomato paste
- 2 sweet potatoes
- 2 medium Zucchini
- 3 stems/basil
- 100g of feta

Directions:

1. Peel onions and garlic, finely dice. Heat 1 tablespoon of oil in a wide saucepan. Fry onions and garlic for a short time. Season with salt, pepper, and ½ teaspoon cinnamon. Stir in harissa and tomato paste.
2. Add tomatoes and 200 ml of water, bring to the boil and simmer for about 15 minutes with occasional stirring. Peel sweet potatoes and zucchini or clean and wash. Cut vegetables into spaghetti with a spiral cutter.
3. Heat 2-3 tablespoons of oil in a large pan. Braise sweet potato spaghetti in it for about 3 minutes. Add the zucchini spaghetti and continue to simmer for 3-4 minutes while turning.
4. Season with salt and pepper. Wash the basil, shake dry and peel off the leaves. Garnish vegetable spaghetti and Bolognese on plates. Feta crumbles over. Sprinkle with basil.

Nutrition:
Calories: 452, Fat: 22.3g, Protein: 37.1g, Sodium: 253mg, Carbohydrates: 27.6g, Potassium: 106mg.

275. Curry Vegetable Noodles with Chicken

Preparation Time: 15 minutes
Cooking Time: 15 minutes
Servings: 2
Ingredients:

- 600g of zucchini
- 500g chicken fillet
- Pinch of salt and pepper
- 2 tbsp. oil
- 150 g of red and yellow cherry tomatoes
- 1 teaspoon curry powder
- 150g, fat-free cheese
- 200 ml vegetable broth
- 4 stalk (s) of fresh basil

Directions:

1. Wash the zucchini, clean them and cut them into long thin strips with a spiral cutter. Wash the flesh, dry and season with salt. Heat 1 tablespoon of oil in a frying pan. Roast the chicken in it for about 10 minutes until browned.

2. Wash the cherry tomatoes and cut them in half. Approximately 3 minutes before the end of the cooking time to the chicken in the pan. Heat 1 tablespoon of oil in another skillet. Sweat the curry powder in it and then stir in the cream cheese and broth. Flavor the sauce with salt plus pepper and simmer for about 4 minutes.
3. Wash the basil, shake it dry and pluck the leaves from the stems. Cut small leaves of 3 stems. Remove meat from the pan and cut it into strips. Add tomatoes, basil, and zucchini to the sauce and heat for 2-3 minutes. Serve vegetable noodles and meat on plates and garnish with basil.

Nutrition:
Calories: 376, Fat: 17.2g, Protein: 44.9g, Sodium: 352mg, Carbohydrates: 9.5, Cholesterol: 53mg, Potassium: 123mg.

276. Sweet and Sour Vegetable Noodles

Preparation Time: 15 minutes
Cooking Time: 30 minutes
Servings: 4
Ingredients:

- 4 chicken fillets (75 g each)
- 300g of whole-wheat spaghetti
- 750g carrots
- ½ liter clear chicken broth (instant)
- 1 tablespoon sugar
- 1 tbsp. of green peppercorns
- 2-3 tbsp. balsamic vinegar
- Capuchin flowers
- Pinch of salt

Directions:

1. Cook spaghetti in boiling water for about 8 minutes. Then drain. In the meantime, peel and wash carrots. Cut into long strips (best with a special grater). Blanch within 2 minutes in boiling salted water, drain. Wash chicken fillets. Add to the boiling chicken soup and cook for about 15 minutes.
2. Melt the sugar until golden brown. Measure 1/4 liter of chicken stock and deglaze the sugar with it. Add peppercorns and cook for 2 minutes. Season with salt and vinegar. Add the fillets, then cut into thin slices. Next, turn the pasta and carrots in the sauce and serve garnished

with capuchin blossoms. Serve and enjoy.

Nutrition:
Calories: 374, Fat: 21g, Protein: 44g, Sodium: 295mg, Carbohydrates: 23.1 Potassium: 386mg.

277. Tuna Sandwich

Preparation Time: 15 minutes
Cooking Time: 0 minutes
Servings: 1
Ingredients:
- 2 slices whole-grain bread
- 1 6-oz. can low sodium tuna in water, in its juice
- 2 tsp. Yogurt (1.5% fat) or low-fat mayonnaise
- 1 medium tomato, diced
- ½ small sweet onion, finely diced
- Lettuce leaves

Directions:
1. Toast whole grain bread slices. Mix tuna, yogurt, or mayonnaise, diced tomato, and onion. Cover a toasted bread with lettuce leaves and spread the tuna mixture on the sandwich. Spread tuna mixed on toasted bread with lettuce leaves. Place another disc as a cover on top. Enjoy the sandwich.

Nutrition:
Calories: 235, Fat: 3g, Protein: 27.8g, Sodium: 350mg, Carbohydrates: 25.9 Potassium: 107mg.

278. Fruited Quinoa Salad

Preparation Time: 15 minutes
Cooking Time: 0 minutes
Servings: 2
Ingredients:
- 2 cups cooked quinoa
- 1 mango, sliced and peeled
- 1 cup strawberry, quartered
- ½ cup blueberries
- 2 tablespoon pine nuts
- Chopped mint leave for garnish

Lemon vinaigrette:
- ¼ cup olive oil
- ¼ cup apple cider vinegar
- Zest of lemon
- 3 tablespoon lemon juice

- 1 teaspoon sugar

Directions:
1. For the lemon vinaigrette, whisk olive oil, apple cider vinegar, lemon zest and juice, and sugar to a bowl; set aside. Combine quinoa, mango strawberries, blueberries, and pine nuts in a large bowl. Stir the lemon vinaigrette and garnish it with mint. Serve and enjoy!

Nutrition:
Calories: 425, Carbohydrates: 76.1g, Proteins: 11.3g, Fat: 10.9, Sodium: 16mg, Potassium: 48mg.

279. Turkey Wrap

Preparation Time: 15 minutes
Cooking Time: 0 minutes
Servings: 2
Ingredients:
- 2 slices of low-fat Turkey breast (deli-style)
- 4 tablespoon non-fat cream cheese
- ½ cup lettuce leaves
- ½ cup carrots, slice into a stick
- 2 Homemade wraps or store-bought whole-wheat tortilla wrap

Directions:
1. Prepare all the ingredients. Spread 2 tablespoons of non-fat cream cheese on each wrap. Arrange lettuce leaves, then add a slice of turkey breast; a slice of carrots stick on top. Roll and cut it in half. Serve and enjoy!

Nutrition:
Calories: 224, Carbohydrates: 35g, Protein: 10.3g, Fat: 3.8g, Sodium: 293mg, Potassium: 153mg.

280. Chicken Wrap

Preparation Time: 15 minutes
Cooking Time: 15 minutes
Servings: 2
Ingredients:
- 1 tablespoon extra-virgin olive oil
- Lemon juice, divided into 3 parts
- 2 cloves garlic, minced
- 1 lb. boneless skinless chicken breasts
- ½ cup non-fat plain Greek yogurt
- ½ teaspoon paprika
- Pinch of salt and pepper

- Hot sauce to taste
- Pita bread
- Tomato slice

Directions:
1. For the marinade, whisk 1 tablespoon of olive oil, juice of 2 lemons, garlic, salt, and pepper in a bowl. Add chicken breasts to the marinade and place it into a large Ziploc. Let marinate for 30 mins. to 4 hours.
2. For the yogurt sauce, mix yogurt, hot sauce, and the remaining lemon juice season with paprika and a pinch of salt and pepper.
3. Warm skillet over medium heat and coat it with oil. Add chicken breast and cook until golden brown and cook about 8 minutes per side. Remove from pan and rest for few minutes, then slice.
4. To a piece of pita bread, add lettuce, tomato, and chicken slices. Drizzle with the prepared spicy yogurt sauce. Serve and enjoy!

Nutrition:
Calories: 348, Carbohydrates: 8.7g, Proteins: 56g, Fat: 10.2g, Sodium: 198mg, Potassium: 64mg.

281. Veggie Wrap

Preparation Time: 15 minutes
Cooking Time: 0 minutes
Servings: 2
Ingredients:
- 2 homemade wraps or any flour tortillas
- ½ cup spinach
- 1/2 cup alfalfa sprouts
- ½ cup avocado, sliced thinly
- 1 medium tomato, sliced thinly
- ½ cup cucumber, sliced thinly
- Pinch of salt and pepper

Directions:
1. Put 2 tablespoons of cream cheese on each tortilla. Layer each veggie according to your liking. Pinch of salt and pepper. Roll and cut it in half. Serve and enjoy!

Nutrition:
Calories: 249, Carbohydrates: 12.3g, Protein: 5.7g, Fat: 21.5g, Sodium: 169mg, Potassium: 85mg.

282. Salmon Wrap

Preparation Time: 15 minutes

Cooking Time: 0 minutes
Servings: 1
Ingredients:

- 2 oz. smoked salmon
- 2 teaspoon low-fat cream cheese
- ½ medium-size red onion, finely sliced
- ½ teaspoon fresh basil or dried basil
- Pinch of pepper
- Arugula leaves
- 1 Homemade wrap or any whole-meal tortilla

Directions:

1. Warm wraps or tortillas into a heated pan or oven. Combine cream cheese, basil, pepper, and spread into the tortilla. Top with salmon, arugula, and sliced onion. Roll up and slice. Serve and enjoy!

Nutrition:
Calories: 151, Carbohydrates: 19.2g, Protein: 10.4g, Fat: 3.4g, Sodium: 316mg, Potassium: 96mg.

283. Dill Chicken Salad

Preparation Time: 15 minutes
Cooking Time: 15 minutes
Servings: 3
Ingredients:

- 1 tablespoon unsalted butter
- 1 small onion, diced
- 2 cloves garlic, minced
- 500g boneless skinless chicken breasts

Salad:

- 2/3 cup fat-free yogurt
- ¼ cup mayonnaise light
- 2 large shallots, minced
- ½ cup fresh dill, finely chopped

Directions:

1. Dissolve the butter over medium heat in a wide pan. Sauté onion and garlic in the butter and chicken breasts. Put water to cover the chicken breasts by 1-inch. Bring to boil. Cover and reduce the heat to a bare simmer.
2. Cook within 8 to 10 minutes or until the chicken is cooked through. Cool thoroughly. Shred the chicken finely using 2 forks. Set aside. Whisk yogurt and mayonnaise. Then toss with the chicken. Add shallots and dill. Mix again all. Serve and enjoy!

Nutrition:

Calories: 253, Carbohydrates: 9g, Protein: 33.1g, Fat: 9.5g, Sodium: 236mg, Potassium: 54mg.

284. Spinach Rolls

Preparation Time: 10 minutes
Cooking Time: 10 minutes
Servings: 4
Ingredients:

- 4 eggs, whisked
- 1/3 cup organic almond milk
- ½ teaspoon salt
- ½ teaspoon white pepper
- 1 teaspoon butter
- 9 oz. chicken breast, boneless, skinless, cooked
- 2 cups spinach
- 2 tablespoon heavy cream

Directions:

1. Mix whisked eggs with almond milk and salt.
2. Preheat the skillet well and toss the butter in it.
3. Melt it.
4. Cook 4 crepes in the preheated skillet.
5. Meanwhile, chop the spinach and chicken breast.
6. Fill every egg crepe with chopped spinach, chicken breast, and heavy cream.
7. Roll the crepes and transfer them to the serving plate.

Nutrition:
Calories: 220, Fat: 14.5g, Fiber: 0.8g, Carbs: 2.4g, Protein: 20.1g, Sodium: 53mg, Potassium: 123mg.

285. Goat Cheese Fold-Overs

Preparation Time: 15 minutes
Cooking Time: 8 minutes
Servings: 4
Ingredients:

- 8 oz. goat cheese, crumbled
- 5 oz. ham, sliced
- 1 cup almond flour
- ¼ cup of coconut milk
- 1 teaspoon olive oil
- ½ teaspoon dried dill
- 1 teaspoon Italian seasoning
- ½ teaspoon salt

Directions:

1. In the mixing bowl, mix almond flour, coconut milk, olive oil, and salt. You will get a smooth batter.
2. Preheat the non-stick skillet.
3. Separate batter into 4 parts. Pour first batter part into the

preheated skillet and cook it for 1 minute from each side.

4. Repeat the same steps with all batter.
5. After this, mix crumbled goat cheese, dried dill, and Italian seasoning.
6. Spread every almond flour pancake with goat cheese mixture. Add sliced ham and fold them.

Nutrition:
Calories: 402 Fat: 31.8g, Fiber: 1.6g, Carbs: 5.1g, Protein: 25.1g, Sodium: 63mg, Potassium: 113mg.

286. Crepe Pie

Preparation Time: 10 minutes
Cooking Time: 15 minutes
Servings: 8
Ingredients:

- 1 cup almond flour
- 1 cup coconut flour
- ½ cup heavy cream
- 1 teaspoon baking powder
- ½ teaspoon salt
- 10 oz. ham, sliced
- ½ cup cream cheese
- 1 teaspoon chili flakes
- 1 tablespoon fresh cilantro, chopped
- 4 oz. Cheddar cheese, shredded

Directions:

1. Make crepes: in the mixing bowl, mix almond flour, coconut flour, heavy cream, salt, and baking powder. Whisk the mixture.
2. Preheat the non-stick skillet well and ladle 1 portion of the crepe batter in it.
3. Make the crepes: cook them for 1 minute from each side over medium heat.
4. Mix cream cheese, chili flakes, cilantro, and shredded Cheddar cheese.
5. After this, transfer first crepe to the plate. Spread it with the cream cheese mixture. Add ham.
6. Repeat the steps until you use all the ingredients.
7. Bake the crepe cake for 5 minutes in a preheated oven at 365F.
8. Cut it into the serving and serve hot.

Nutrition:
Calories: 272, Fat: 18.8g, Fiber: 6.9g, Carbs: 13.2g, Protein: 13.4g, Sodium: 53mg, Potassium: 133mg.

287. Coconut Soup

Preparation Time: 15 minutes
Cooking Time: 25 minutes
Servings: 4
Ingredients:

- 1 cup of coconut milk
- 2 cups of water
- 1 teaspoon curry paste
- 4 chicken thighs
- ½ teaspoon fresh ginger, grated
- 1 garlic clove, diced
- 1 teaspoon butter
- 1 teaspoon chili flakes
- 1 tablespoon lemon juice

Directions:

1. Toss the butter in the skillet and melt it.
2. Add diced garlic and grated ginger. Cook the ingredients for 1 minute. Stir them constantly.
3. Pour water into the saucepan. Add coconut milk and curry paste. Mix the liquid until homogenous.
4. Add chicken thighs, chili flakes, and cooked ginger mixture.
5. Close the lid and cook soup for 15 minutes.
6. Then start to whisk soup with the hand whisker and add lemon juice.
7. When all the lemon juice is added, stop whisking.
8. Close the lid and cook soup for 5 minutes more over medium heat.
9. Then remove soup from the heat and let it rest for 15 minutes.

Nutrition:

Calories: 318, Fat: 26g, Fiber: 1.4g, Carbs: 4.2g, Protein: 20.6g, Sodium: 63mg, Potassium: 113mg.

288. Fish Tacos

Preparation Time: 10 minutes
Cooking Time: 5 minutes
Servings: 4
Ingredients:

- 4 lettuce leaves
- ½ red onion, diced
- ½ jalapeno pepper, minced
- 1 tablespoon olive oil
- 1-pound cod fillet
- 1 tablespoon lemon juice
- ¼ teaspoon ground coriander

Directions:

1. Sprinkle cod fillet with a ½ tablespoon of olive oil and ground coriander.
2. Preheat the grill well.
3. Grill the fish for 2 minutes from each side. The cooked fish has a light brown color.
4. After this, mix diced red onion, minced jalapeno pepper, remaining olive oil, and lemon juice.
5. Cut the grilled cod fillet into 4 pieces.
6. Place the fish in the lettuce leaves. Add mixed red onion mixture over the fish and transfer the tacos to the serving plates.

Nutrition:

Calories: 157, Fat: 4.5g, Fiber: 0.4g, Carbs: 1.6g, Protein: 26.1g, Sodium: 63mg. Potassium: 113mg.

289. Cheese Soup

Preparation Time: 10 minutes
Cooking Time: 15 minutes
Servings: 3
Ingredients:

- 2 white onions, peeled, diced
- 1 cup Cheddar cheese, shredded
- ½ cup heavy cream
- ½ cup of water
- 1 teaspoon ground black pepper
- 1 tablespoon butter
- ½ teaspoon salt

Directions:

1. Pour water and heavy cream into the saucepan.
2. Bring it to boil.
3. Meanwhile, toss the butter in the pan, add diced onions and sauté them.
4. When the onions are translucent, transfer them to the boiling liquid.
5. Add ground black pepper, salt, and cheese. Cook the soup for 5 minutes.
6. Then let it chill a little and ladle it into the bowls.

Nutrition:

Calories: 286, Fat: 23.8g, Fiber: 1.8g, Carbs: 8.3g, Protein: 10.7g, Sodium: 55mg, Potassium: 112mg.

290. Tuna Tartare

Preparation Time: 10 minutes
Cooking Time: 0 minutes
Servings: 4
Ingredients:

- 1-pound tuna steak
- 1 tablespoon mayonnaise
- 3 oz. avocado, chopped
- 1 cucumber, chopped
- 1 tablespoon lemon juice
- 1 teaspoon cayenne pepper
- 1 teaspoon soy sauce
- 1 teaspoon chives
- ½ teaspoon cumin seeds
- 1 teaspoon canola oil

Directions:

1. Chop tuna steak and place it in the big bowl.
2. Add avocado, cucumber, and chives.
3. Mix lemon juice, cayenne pepper, soy sauce, cumin seeds, and canola oil.
4. Add mixed liquid to the tuna mixture and mix well.
5. Place tuna Tartare on the serving plates.

Nutrition:

Calories: 292, Fat: 13.9g, Fiber: 2g, Carbs: 6g, Protein: 35.1g, Sodium: 63mg, Potassium: 113mg.

291. Clam Chowder

Preparation Time: 5 minutes
Cooking Time: 15 minutes
Servings: 3
Ingredients:

- 1 cup of coconut milk
- 1 cup of water
- 6 oz. clam, chopped
- 1 teaspoon chives
- ½ teaspoon white pepper
- ¾ teaspoon chili flakes
- ½ teaspoon salt
- 1 cup broccoli florets, chopped

Directions:

1. Pour coconut milk and water into the saucepan.
2. Add chopped clams, chives, white pepper, chili flakes, salt, and broccoli florets.
3. Close the lid and cook chowder over medium-low heat for 15 minutes or until all the ingredients are soft.
4. It is recommended to serve the soup hot.

Nutrition:

Calories: 139, Fat: 9.8g, Fiber: 1.1g, Carbs: 10.8g, Protein: 2.4g, Sodium: 63mg, Potassium: 132mg.

292. Asian Beef Salad

Preparation Time: 10 minutes
Cooking Time: 25 minutes
Servings: 4

Ingredients:

- 14 oz. beef brisket
- 1 teaspoon sesame seeds
- ½ teaspoon cumin seeds
- 1 tablespoon apple cider vinegar
- 1 tablespoon avocado oil
- 1 red bell pepper, sliced
- 1 white onion, sliced
- 1 teaspoon butter
- 1 teaspoon ground black pepper
- 1 teaspoon soy sauce
- 1 garlic clove, sliced
- 1 cup water for cooking

Directions:

1. Slice beef brisket and place it in the pan. Add water and close the lid.
2. Cook the beef for 25 minutes.
3. Then drain water and transfer beef brisket to the pan.
4. Add butter and roast it for 5 minutes.
5. Put the cooked beef brisket in the salad bowl.
6. Add sesame seeds, cumin seeds, apple cider vinegar, avocado oil, sliced bell pepper, onion, ground black pepper, and soy sauce.
7. Sprinkle the salad with garlic and mix it up.

Nutrition:

Calories: 227, Fat: 8.1g, Fiber: 1.4g, Carbs: 6g, Protein: 31.1g, Sodium: 44mg, Potassium: 133mg.

293. Carbonara

Preparation Time: 10 minutes
Cooking Time: 25 minutes
Servings: 6
Ingredients:

- 3 zucchinis, trimmed
- 1 cup heavy cream
- 5 oz. bacon, chopped
- 2 egg yolks
- 4 oz. Cheddar cheese, grated
- 1 tablespoon butter
- 1 teaspoon chili flakes
- 1 teaspoon salt
- ½ cup water for cooking

Directions:

1. Make the zucchini noodles with the help of the spiralizer.
2. Toss bacon in the skillet and roast it for 5 minutes on medium heat. Stir it from time to time.
3. Meanwhile, in the saucepan, mix heavy cream, butter, salt, and chili flakes.
4. Add egg yolk and whisk the mixture until smooth.

5. Start to preheat the liquid, stir it constantly.
6. When the liquid starts to boil, add grated cheese and fried bacon. Mix it up and close the lid. Sauté it on low heat for 5 minutes.
7. Meanwhile, place the zucchini noodles in the skillet where bacon was and roast it for 3 minutes.
8. Then pour heavy cream mixture over zucchini and mix well. Cook it for 1 minute more and transfer it to the serving plates.

Nutrition:

Calories: 324, Fat: 27.1g, Fiber: 1.1g, Carbs: 4.6g, Protein: 16g, Sodium: 163mg, Potassium: 153mg.

294. Cauliflower Soup with Seeds

Preparation Time: 10 minutes
Cooking Time: 20 minutes
Servings: 4
Ingredients:

- 2 cups cauliflower
- 1 tablespoon pumpkin seeds
- 1 tablespoon chia seeds
- ½ teaspoon salt
- 1 teaspoon butter
- ¼ white onion, diced
- ½ cup coconut cream
- 1 cup of water
- 4 oz. Parmesan, grated
- 1 teaspoon paprika
- 1 tablespoon dried cilantro

Directions:

1. Chop the cauliflower and put it in the pan.
2. Add the salt, butter, chopped onion, paprika and dried coriander.
3. Cook the cauliflower over medium heat for 5 minutes.
4. Then add the coconut cream and water.
5. Close the lid and boil the soup for 15 minutes.
6. Then puree the soup with the help of a hand blender.
7. Bring back to a boil.
8. Add the grated cheese and mix well.
9. Serve the soup in bowls and top each bowl with pumpkin and chia seeds.

Nutrition:

Calories: 214, Fat: 16.4g, Fiber: 3.6g, Carbs: 8.1g, Protein: 12.1g,

Sodium: 63mg, Potassium: 113mg.

295. Prosciutto-Wrapped Asparagus

Preparation Time: 15 minutes
Cooking Time: 20 minutes
Servings: 6
Ingredients:

- 2-pound asparagus
- 8 oz. prosciutto, sliced
- 1 tablespoon butter, melted
- ½ teaspoon ground black pepper
- 4 tablespoon heavy cream
- 1 tablespoon lemon juice

Directions:

1. Slice prosciutto slices into strips.
2. Wrap asparagus into prosciutto strips and place it on the tray.
3. Sprinkle the vegetables with ground black pepper, heavy cream, and lemon juice. Add butter.
4. Preheat the oven to 365F.
5. Place the tray with asparagus in the oven and cook for 20 minutes.
6. Serve the cooked meal only hot.

Nutrition:

Calories: 138, Fat: 7.9g, Fiber: 3.2g, Carbs: 6.9g, Protein: 11.5g, Sodium: 63mg, Potassium: 113mg.

296. Stuffed Bell Peppers

Preparation Time: 10 minutes
Cooking Time: 25 minutes
Servings: 4
Ingredients:

- 4 bell peppers
- 1 ½ cup ground beef
- 1 zucchini, grated
- 1 white onion, diced
- ½ teaspoon ground nutmeg
- 1 tablespoon olive oil
- 1 teaspoon ground black pepper
- ½ teaspoon salt
- 3 oz. Parmesan, grated

Directions:

1. Cut the bell peppers into halves and remove seeds.
2. Place ground beef in the skillet.
3. Add grated zucchini, diced onion, ground nutmeg, olive oil, ground black pepper, and salt.
4. Roast the mixture for 5 minutes.

5. Place bell pepper halves in the tray.
6. Fill every pepper half with ground beef mixture and top with grated Parmesan.
7. Cover the tray with foil and secure the edges.
8. Cook the stuffed bell peppers for 20 minutes at 360F.

Nutrition:
Calories: 241, Fat: 14.6g, Fiber: 3.4g, Carbs: 11g, Protein: 18.6g, Sodium: 63mg, Potassium: 123mg.

297. Stuffed Eggplants with Goat Cheese

Preparation Time: 15 minutes
Cooking Time: 25 minutes
Servings: 4
Ingredients:
- 1 large eggplant, trimmed
- 1 tomato, crushed
- 1 garlic clove, diced
- ½ teaspoon ground black pepper
- ½ teaspoon smoked paprika
- 1 cup spinach, chopped
- 4 oz. goat cheese, crumbled
- 1 teaspoon butter
- 2 oz. Cheddar cheese, shredded

Directions:
1. Cut the eggplants into halves and then cut every half into 2 parts.
2. Remove the flesh from the eggplants to get eggplant boards.
3. Mix crushed tomato, diced garlic, ground black pepper, smoked paprika, chopped spinach, crumbled goat cheese, and butter.
4. Fill the eggplants with this mixture.
5. Top every eggplant board with shredded Cheddar cheese.
6. Put the eggplants in the tray.
7. Preheat the oven to 365F.
8. Place the tray with eggplants in the oven and cook for 25 minutes.

Nutrition:
Calories: 229, Fat: 16.1g, Fiber: 4.6g, Carbs: 9g, Protein: 13.8g, Sodium: 63mg, Potassium: 123mg.

298. Korma Curry

Preparation Time: 10 minutes
Cooking Time: 25 minutes
Servings: 6
Ingredients:
- 3-pound chicken breast, skinless, boneless
- 1 teaspoon garam masala
- 1 teaspoon curry powder
- 1 tablespoon apple cider vinegar
- ½ coconut cream
- 1 cup organic almond milk
- 1 teaspoon ground coriander
- ¾ teaspoon ground cardamom
- ½ teaspoon ginger powder
- ¼ teaspoon cayenne pepper
- ¾ teaspoon ground cinnamon
- 1 tomato, diced
- 1 teaspoon avocado oil
- ½ cup of water

Directions:
1. Chop the chicken breast and put it in the saucepan.
2. Add avocado oil and start to cook it over medium heat.
3. Sprinkle the chicken with garam masala, curry powder, apple cider vinegar, ground coriander, cardamom, ginger powder, cayenne pepper, ground cinnamon, and diced tomato. Mix the ingredients carefully. Cook them for 10 minutes.
4. Add water, coconut cream, and almond milk. Sauté the meal for 10 minutes more.

Nutrition:
Calories: 411, Fat: 19.3g, Fiber: 0.9g, Carbs: 6g, Protein: 49.9g, Sodium: 63mg, Potassium: 123mg.

299. Zucchini Bars

Preparation Time: 10 minutes
Cooking Time: 15 minutes
Servings: 8
Ingredients:
- 3 zucchinis, grated
- ½ white onion, diced
- 2 teaspoons butter
- 3 eggs, whisked
- 4 tablespoons coconut flour
- 1 teaspoon salt
- ½ teaspoon ground black pepper
- 5 oz. goat cheese, crumbled
- 4 oz. Swiss cheese, shredded
- ½ cup spinach, chopped
- 1 teaspoon baking powder
- ½ teaspoon lemon juice

Directions:
1. In the mixing bowl, mix grated zucchini, diced onion, eggs, coconut flour, salt, ground black pepper, crumbled cheese, chopped spinach, baking powder, and lemon juice.
2. Add butter and churn the mixture until homogenous.
3. Line the baking dish with baking paper.
4. Transfer the zucchini mixture to the baking dish and flatten it.
5. Preheat the oven to 365F and put the dish inside.
6. Cook it for 15 minutes. Then chill the meal well.
7. Cut it into bars.

Nutrition:
Calories: 199, Fat: 1316g, Fiber: 215g, Carbs: 7.1g, Protein: 13.1g, Sodium: 63mg, Potassium: 123mg.

300. Mushroom Soup

Preparation Time: 10 minutes
Cooking Time: 25 minutes
Servings: 4
Ingredients:
- 1 cup of water
- 1 cup of coconut milk
- 1 cup white mushrooms, chopped
- ½ carrot, chopped
- ¼ white onion, diced
- 1 tablespoon butter
- 2 oz. turnip, chopped
- 1 teaspoon dried dill
- ½ teaspoon ground black pepper
- ¾ teaspoon smoked paprika
- 1 oz. celery stalk, chopped

Directions:
1. Pour water and coconut milk into the saucepan. Bring the liquid to a boil.
2. Add chopped mushrooms, carrot, and turnip. Close the lid and boil for 10 minutes.
3. Meanwhile, put butter in the skillet. Add diced onion. Sprinkle it with dill, ground black pepper, and smoked paprika. Roast the onion for 3 minutes.
4. Add the roasted onion to the soup mixture.
5. Next, add chopped celery stalk. Close the lid.
6. Cook soup for 10 minutes.
7. Finally, ladle it into the serving bowls.

Nutrition:

Calories: 181, Fat: 17.3g, Fiber: 2.5g, Carbs: 6.9g, Protein: 2.4g, Sodium: 63mg, Potassium: 164mg.

301. Stuffed Portobello Mushrooms

Preparation Time: 10 minutes
Cooking Time: 10 minutes
Servings: 4
Ingredients:

- 2 portobello mushrooms
- 1 cup spinach, chopped, steamed
- 2 oz. artichoke hearts, drained, chopped
- 1 tablespoon coconut cream
- 1 tablespoon cream cheese
- 1 teaspoon minced garlic
- 1 tablespoon fresh cilantro, chopped
- 3 oz. Cheddar cheese, grated
- ½ teaspoon ground black pepper
- 2 tablespoons olive oil
- ½ teaspoon salt

Directions:

1. Sprinkle mushrooms with olive oil and place them in the tray.
2. Transfer the tray in the preheated to 360F oven and broil them for 5 minutes.
3. Meanwhile, blend artichoke hearts, coconut cream, cream cheese, minced garlic, and chopped cilantro.
4. Add grated cheese in the mixture and sprinkle with ground black pepper and salt.
5. Fill the broiled mushrooms with the cheese mixture and cook them for 5 minutes more. Serve the mushrooms only hot.

Nutrition:
Calories: 183, Fat: 16.3g, Fiber: 1.9g, Carbs: 3g, Protein: 7.7g, Sodium: 63mg, Potassium: 123mg.

302. Lettuce Salad

Preparation Time: 10 minutes
Cooking Time: 10 minutes
Servings: 1
Ingredients:

- 1 cup Romaine lettuce, roughly chopped
- 3 oz. Seitan, chopped
- 1 tablespoon avocado oil
- 1 teaspoon sunflower seeds
- 1 teaspoon lemon juice

- 1 egg, boiled, peeled
- 2 oz. Cheddar cheese, shredded

Directions:

1. Place lettuce in the salad bowl. Add chopped Seitan and shredded cheese.
2. Then chop the egg roughly and add it to the salad bowl too.
3. Mix lemon juice with avocado oil.
4. Sprinkle the salad with the oil mixture and sunflower seeds. Don't stir the salad before serving.

Nutrition:
Calories: 663, Fat: 29.5g, Fiber: 4.7g, Carbs: 3.8g, Protein: 84.2g, Sodium: 63mg, Potassium: 123mg.

303. Onion Soup

Preparation Time: 10 minutes
Cooking Time: 25 minutes
Servings: 6
Ingredients:

- 2 cups white onion, diced
- 4 tablespoon butter
- ½ cup white mushrooms, chopped
- 3 cups of water
- 1 cup heavy cream
- 1 teaspoon salt
- 1 teaspoon chili flakes
- 1 teaspoon garlic powder

Directions:

1. Put butter in the saucepan and melt it.
2. Add diced white onion, chili flakes, and garlic powder. Mix it up and sauté for 10 minutes over medium-low heat.
3. Then add water, heavy cream, and chopped mushrooms. Close the lid.
4. Cook the soup for 15 minutes more.
5. Then blend the soup until you get the creamy texture. Ladle it in the bowls.

Nutrition:
Calories: 155, Fat: 15.1g, Fiber: 0.9g, Carbs: 4.7g, Protein: 1.2g, Sodium: 44mg, Potassium: 125mg.

304. Asparagus Salad

Preparation Time: 10 minutes
Cooking Time: 15 minutes
Servings: 3
Ingredients:

- 10 oz. asparagus
- 1 tablespoon olive oil

- ½ teaspoon white pepper
- 4 oz. Feta cheese, crumbled
- 1 cup lettuce, chopped
- 1 tablespoon canola oil
- 1 teaspoon apple cider vinegar
- 1 tomato, diced

Directions:

1. Preheat the oven to 365F.
2. Place asparagus in the tray, sprinkle with olive oil and white pepper and transfer in the preheated oven. Cook it for 15 minutes.
3. Meanwhile, put crumbled Feta in the salad bowl.
4. Add chopped lettuce and diced tomato.
5. Sprinkle the ingredients with apple cider vinegar.
6. Chill the cooked asparagus to room temperature and add in the salad.
7. Shake the salad gently before serving.

Nutrition:
Calories: 207, Fat: 17.6g, Fiber: 2.4g, Carbs: 6.8g, Protein: 7.8g, Sodium: 44mg, Potassium: 113mg.

305. Cauliflower Tabbouleh

Preparation Time: 10 minutes
Cooking Time: 4 minutes
Servings: 4
Ingredients:

- 1-pound cauliflower head
- 1 cucumber, chopped
- 2 tablespoons lemon juice
- 2 tablespoons olive oil
- ½ cup fresh parsley
- 1 garlic clove, diced
- 1 oz. scallions, chopped
- 1 teaspoon mint

Directions:

1. Trim and chop the cauliflower head. Transfer to food processor and pulse until cauliflower rice is obtained.
2. Place the cauliflower rice in the glass mixing bowl. Add the lemon juice and chopped scallions. Stir the mixture.
3. Microwave during 4 minutes.
4. Meanwhile, mix the olive oil, parsley and minced garlic.
5. Toss the cooked cauliflower rice with the parsley mixture. Add the mint and chopped cucumbers.
6. Mix and transfer to serving plates.

Nutrition:

Calories: 108, Fat: 7.3g, Fiber: 3.7g, Carbs: 10.2g, Protein: 3.2g, Sodium: 34mg, Potassium: 113mg.

306. Stuffed Artichoke

Preparation Time: 10 minutes
Cooking Time: 15 minutes
Servings: 4
Ingredients:
- 2 artichokes
- 4 tablespoon Parmesan, grated
- 2 teaspoon almond flour
- 1 teaspoon minced garlic
- 3 tablespoons sour cream
- 1 teaspoon avocado oil
- 1 cup water for cooking

Directions:
1. Pour water into the saucepan and bring it to a boil.
2. When the water is boiling, add artichokes and boil them for 5 minutes.
3. Drain water from artichokes and trim them.
4. Remove the artichoke hearts.
5. Preheat the oven to 365F.
6. Mix almond flour, grated Parmesan, minced garlic, sour cream, and avocado oil.
7. Fill the artichokes with cheese mixture and place them on the baking tray.
8. Cook the vegetables for 10 minutes.
9. Then cut every artichoke into halves and transfer it to the serving plates.

Nutrition:
Calories: 162, Fat: 10.7g, Fiber: 5.9g, Carbs: 12.4g, Protein: 8.2g, Sodium: 43mg, Potassium: 113mg.

307. Beef Salpicao

Preparation Time: 10 minutes
Cooking Time: 18 minutes

Servings: 2
Ingredients:
- 1-pound rib eye, boneless
- 2 garlic cloves, peeled, diced
- 2 tablespoons butter
- 1 tablespoon sour cream
- ½ teaspoon salt
- ½ teaspoon chili pepper
- 1 tablespoon lime juice

Directions:
1. Cut rib eye into the strips.
2. Sprinkle the meat with salt, chili pepper, and lime juice.
3. Toss butter in the skillet. Add diced garlic and roast it for 2 minutes over medium heat.
4. Then add meat strips and roast them over high heat for 2 minutes from each side.
5. Add sour cream and close the lid. Cook the meal for 10 minutes more over medium heat. Stir it from time to time.
6. Transfer cooked beef Salpicao on the serving plates.

Nutrition:
Calories: 641, Fat: 52.8g, Fiber: 0.1g, Carbs: 1.9g, Protein: 42.5g, Sodium: 63mg, Potassium: 113mg.

308. Cream Dredged Corn Platter

Preparation Time: 10 minutes
Cooking Time: 4 hours
Servings: 3
Ingredients:
- 3 cups corn
- 2 ounces cream cheese, cubed
- 2 tablespoons milk
- 2 tablespoons whipping cream
- 2 tablespoons butter, melted
- Salt and pepper as needed
- 1 tablespoon green onion, chopped

Directions:

1. Add corn, cream cheese, milk, whipping cream, butter, salt and pepper to your Slow Cooker.
2. Give it a nice toss to mix everything well. Place lid and cook on LOW for 4 hours.
3. Divide the mixture into serving trays. Serve and enjoy!

Nutrition:
Calories: 641, Fat: 52.8g, Fiber: 0.1g, Carbs: 1.9g, Protein: 42.5g, Sodium: 63mg, Potassium: 123mg.

309. Ethiopian Cabbage Delight

Preparation Time: 15 minutes
Cooking Time: 6- 8 hours
Servings: 6
Ingredients:
- ½ cup water
- 1 head green cabbage, cored and chopped
- 1 pound sweet potatoes, peeled and chopped
- 3 carrots, peeled and chopped
- 1 onion, sliced
- 1 teaspoon extra virgin olive oil
- ½ teaspoon ground turmeric
- ½ teaspoon ground cumin
- ¼ teaspoon ground ginger

Directions:
1. Add water to your Slow Cooker. Take a medium bowl and add cabbage, carrots, sweet potatoes, onion and mix.
2. Add olive oil, turmeric, ginger, cumin and toss until the veggies are fully coated.
3. Transfer veggie mix to your Slow Cooker. Cover and cook on LOW for 6-8 hours. Serve and enjoy!

Nutrition:
Calories: 641, Fat: 52.8g, Fiber: 0.1g, Carbs: 1.9g, Protein: 42.5g, Sodium: 103mg, Potassium: 123mg.

Chapter 9. Dinner

310. Shrimp Cocktail

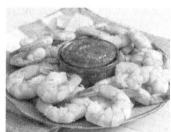

Preparation Time: 10 minutes
Cooking Time: 5 minutes
Servings: 8
Ingredients:

- 2 pounds big shrimp, deveined
- 4 cups of water
- 2 bay leaves
- 1 small lemon, halved
- Ice for cooling the shrimp
- Ice for serving
- 1 medium lemon sliced for serving
- ¾ cup tomato passata
- 2 and ½ tablespoons horseradish, prepared
- ¼ teaspoon chili powder
- 2 tablespoons lemon juice

Directions:

1. Pour the 4 cups water into a large pot, add lemon and bay leaves. Boil over medium-high heat, reduce temperature and boil for 10 minutes. Put shrimp, stir and cook within 2 minutes. Move the shrimp to a bowl filled with ice and leave aside for 5 minutes.
2. In a bowl, mix tomato passata with horseradish, chili powder, and lemon juice and stir well. Place shrimp in a serving bowl filled with ice and lemon slices, and serve with the cocktail sauce you've prepared.

Nutrition:
Calories: 276, Carbs: 0g, Fat: 8g, Protein: 25g, Sodium: 182mg, Potassium: 65mg.

311. Squid and Shrimp Salad

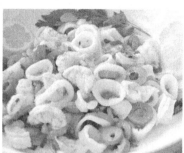

Preparation Time: 10 minutes
Cooking Time: 15 minutes
Servings: 4
Ingredients:

- 8 ounces squid, cut into medium pieces
- 8 ounces shrimp, peeled and deveined
- 1 red onion, sliced
- 1 cucumber, chopped
- 2 tomatoes, cut into medium wedges
- 2 tablespoons cilantro, chopped
- 1 hot jalapeno pepper, cut in rounds
- 3 tablespoons rice vinegar
- 3 tablespoons dark sesame oil
- Black pepper to the taste

Directions:

1. In a bowl, mix the onion with cucumber, tomatoes, pepper, cilantro, shrimp, and squid and stir well. Cut a big parchment paper in half, fold it in half heart shape and open. Place the seafood mixture in this parchment piece, fold over, seal edges, place on a baking sheet, and introduce in the oven at 400 degrees F for 15 minutes.
2. Meanwhile, in a small bowl, mix sesame oil with rice vinegar and black pepper and stir very well. Take the salad out of the oven, leave to cool down for a few minutes, and transfer to a serving plate. Put the dressing over the salad and serve right away.

Nutrition:
Calories: 235, Carbs: 9g, Fat: 8g, Protein: 30g, Sodium: 165mg, Potassium: 89mg.

312. Parsley Seafood Cocktail

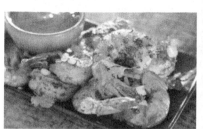

Preparation Time: 2 hours and 10 minutes
Cooking Time: 1 hour and 30 minutes
Servings: 4
Ingredients:

- 1 big octopus, cleaned
- 1-pound mussels
- 2 pounds clams
- 1 big squid cut in rings
- 3 garlic cloves, chopped
- 1 celery rib, cut crosswise into thirds
- ½ cup celery rib, sliced
- 1 carrot, cut crosswise into 3 pieces
- 1 small white onion, chopped
- 1 bay leaf
- ¾ cup white wine
- 2 cups radicchio, sliced
- 1 red onion, sliced
- 1 cup parsley, chopped
- 1 cup olive oil
- 1 cup red wine vinegar
- Black pepper to the taste

Directions:

1. Put the octopus in a pot with celery rib cut in thirds, garlic, carrot, bay leaf, white onion, and white wine. Add water to cover the octopus, cover with a lid, bring to a boil over high heat, reduce to low, and simmer within 1 and ½ hours.
2. Drain octopus, reserve boiling liquid, and leave aside to cool down. Put ¼ cup octopus cooking liquid in another pot. Add mussels, and heat over medium-high heat, cook until they open. Transfer to a bowl, and leave aside.
3. Add clams to the pan, cover, cook over medium-high heat until they open. Transfer to the

bowl with mussels, and leave aside. Add squid to the pan, cover and cook over medium-high heat for 3 minutes. Transfer to the bowl with mussels and clams.

4. Meanwhile, slice octopus into small pieces and mix with the rest of the seafood. Add sliced celery, radicchio, red onion, vinegar, olive oil, parsley, salt, and pepper. Stir gently and leave aside in the fridge within 2 hours before serving.

Nutrition:
Calories: 102, Carbs: 7g, Fat: 1g, Protein: 16g, Sodium: 0mg, Potassium: 134mg.

313. Shrimp and Onion Ginger Dressing

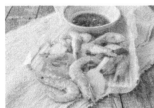

Preparation Time: 10 minutes
Cooking Time: 5 minutes
Servings: 2
Ingredients:
- 8 medium shrimps, peeled and deveined
- 12 ounces package mixed salad leaves
- 10 cherry tomatoes, halved
- 2 green onions, sliced
- 2 medium mushrooms, sliced
- 1/3 cup rice vinegar
- ¼ cup sesame seeds, toasted
- 1 tablespoon low-sodium soy sauce
- 2 teaspoons ginger, grated
- 2 teaspoons garlic, minced
- 2/3 cup canola oil
- 1/3 cup sesame oil

Directions:
1. In a bowl, mix rice vinegar with sesame seeds, soy sauce, garlic, ginger, and stir well. Pour this into your kitchen blender, add canola oil and sesame oil, pulse very well, and leave aside. Brush shrimp with 3 tablespoons of the ginger dressing you've prepared.
2. Heat your kitchen grill over high fire. Add shrimp and cook for 3 minutes, flipping once. In a

salad bowl, mix salad leaves with grilled shrimp, mushrooms, green onions, and tomatoes. Drizzle ginger dressing on top and serve right away!

Nutrition:
Calories: 360, Carbs: 14g, Fat: 11g, Protein: 49g, Sodium: 469mg, Potassium: 45mg.

314. Fruit Shrimp Soup

Preparation Time: 10 minutes
Cooking Time: 25 minutes
Servings: 6
Ingredients:
- 8 ounces shrimp, peeled and deveined
- 1 stalk lemongrass, smashed
- 2 small ginger pieces, grated
- 6 cup chicken stock
- 2 jalapenos, chopped
- 4 lime leaves
- 1 and ½ cups pineapple, chopped
- 1 cup shiitake mushroom caps, chopped
- 1 tomato, chopped
- ½ bell pepper, cubed
- 2 tablespoons fish sauce
- 1 teaspoon sugar
- ¼ cup lime juice
- 1/3 cup cilantro, chopped
- 2 scallions, sliced

Directions:
1. In a pot, mix ginger with lemongrass, stock, jalapenos, and lime leaves, stir, boil over medium heat, cook within 15 minutes. Strain liquid in a bowl and discard solids.
2. Return soup to the pot again. Add pineapple, tomato, mushrooms, bell pepper, sugar, and fish sauce. Stir, boil over medium heat and cook for 5 minutes. Add shrimp and cook for 3 more minutes. Remove from heat. Add lime juice, cilantro, and scallions, stir, ladle into soup bowls and serve.

Nutrition:
Calories: 290, Carbs: 39g, Fat: 12g, Protein: 7g, Sodium: 21mg, Potassium: 75mg.

315. Mussels and Chickpea Soup

Preparation Time: 10 minutes
Cooking Time: 10 minutes

Servings: 6
Ingredients:
- 3 garlic cloves, minced
- 2 tablespoons olive oil
- A pinch of chili flakes
- 1 and ½ tablespoons fresh mussels, scrubbed
- 1 cup white wine
- 1 cup chickpeas, rinsed
- 1 small fennel bulb, sliced
- Black pepper to the taste
- Juice of 1 lemon
- 3 tablespoons parsley, chopped

Directions:
1. Heat a big saucepan with the olive oil over medium-high fire, add garlic and chili flakes, stir and cook within a couple of minutes. Add white wine and mussels, stir, cover, and cook for 3-4 minutes until mussels open.
2. Transfer mussels to a baking dish. Add some of the cooking liquid over them and fridge until they are cold enough. Take mussels out of the fridge and discard shells.
3. Heat another pan over medium-high heat. Add mussels, reserved cooking liquid, chickpeas, and fennel. Stir well, and heat them. Add black pepper to the taste, lemon juice, and parsley, stir again, divide between plates and serve.

Nutrition:
Calories: 286, Carbs: 49g, Fat: 4g, Protein: 14g, Sodium: 145mg, Potassium: 80mg.

316. Fish Stew

Preparation Time: 10 minutes
Cooking Time: 30 minutes
Servings: 4
Ingredients:
- 1 red onion, sliced
- 2 tablespoons olive oil
- 1-pound white fish fillets, boneless, skinless, and cubed
- 1 avocado, pitted and chopped
- 1 tablespoon oregano, chopped
- 1 cup chicken stock
- 2 tomatoes, cubed
- 1 teaspoon sweet paprika
- A pinch of salt and black pepper
- 1 tablespoon parsley, chopped
- Juice of 1 lime

Directions:
1. Heat the oil in a pot over medium heat. Add the onion, and sauté within 5 minutes. Add the fish, the avocado, and the other ingredients, toss and cook

over medium heat for 25 minutes more. Divide into bowls and serve for lunch.

Nutrition:
Calories: 78, Carbs: 8g, Fat: 1g, Protein: 11g, Sodium: 151mg, Potassium: 0mg.

317. Shrimp and Broccoli Soup

Preparation Time: 5 minutes
Cooking Time: 25 minutes
Servings: 4
Ingredients:
- 2 tablespoons olive oil
- 1 yellow onion, chopped
- 4 cups chicken stock
- Juice of 1 lime
- 1-pound shrimp, peeled and deveined
- ½ cup coconut cream
- ½ pound broccoli florets
- 1 tablespoon parsley, chopped

Directions:
1. Heat a pot with the oil over medium heat. Add the onion and sauté for 5 minutes. Add the shrimp and the other ingredients, simmer over medium heat for 20 minutes more. Ladle the soup into bowls and serve.

Nutrition:
Calories: 220, Carbs: 12g, Fat: 7g, Protein: 26g, Sodium: 577mg, Potassium: 34mg.

318. Coconut Turkey Mix

Preparation Time: 10 minutes
Cooking Time: 30 minutes
Servings: 4
Ingredients:
- 1 yellow onion, chopped
- 1-pound turkey breast, skinless, boneless, and cubed
- 2 tablespoons olive oil
- 2 garlic cloves, minced
- 1 zucchini, sliced
- 1 cup coconut cream
- A pinch of sea salt
- black pepper

Directions:
1. Bring the pan to medium heat. Add the onion and the garlic and sauté for 5 minutes. Put the meat and brown within 5 minutes more. Add the rest of the ingredients, toss, bring to a simmer and cook over medium

heat for 20 minutes more. Serve for lunch.

Nutrition:
Calories 200, Fat 4g, Fiber: 2g, Carbs 14g, Protein 7g, Sodium 111mg, Potassium: 42mg.

319. Lime Shrimp and Kale

Preparation Time: 10 minutes
Cooking Time: 20 minutes
Servings: 4
Ingredients:
- 1-pound shrimp, peeled and deveined
- 4 scallions, chopped
- 1 teaspoon sweet paprika
- 1 tablespoon olive oil
- Juice of 1 lime
- Zest of 1 lime, grated
- A pinch of salt and black pepper
- 2 tablespoons parsley, chopped

Directions:
1. Bring the pan to medium heat. Add the scallions and sauté for 5 minutes. Add the shrimp and the other ingredients. Toss, cook over medium heat for 15 minutes more, divide into bowls and serve.

Nutrition:
Calories: 149, Carbs: 12g, Fat: 4g, Protein: 21g, Sodium: 250mg, Potassium: 123mg.

320. Parsley Cod Mix

Preparation Time: 10 minutes
Cooking Time: 20 minutes
Servings: 4
Ingredients:
- 1 tablespoon olive oil
- 2 shallots, chopped
- 4 cod fillets, boneless and skinless
- 2 garlic cloves, minced
- 2 tablespoons lemon juice
- 1 cup chicken stock
- A pinch of salt and black pepper

Directions:
1. Bring the pan to medium heat - high heat. Add the shallots and the garlic and sauté for 5 minutes. Add the cod and the other ingredients; cook everything for 15 minutes more, divide between plates and serve for lunch.

Nutrition:

Calories: 216, Carbs: 7g, Fat: 5g, Protein: 34g, Sodium: 380mg, Potassium: 217mg.

321. Salmon and Cabbage Mix

Preparation Time: 5 minutes
Cooking Time: 25 minutes
Servings: 4
Ingredients:
- 4 salmon fillets, boneless
- 1 yellow onion, chopped
- 2 tablespoons olive oil
- 1 cup red cabbage, shredded
- 1 red bell pepper, chopped
- 1 tablespoon rosemary, chopped
- 1 tablespoon coriander, ground
- 1 cup tomato sauce
- A pinch of sea salt
- black pepper

Directions:
1. Bring the pan to medium heat. Add the onion and sauté for 5 minutes. Put the fish and sear it within 2 minutes on each side. Add the cabbage and the remaining ingredients. Toss, cook over medium heat for 20 minutes more, divide between plates and serve.

Nutrition:
Calories: 130, Carbs: 8g, Fat: 6g, Protein: 12g, Sodium: 345mg, Potassium: 43mg.

322. Decent Beef and Onion Stew

Preparation Time: 10 minutes
Cooking Time: 1-2 hours
Servings: 4
Ingredients:
- 2 pounds lean beef, cubed
- 3 pounds shallots, peeled
- 5 garlic cloves, peeled, whole
- 3 tablespoons tomato paste
- 1 bay leaves
- ¼ cup olive oil
- 3 tablespoons lemon juice

Directions:
1. Take a stew pot and place it over medium heat.
2. Add olive oil and let it heat.
3. Add meat and brown.
4. Add remaining ingredients and cover with water.
5. Bring the whole mix to a boil.
6. Reduce heat to low and cover the pot.
7. Simmer for 1-2 hours until beef is cooked thoroughly.
8. Serve hot!

Nutrition:
Calories: 136, Fat: 3g, Carbohydrates: 0.9g, Protein: 24g, Sodium: 63mg, Potassium: 123mg.

323. Clean Parsley and Chicken Breast

Preparation Time: 10 minutes
Cooking Time: 40 minutes
Servings: 2
Ingredients:

- 1/2 tablespoon dry parsley
- 1/2 tablespoon dry basil
- 2 chicken breast halves, boneless and skinless
- 1/4 teaspoon sunflower seeds
- 1/4 teaspoon red pepper flakes, crushed
- 1 tomato, sliced

Directions:

1. Preheat your oven to 350 degrees F.
2. Take a 9x13 inch baking dish and grease it up with cooking spray.
3. Sprinkle 1 tablespoon of parsley, 1 teaspoon of basil and spread the mixture over your baking dish.
4. Arrange the chicken breast halves over the dish and sprinkle garlic slices on top.
5. Take a small bowl and add 1 teaspoon parsley, 1 teaspoon of basil, sunflower seeds, basil, and red pepper and mix well. Pour the mixture over the chicken breast.
6. Top with tomato slices and cover, bake for 25 minutes.
7. Remove the cover and bake for 15 minutes more.
8. Serve and enjoy!

Nutrition:
Calories: 150, Fat: 4g, Carbohydrates: 4g, Protein: 25g, Sodium: 63mg, Potassium: 129mg.

324. Zucchini Beef Sauté with Coriander Greens

Preparation Time: 10 minutes
Cooking Time: 10 minutes
Servings: 4
Ingredients:

- 10 ounces beef, sliced into 1–2-inch strips

- 1 zucchini, cut into 2-inch strips
- 1/4 cup parsley, chopped
- 3 garlic cloves, minced
- 2 tablespoons tamari sauce
- 4 tablespoons avocado oil

Directions:

1. Add 2 tablespoons of avocado oil in a frying pan over high heat.
2. Place strips of beef and brown for a few minutes on high heat.
3. Once the meat is brown, add zucchini strips and sauté until tender.
4. Once tender, add tamari sauce, garlic, parsley and let them sit for a few minutes more.
5. Serve immediately and enjoy!

Nutrition:
Calories: 500, Fat: 40g, Carbohydrates: 5g, Protein: 31g, Sodium: 63mg, Potassium: 120mg.

325. Hearty Lemon and Pepper Chicken

Preparation Time: 5 minutes
Cooking Time: 15 minutes
Servings: 4
Ingredients:

- 2 teaspoons olive oil
- 1 1/4 pounds skinless chicken cutlets
- 2 whole eggs
- 1/4 cup panko crumbs
- 1 tablespoon lemon pepper
- Sunflower seeds and pepper to taste
- 3 cups green beans
- 1/4 cup parmesan cheese
- 1/4 teaspoon garlic powder

Directions:

1. Preheat your oven to 425 degrees F.
2. Take a bowl and stir in seasoning, parmesan, lemon pepper, garlic powder, panko.
3. Whisk eggs in another bowl.
4. Coat cutlets in eggs and press into panko mix.
5. Transfer coated chicken to a parchment-lined baking sheet.
6. Toss the beans in oil, pepper, add sunflower seeds, and lay them on the side of the baking sheet.
7. Bake for 15 minutes.
8. Enjoy!

Nutrition:
Calorie: 299, Fat: 10g, Carbohydrates: 10g, Protein:

43g, Sodium: 63mg, Potassium: 73mg.

326. Walnuts and Asparagus Delight

Preparation Time: 5 minutes
Cooking Time: 5 minutes
Servings: 4
Ingredients:

- 1 1/2 tablespoons olive oil
- 3/4 pound asparagus, trimmed
- 1/4 cup walnuts, chopped
- Sunflower seeds and pepper to taste

Directions:

1. Place a skillet over medium heat. Add olive oil and let it heat.
2. Add asparagus, sauté for 5 minutes until browned.
3. Season with sunflower seeds and pepper.
4. Remove heat.
5. Add walnuts and toss.
6. Serve warm!

Nutrition:
Calories: 124, Fat: 12g, Carbohydrates: 2g, Protein: 3g, Sodium: 55mg, Potassium: 113mg.

327. Healthy Carrot Chips

Preparation Time: 10 minutes
Cooking Time: 10 minutes
Servings: 4
Ingredients:

- 3 cups carrots, sliced paper-thin rounds
- 2 tablespoons olive oil
- 2 teaspoons ground cumin
- 1/2 teaspoon smoked paprika
- Pinch of sunflower seeds

Directions:

1. Preheat your oven to 400 degrees F.
2. Cut the carrot into paper-like coins with a peeler.
3. Place the slices in a bowl and toss with oil and spices.
4. Place the slices on a baking sheet lined with parchment paper in a single layer.
5. Sprinkle sunflower seeds.
6. Transfer to oven and bake for 8-10 minutes.
7. Remove and serve.
8. Enjoy!

Nutrition:

Calories: 434, Fat: 35g, Carbohydrates: 31g, Protein: 2g, Sodium: 63mg, Potassium: 123mg.

328. Beef Soup

Preparation Time: 10 minutes
Cooking Time: 40 minutes
Servings: 4
Ingredients:
- 1 pound ground beef, lean
- 1 cup mixed vegetables, frozen
- 1 yellow onion, chopped
- 6 cups vegetable broth
- 1 cup low-fat cream
- Pepper to taste

Directions:
1. Take a stockpot and add all the ingredients except heavy cream, salt, and black pepper.
2. Bring to a boil.
3. Reduce heat to simmer.
4. Cook for 40 minutes.
5. Once cooked, warm the heavy cream.
6. Then add once the soup is cooked.
7. Blend the soup till smooth by using an immersion blender.
8. Season with salt and black pepper.
9. Serve and enjoy!

Nutrition:
Calories: 270, Fat: 14g, Carbohydrates: 6g, Protein: 29g, Sodium: 63mg.

329. Amazing Grilled Chicken and Blueberry Salad

Preparation Time: 10 minutes
Cooking Time: 25 minutes
Servings: 5
Ingredients:
- 5 cups mixed greens
- 1 cup blueberries
- ¼ cup slivered almonds
- 2 cups chicken breasts, cooked and cubed

For dressing
- ¼ cup olive oil
- ¼ cup apple cider vinegar
- ¼ cup blueberries
- 2 tablespoons honey
- Sunflower seeds and pepper to taste

Directions:

1. Take a bowl and add greens, berries, almonds, chicken cubes and mix well.
2. Take a bowl and mix the dressing ingredients, pour the mix into a blender and blitz until smooth.
3. Add dressing on top of the chicken cubes and toss well.
4. Season more and enjoy!

Nutrition:
Calories: 266, Fat: 17g, Carbohydrates: 18g, Protein: 10g, Sodium: 44mg, Potassium: 83mg.

330. Clean Chicken and Mushroom Stew

Preparation Time: 10 minutes
Cooking Time: 35 minutes
Servings: 4
Ingredients:
- 4 chicken breast halves, cut into bite-sized pieces
- 1 pound mushrooms, sliced (5-6 cups)
- 1 bunch spring onion, chopped
- 4 tablespoons olive oil
- 1 teaspoon thyme
- Sunflower seeds and pepper as needed

Directions:
1. Take a large deep-frying pan and place it over medium-high heat.
2. Add oil and let it heat.
3. Add chicken and cook for 4-5 minutes per side until slightly browned.
4. Add spring onions and mushrooms, season with sunflower seeds and pepper according to your taste.
5. Stir.
6. Cover with lid and bring the mix to a boil.
7. Reduce heat and simmer for 25 minutes.
8. Serve!

Nutrition:
Calories: 247, Fat: 12g, Carbohydrates: 10g, Protein: 23g, Sodium: 63mg, Potassium: 76mg.

331. Elegant Pumpkin Chili Dish

Preparation Time: 10 minutes

Cooking Time: 15 minutes
Servings: 4
Ingredients:
- 3 cups yellow onion, chopped
- 8 garlic cloves, chopped
- 1 pound turkey, ground
- 2 cans (15 ounces each) fire roasted tomatoes
- 2 cups pumpkin puree
- 1 cup chicken broth
- 4 teaspoons chili spice
- 1 teaspoon ground cinnamon
- 1 teaspoon sea sunflower seeds

Directions:
1. Take a large-sized pot and place it over medium-high heat.
2. Add coconut oil and let the oil heat.
3. Add onion and garlic, sauté for 5 minutes.
4. Add ground turkey and break it while cooking, cook for 5 minutes.
5. Add remaining ingredients and bring the mix to simmer.
6. Simmer for 15 minutes over low heat (lid off).
7. Pour chicken broth.
8. Serve with desired salad.
9. Enjoy!

Nutrition:
Calories: 312, Fat: 16g, Carbohydrates: 14g, Protein: 27g, Sodium: 63mg, Potassium: 79mg.

332. Tasty Roasted Broccoli

Preparation Time: 5 minutes
Cooking Time: 20 minutes
Servings: 4
Ingredients:
- 4 cups broccoli florets
- 1 tablespoon olive oil
- Sunflower seeds and pepper to taste

Directions:
1. Preheat your oven to 400 degrees F.
2. Add broccoli in a zip bag alongside oil and shake until coated.
3. Add seasoning and shake again.
4. Spread broccoli out on a baking sheet, bake for 20 minutes.
5. Let it cool and serve.
6. Enjoy!

Nutrition:
Calories: 62, Fat: 4g, Carbohydrates: 4g, Protein: 4g,

Sodium: 63mg, Potassium: 24mg.

333. The Almond Breaded Chicken Goodness

Preparation Time: 15 minutes
Cooking Time: 15 minutes
Servings: 3
Ingredients:
- 2 large chicken breasts, boneless and skinless
- 1/3 cup lemon juice
- 1 ½ cups seasoned almond meal
- 2 tablespoons coconut oil
- Lemon pepper to taste
- Parsley for decoration

Directions:
1. Slice chicken breast in half.
2. Pound out each half until ¼ inch thick.
3. Take a pan and place it over medium heat. Add oil and heat it.
4. Dip each chicken breast slice into lemon juice and let it sit for 2 minutes.
5. Turn over and let the other side sit for 2 minutes as well.
6. Transfer to almond meal and coat both sides.
7. Add coated chicken to the oil and fry for 4 minutes per side, making sure to sprinkle lemon pepper liberally.
8. Transfer to a paper-lined sheet and repeat until all chicken is fried.
9. Garnish with parsley and enjoy!

Nutrition:
Calories: 325, Fat: 24g, Carbohydrates: 3g, Protein: 16g, Sodium: 63mg, Potassium: 89mg.

334. South-Western Pork Chops

Preparation Time: 10 minutes
Cooking Time: 15 minutes
Servings: 4
Ingredients:
- Cooking spray as needed
- 4-ounce pork loin chop, boneless and fat rimmed
- 1/3 cup salsa
- 2 tablespoons fresh lime juice
- ¼ cup fresh cilantro, chopped

Directions:

1. Take a large-sized non-stick skillet and spray it with cooking spray.
2. Heat until hot over high heat.
3. Press the chops with your palm to flatten them slightly.
4. Add them to the skillet and cook for 1 minute for each side until they are nicely browned.
5. Lower the heat to medium-low.
6. Combine the salsa and lime juice.
7. Pour the mix over the chops.
8. Simmer uncovered for about 8 minutes until the chops are perfectly done.
9. If needed, sprinkle some cilantro on top.
10. Serve!

Nutrition:
Calorie: 184, Fat: 4g, Carbohydrates: 4g, Protein: 0.5g, Sodium: 63mg, Potassium: 50mg.

335. Almond butter Pork Chops

Preparation Time: 5 minutes
Cooking Time: 25 minutes
Servings: 2
Ingredients:
- 1 tablespoon almond butter, divided
- 2 boneless pork chops
- Pepper to taste
- 1 tablespoon dried Italian seasoning, low fat and low sodium
- 1 tablespoon olive oil

Directions:
1. Preheat your oven to 350 degrees F.
2. Pat pork chops dry with a paper towel and place them in a baking dish.
3. Season with pepper and Italian seasoning.
4. Drizzle olive oil over pork chops.
5. Top each chop with ½ tablespoon almond butter.
6. Bake for 25 minutes.
7. Transfer pork chops on two plates and top with almond butter juice.
8. Serve and enjoy!

Nutrition:
Calories: 333, Fat: 23g, Carbohydrates: 1g, Protein: 31g, Sodium: 63mg, Potassium: 80mg.

336. Chicken Salsa

Preparation Time: 4 minutes
Cooking Time: 14 minutes
Servings: 1
Ingredients:
- 2 chicken breasts
- 1 cup salsa
- 1 taco seasoning mix
- 1 cup plain Greek Yogurt
- ½ cup of kite ricotta/cashew cheese, cubed

Directions:
1. Take a skillet and place it over medium heat.
2. Add chicken breast, ½ cup of salsa and taco seasoning.
3. Mix well and cook for 12-15 minutes until the chicken is done.
4. Take the chicken out and cube them.
5. Place the cubes on a toothpick and top with cheddar.
6. Place yogurt and remaining salsa in cups and use as dips.
7. Enjoy!

Nutrition:
Calories: 359, Fat: 14g, Net Carbohydrates: 14g, Protein: 43g, Sodium: 63mg, Potassium: 53mg.

337. Healthy Mediterranean Lamb Chops

Preparation Time: 10 minutes
Cooking Time: 10 minutes
Servings: 4
Ingredients:
- 4 lamb shoulder chops, 8 ounces each
- 2 tablespoons Dijon mustard
- 2 tablespoons Balsamic vinegar
- ½ cup olive oil
- 2 tablespoons shredded fresh basil

Directions:
1. Pat your lamb chop dry using a kitchen towel and arrange them on a shallow glass baking dish.
2. Take a bowl and whisk in Dijon mustard, balsamic vinegar, pepper and mix them well.
3. Whisk in the oil very slowly into the marinade until the mixture is smooth
4. Stir in basil.
5. Pour the marinade over the lamb chops and stir to coat both sides well.

6. Cover the chops and allow them to marinate for 1-4 hours (chilled).
7. Take the chops out and leave them for 30 minutes to allow the temperature to reach a normal level.
8. Preheat your grill to medium heat and add oil to the grate.
9. Grill the lamb chops for 5-10 minutes per side until both sides are browned.
10. Once the center reads 145 degrees F, the chops are ready, serve and enjoy!

Nutrition:
Calories: 521, Fat: 45g, Carbohydrates: 3.5g, Protein: 22g, Sodium: 63mg, Potassium: 53mg.

338. Amazing Sesame Breadsticks

Preparation Time: 10 minutes
Cooking Time: 20 minutes
Servings: 5
Ingredients:
- 1 egg white
- 2 tablespoons almond flour
- 1 teaspoon Himalayan pink sunflower seeds
- 1 tablespoon extra-virgin olive oil
- ½ teaspoon sesame seeds

Directions:
1. Preheat your oven to 320 degrees F.
2. Line a baking sheet with parchment paper and keep it on the side.
3. Take a bowl and whisk in egg whites, add flour and half of sunflower seeds and olive oil.
4. Knead until you have a smooth dough.
5. Divide into 4 pieces and roll into breadsticks.
6. Place on prepared sheet and brush with olive oil, sprinkle sesame seeds and remaining sunflower seeds.
7. Bake for 20 minutes.
8. Serve and enjoy!

Nutrition:
Total Carbs: 1.1g, Fiber: 1g, Protein: 1.6g, Fat: 5g, Sodium: 63mg, Potassium: 73mg.

339. Brown Butter Duck Breast

Preparation Time: 5 minutes
Cooking Time: 25 minutes

Servings: 3
Ingredients:
- 1 whole 6-ounce duck breast, skin on
- Pepper to taste
- 1 head radicchio, 4 ounces, core removed
- ¼ cup unsalted butter
- 6 fresh sage leaves, sliced

Directions:
1. Preheat your oven to 400 degrees F.
2. Pat duck breast dry with a paper towel.
3. Season with pepper.
4. Place duck breast in skillet and place it over medium heat, sear for 3-4 minutes on each side.
5. Turn the breast over and transfer the skillet to the oven.
6. Roast for 10 minutes (uncovered).
7. Cut radicchio in half.
8. Remove and discard the woody white core and thinly slice the leaves.
9. Keep them on the side.
10. Remove skillet from oven.
11. Transfer duck breast, fat side up to cutting board and let it rest.
12. Re-heat your skillet over medium heat.
13. Add unsalted butter, sage and cook for 3-4 minutes.
14. Cut the duck into 6 equal slices.
15. Divide radicchio between 2 plates, top with slices of duck breast and drizzle browned butter and sage.
16. Enjoy!

Nutrition:
Calories: 393, Fat: 33g, Carbohydrates: 2g, Protein: 22g, Sodium: 63mg, Potassium: 70mg.

340. Generous Garlic Bread Stick

Preparation Time: 15 minutes
Cooking Time: 15 minutes
Servings: 8
Ingredients:
- ¼ cup almond butter, softened
- 1 teaspoon garlic powder
- 2 cups almond flour
- ½ tablespoon baking powder
- 1 tablespoon Psyllium husk powder
- ¼ teaspoon sunflower seeds
- 3 tablespoons almond butter, melted
- 1 egg

- ¼ cup boiling water

Directions:
1. Preheat your oven to 400 degrees F.
2. Line the baking sheet with parchment paper and keep it on the side.
3. Beat almond butter with garlic powder and keep it on the side.
4. Add almond flour, baking powder, husk, sunflower seeds in a bowl and mix in almond butter and egg, mix well.
5. Pour boiling water into the mix and stir until you have a nice dough.
6. Divide the dough into 8 balls and roll into breadsticks.
7. Place on a baking sheet and bake for 15 minutes.
8. Brush each stick with garlic almond butter and bake for 5 minutes more.
9. Serve and enjoy!

Nutrition:
Total Carbs: 7g, Fiber: 2g, Protein: 7g, Fat: 24g, Sodium: 63mg, Potassium: 70mg.

341. Cauliflower Bread Stick

Preparation Time: 10 minutes
Cooking Time: 48 minutes
Servings: 5
Ingredients:
- 1 cup cashew cheese/ kite ricotta cheese
- 1 tablespoon organic almond butter
- 1 whole egg
- ½ teaspoon Italian seasoning
- ¼ teaspoon red pepper flakes
- 1/8 teaspoon kosher sunflower seeds
- 2 cups cauliflower rice, cooked for 3 minutes in a microwave
- 3 teaspoons garlic, minced
- Parmesan cheese, grated

Directions:
1. Preheat your oven to 350 degrees F.
2. Add almond butter to a small pan and melt over low heat.
3. Add red pepper flakes, garlic to the almond butter and cook for 2-3 minutes.
4. Add garlic and almond butter mix to the bowl with cooked cauliflower and add the Italian seasoning.
5. Season with sunflower seeds and mix, refrigerate for 10 minutes.

6. Add cheese and eggs to the bowl and mix.
7. Place a layer of parchment paper at the bottom of a 9 x 9 baking dish and grease with cooking spray, add egg and mozzarella cheese mix to the cauliflower mix.
8. Add mix to the pan and smooth to a thin layer with the palms of your hand.
9. Bake for 30 minutes, take out from oven and top with few shakes of parmesan and mozzarella.
10. Cook for 8 minutes more.
11. Enjoy!

Nutrition:
Total Carbs: 11.5g, Fiber: 2g, Protein: 10.7g, Fat: 20g, Sodium: 63mg, Potassium: 52mg.

342. Bacon and Chicken Garlic Wrap

Preparation Time: 15 minutes
Cooking Time: 10 minutes
Servings: 4
Ingredients:
- 1 chicken fillet, cut into small cubes
- 8-9 thin slices bacon, cut to fit cubes
- 6 garlic cloves, minced

Directions:
1. Preheat your oven to 400 degrees F.
2. Line a baking tray with aluminum foil.
3. Add minced garlic to a bowl and rub each chicken piece with it.
4. Wrap a bacon piece around each garlic chicken bite.
5. Secure with a toothpick.
6. Transfer bites to baking sheet, keeping a little bit of space between them.
7. Bake for about 15-20 minutes until crispy.
8. Serve and enjoy!

Nutrition:
Calories: 260, Fat: 19g, Carbohydrates: 5g, Protein: 22g, Sodium: 63mg, Potassium: 84mg.

343. Chipotle Lettuce Chicken

Preparation Time: 10 minutes
Cooking Time: 25 minutes

Servings: 6
Ingredients:
- 1 pound chicken breast, cut into strips
- Splash of olive oil
- 1 red onion, finely sliced
- 14 ounces tomatoes
- 1 teaspoon chipotle, chopped
- ½ teaspoon cumin
- Lettuce as needed
- Fresh coriander leaves
- Jalapeno chilies, sliced
- Fresh tomato slices for garnish
- Lime wedges

Directions:
1. Take a non-stick frying pan and place it over medium heat.
2. Add oil and heat it.
3. Add chicken and cook until brown.
4. Keep the chicken on the side.
5. Add tomatoes, sugar, chipotle, cumin to the same pan and simmer for 25 minutes until you have a nice sauce.
6. Add chicken into the sauce and cook for 5 minutes.
7. Transfer the mix to another place.
8. Use lettuce wraps to take a portion of the mixture and serve with a squeeze of lemon.
9. Enjoy!

Nutrition:
Calories: 332, Fat: 15g, Carbohydrates: 13g, Protein: 34g, Sodium: 63mg, Potassium: 53mg.

344. Balsamic Chicken and Vegetables

Preparation Time: 15 minutes
Cooking Time: 25 minutes
Servings: 2
Ingredients:
- 4 chicken thighs, boneless and skinless
- 5 stalks of asparagus, halved
- 1 pepper, cut in chunks
- 1/2 red onion, diced
- ½ cup carrots, sliced
- 1 garlic clove, minced
- 2-ounces mushrooms, diced
- ¼ cup balsamic vinegar
- 1 tablespoon olive oil
- ½ teaspoon stevia
- ½ tablespoon oregano
- Sunflower seeds and pepper as needed

Directions:

1. Preheat your oven to 425 degrees F.
2. Take a bowl and add all the vegetables and mix.
3. Add spices and oil and mix.
4. Dip the chicken pieces into the spice mix and coat them well.
5. Place the veggies and chicken onto a pan in a single layer.
6. Cook for 25 minutes.
7. Serve and enjoy!

Nutrition:
Calories: 401, Fat: 17g, Net Carbohydrates: 11g, Protein: 48g, Sodium: 63mg, Potassium: 41mg.

345. Exuberant Sweet Potatoes

Preparation Time: 5 minutes
Cooking Time: 7-8 hours
Servings: 4
Ingredients:
- 6 sweet potatoes, washed and dried

Directions:
1. Roll 7-8 pieces of aluminum foil into a ball in the bottom of your Slow Cooker, covering about half of the surface.
2. Prick each potato 6-8 times using a fork.
3. Wrap each potato with foil and seal them.
4. Place wrapped potatoes in the cooker on top of the foil bed.
5. Place lid and cook on LOW for 7-8 hours.
6. Use tongs to remove the potatoes and unwrap them.
7. Serve and enjoy!

Nutrition:
Calories: 129, Fat: 0g, Carbohydrates: 30g, Protein: 2g, Sodium: 63mg, Potassium: 175mg.

346. The Vegan Lovers Refried Beans

Preparation Time: 5 minutes
Cooking Time: 10 hours
Servings: 12
Ingredients:
- 4 cups vegetable broth
- 4 cups water
- 3 cups dried pinto beans
- 1 onion, chopped
- 2 jalapeno peppers, minced
- 4 garlic cloves, minced
- 1 tablespoon chili powder

- 2 teaspoon ground cumin
- 1 teaspoon sweet paprika
- 1 teaspoon salt
- ½ teaspoon fresh ground black pepper

Directions:
1. Add the listed ingredients to your Slow Cooker.
2. Cover and cook on HIGH for 10 hours.
3. If there's any extra liquid, ladle the liquid up and reserve it in a bowl.
4. Use an immersion blender to blend the mixture (in the Slow Cooker) until smooth.
5. Add the reserved liquid.
6. Serve hot and enjoy!

Nutrition:
Calories: 91, Fat: 0g, Carbohydrates: 16g, Protein: 5g, Sodium: 176mg, Potassium: 203mg.

347. Cool Apple and Carrot Harmony

Preparation Time: 10 minutes
Cooking Time: 10 minutes
Servings: 6
Ingredients:
- 1 cup apple juice
- 1 pound baby carrots
- 1 tablespoon cornstarch
- 1 tablespoon mint, chopped

Directions:
1. Add apple juice, carrots, cornstarch and mint to your Instant Pot.
2. Stir and lock the lid.
3. Cook on HIGH pressure for 10 minutes.
4. Perform a quick release.
5. Divide the mix amongst plates and serve.
6. Enjoy!

Nutrition:
Calories: 161, Fat: 2g, Carbohydrates: 9g, Protein: 8g, Sodium: 63mg, Potassium: 19mg.

348. Mac and Chokes

Preparation Time: 5 minutes
Cooking Time: 20 minutes
Servings: 6
Ingredients:
- 1 tablespoon of olive oil
- 1 large-sized diced onion
- 10 minced garlic cloves

- 1 can artichoke hearts
- 1 pound uncooked macaroni shells
- 12-ounce baby spinach
- 4 cups vegetable broth
- 1 teaspoon red pepper flakes
- 4 ounces vegan cheese
- ¼ cup cashew cream

Directions:
1. Set the pot to Sauté mode and add oil, allow the oil to heat and add onions.
2. Cook for 2 minutes.
3. Add garlic and stir well.
4. Add artichoke hearts and sauté for 1 minute more.
5. Add uncooked pasta and 3 cups of broth alongside 2 cups of water.
6. Mix well.
7. Lock the lid and cook on HIGH pressure for 4 minutes.
8. Quick release the pressure.
9. Open the pot and stir.
10. Add extra water, fold in spinach and cook on Sauté mode for a few minutes.
11. Add cashew cream and grated vegan cheese.
12. Add pepper flakes and mix well.
13. Enjoy!

Nutrition:
Calories: 649, Fat: 29g, Carbohydrates: 64g, Protein: 34g, Sodium: 63mg, Potassium: 154mg.

349. Black Eyed Peas and Spinach Platter

Preparation Time: 10 minutes
Cooking Time: 8 hours
Servings: 4
Ingredients:
- 1 cup black eyed peas, soaked overnight and drained
- 2 cups low-sodium vegetable broth
- 1 can (15 ounces) tomatoes, diced with juice
- 8 ounces ham, chopped
- 1 onion, chopped
- 2 garlic cloves, minced
- 1 teaspoon dried oregano
- 1 teaspoon salt
- ½ teaspoon freshly ground black pepper
- ½ teaspoon ground mustard
- 1 bay leaf

Directions:
1. Add the listed ingredients to your Slow Cooker and stir.

2. Place lid and cook on LOW for 8 hours.
3. Discard the bay leaf.
4. Serve and enjoy!

Nutrition:
Calories: 209, Fat: 6g, Carbohydrates: 22g, Protein: 17g, Sodium: 53mg, Potassium: 197mg.

350. Humble Mushroom Rice

Preparation Time: 10 minutes
Cooking Time: 3 hours
Servings: 3
Ingredients:
- ½ cup rice
- 2 green onions chopped
- 1 garlic clove, minced
- ¼ pound baby Portobello mushrooms, sliced
- 1 cup vegetable stock

Directions:
1. Add rice, onions, garlic, mushrooms, and stock to your Slow Cooker.
2. Stir well and place the lid.
3. Cook on LOW for 3 hours.
4. Stir and divide amongst serving platters.
5. Enjoy!

Nutrition:
Calories: 200, Fat: 6g, Carbohydrates: 28g, Protein: 5g, Sodium: 63mg, Potassium: 165mg.

351. Sweet and Sour Cabbage and Apples

Preparation Time: 15 minutes
Cooking Time: 8 hours
Servings: 4
Ingredients:
- ¼ cup honey
- ¼ cup apple cider vinegar
- 2 tablespoons Orange Chili-Garlic Sauce
- 1 teaspoon sea salt
- 3 sweet tart apples, peeled, cored and sliced
- 2 heads green cabbage, cored and shredded
- 1 sweet red onion, thinly sliced

Directions:
1. Take a small bowl and whisk in honey, orange-chili garlic sauce, vinegar.
2. Stir well.

3. Add honey mix, apples, onion and cabbage to your Slow Cooker and stir.
4. Close lid and cook on LOW for 8 hours.
5. Serve and enjoy!

Nutrition:
Calories: 164, Fat: 1g, Carbohydrates: 41g, Protein: 4g, Sodium: 45mg, Potassium: 125mg.

352. Delicious Aloo Palak

Preparation Time: 10 minutes
Cooking Time: 6-8 hours
Servings: 6
Ingredients:
- 2 pounds red potatoes, chopped
- 1 small onion, diced
- 1 red bell pepper, seeded and diced
- ¼ cup fresh cilantro, chopped
- 1/3 cup low-sodium veggie broth
- 1 teaspoon salt
- ½ teaspoon Garam masala
- ½ teaspoon ground cumin
- ¼ teaspoon ground turmeric
- ¼ teaspoon ground coriander
- ¼ teaspoon freshly ground black pepper
- 2 pounds fresh spinach, chopped

Directions:
1. Add potatoes, bell pepper, onion, cilantro, broth and seasoning to your Slow Cooker.
2. Mix well.
3. Add spinach on top.
4. Place lid and cook on LOW for 6-8 hours.
5. Stir and serve.
6. Enjoy!

Nutrition:
Calories: 205, Fat: 1g, Carbohydrates: 44g, Protein: 9g, Sodium: 63mg, Potassium: 126mg.

353. Orange and Chili Garlic Sauce

Preparation Time: 15 minutes
Cooking Time: 8 hours
Servings: 5
Ingredients:
- ½ cup apple cider vinegar
- 4 pounds red jalapeno peppers, stems, seeds and ribs removed, chopped

- 10 garlic cloves, chopped
- ½ cup tomato paste
- Juice of 1 orange zest
- ½ cup honey
- 2 tablespoons soy sauce
- 2 teaspoons salt

Directions:
1. Add vinegar, garlic, peppers, tomato paste, orange juice, honey, zest, soy sauce and salt to your Slow Cooker.
2. Stir and close the lid.
3. Cook on LOW for 8 hours.
4. Use as needed!

Nutrition:
Calories: 33, Fat: 1g, Carbohydrates: 8g, Protein: 1g, Sodium: 63mg, Potassium: 142mg.

354. Tantalizing Mushroom Gravy

Preparation Time: 5 minutes
Cooking Time: 5-8 hours
Servings: 2
Ingredients:
- 1 cup button mushrooms, sliced
- ¾ cup low-fat buttermilk
- 1/3 cup water
- 1 medium onion, finely diced
- 2 garlic cloves, minced
- 2 tablespoons extra virgin olive oil
- 2 tablespoons all-purpose flour
- 1 tablespoon fresh rosemary, minced
- Freshly ground black pepper

Directions:
1. Add the listed ingredients to your Slow Cooker.
2. Place lid and cook on LOW for 5-8 hours.
3. Serve warm and use as needed!

Nutrition:
Calories: 54, Fat: 4g, Carbohydrates: 4g, Protein: 2g, Sodium: 63mg, Potassium: 176mg.

355. Everyday Vegetable Stock

Preparation Time: 5 minutes
Cooking Time: 8-12 hours
Servings: 10
Ingredients:
- 2 celery stalks (with leaves), quartered

- 4 ounces mushrooms, with stems
- 2 carrots, unpeeled and quartered
- 1 onion, unpeeled, quartered from pole to pole
- 1 garlic head, unpeeled, halved across the middle
- 2 fresh thyme sprigs
- 10 peppercorns
- ½ teaspoon salt
- Enough water to fill 3 quarters of Slow Cooker

Directions:
1. Add celery, mushrooms, onion, carrots, garlic, thyme, salt, peppercorn and water to your Slow Cooker.
2. Stir and cover.
3. Cook on LOW for 8-12 hours.
4. Strain the stock through a fine mesh cloth/metal mesh and discard solids.
5. Use as needed.

Nutrition:
Calories: 38, Fat: 5g, Carbohydrates: 1g, Protein: 0g, Sodium: 63mg, Potassium: 186mg.

356. Grilled Chicken with Lemon and Fennel

Preparation Time: 5 minutes
Cooking Time: 25 minutes
Servings: 4
Ingredients:
- 2 cups chicken fillets, cut and skewed
- 1 large fennel bulb
- 2 garlic cloves
- 1 jar green olives
- 1 lemon

Directions:
1. Preheat your grill to medium-high.
2. Crush garlic cloves.
3. Take a bowl and add olive oil and season with sunflower seeds and pepper.
4. Coat chicken skewers with the marinade.
5. Transfer them under the grill and grill for 20 minutes, making sure to turn them halfway through until golden.
6. Zest half of the lemon and cut the other half into quarters.

7. Cut the fennel bulb into similarly sized segments.
8. Brush olive oil all over the garlic clove segments and cook for 3-5 minutes.
9. Chop them and add them to the bowl with the marinade.
10. Add lemon zest and olives.
11. Once the meat is ready, serve with the vegetable mix.
12. Enjoy!

Nutrition:
Calories: 649, Fat: 16g, Carbohydrates: 33g, Protein: 18g, Sodium: 56mg, Potassium: 189mg.

357. Caramelized Pork Chops and Onion

Preparation Time: 5 minutes
Cooking Time: 40 minutes
Servings: 4
Ingredients:
- 4-pound chuck roast
- 4 ounces green Chili, chopped
- 2 tablespoons of chili powder
- ½ teaspoon of dried oregano
- ½ teaspoon of cumin, ground
- 2 garlic cloves, minced

Directions:
1. Rub the chops with a seasoning of 1 teaspoon of pepper and 2 teaspoons of sunflower seeds.
2. Take a skillet and place it over medium heat. Add oil and allow the oil to heat.
3. Brown the seasoned chop on both sides.
4. Add water and onion to the skillet and cover, lower the heat to low and simmer for 20 minutes.
5. Turn the chops over and season with more sunflower seeds and pepper.
6. Cover and cook until the water fully evaporates and the beef shows a slightly brown texture.
7. Remove the chops and serve with a topping of the caramelized onion.
8. Serve and enjoy!

Nutrition:
Calorie: 47, Fat: 4g, Carbohydrates: 4g, Protein: 0.5g, Sodium: 63mg, Potassium: 190mg.

358. Hearty Pork Belly Casserole

Preparation Time: 5 minutes
Cooking Time: 25 minutes
Servings: 4
Ingredients:
- 8 pork belly slices, cut into small pieces
- 3 large onions, chopped
- 4 tablespoons lemon
- Juice of 1 lemon
- Seasoning as you needed

Directions:
1. Take a large pressure cooker and place it over medium heat.
2. Add onions and sweat them for 5 minutes.
3. Add pork belly slices and cook until the meat browns and onions become golden.
4. Cover with water and add honey, lemon zest, sunflower seeds, pepper, and close the pressure seal.
5. Pressure cook for 40 minutes.
6. Serve and enjoy with a garnish of fresh chopped parsley if you prefer.

Nutrition:
Calories: 753, Fat: 41g, Carbohydrates: 68g, Protein: 30g, Sodium: 63mg, Potassium: 154mg.

359. Apple Pie Crackers

Preparation Time: 10 minutes
Cooking Time: 120 minutes
Servings: 100 crackers
Ingredients:
- 2 tablespoons + 2 teaspoons avocado oil
- 1 medium Granny Smith apple, roughly chopped
- ¼ cup Erythritol
- 1/4 cup sunflower seeds, ground
- 1 ¾ cups roughly ground flax seeds
- 1/8 teaspoon Ground cloves
- 1/8 teaspoon ground cardamom
- 3 tablespoons nutmeg
- ¼ teaspoon ground ginger

Directions:
1. Preheat your oven to 225 degrees F.
2. Line two baking sheets with parchment paper and keep them on the side.
3. Add oil, apple, Erythritol to a bowl and mix.

4. Transfer to a food processor and add remaining ingredients, process until combined.
5. Transfer batter to baking sheets, spread evenly and cut into crackers.
6. Bake for 1 hour, flip and bake for another hour.
7. Let them cool and serve.
8. Enjoy!

Nutrition:
Total Carbs: 0.9g, Fiber: 0.5g, Protein: 0.4g, Fat: 2.1g, Sodium: 112mg, Potassium: 142mg.

360. Paprika Lamb Chops

Preparation Time: 10 minutes
Cooking Time: 15 minutes
Servings: 4
Ingredients:
- 1 lamb rack, cut into chops
- pepper to taste
- 1 tablespoon paprika
- 1/2 cup cumin powder
- 1/2 teaspoon chili powder

Directions:
1. Take a bowl and add paprika, cumin, chili, pepper, and stir.
2. Add lamb chops and rub the mixture.
3. Heat grill over medium-temperature and add lamb chops, cook for 5 minutes.
4. Flip and cook for 5 minutes more, flip again.
5. Cook for 2 minutes, flip and cook for 2 minutes more.
6. Serve and enjoy!

Nutrition:
Calories: 200, Fat: 5g, Carbohydrates: 4g, Protein: 8g, Sodium: 113mg, Potassium: 133mg.

361. Fennel Sauce Tenderloin

Preparation Time: 10 minutes
Cooking Time: 25 minutes
Servings: 4
Ingredients:
- 1 fennel bulb, cored & sliced
- 1 sweet onion, sliced
- ½ cup dry white wine
- 1 teaspoon fennel seeds
- 4 pork tenderloin fillets
- 2 tablespoons olive oil
- 12 ounces chicken broth, low sodium
- Fennel fronds for garnish
- Orange slices for garnish

Directions:
1. Thin your pork tenderloin by spreading them between parchment sheets and pounding with a mallet.
2. Heat a skillet and add in your oil. Place it over medium heat and cook your fennel seeds for three minutes.
3. Add the pork to the pan, cooking for an additional three minutes per side.
4. Transfer your pork to a platter before setting it to the side and add in your fennel and onion.
5. Cook for five minutes, and then place the vegetables to the side.
6. Pour in your broth and wine and bring it to a boil over high heat. Cook until the liquid has reduced by half.
7. Return your pork to the skillet and cook for another five minutes.
8. Stir in your onion mixture, covering again. Cook for two more minutes and serve warm.

Nutrition:
Calories: 276, Protein: 23.4g, Fat: 24g, Carbs: 14g, Sodium: 647mg, Cholesterol: 49mg, Potassium: 73mg.

362. Beefy Fennel Stew

Preparation Time: 20 minutes
Cooking Time: 1 hour and 20 minutes
Servings: 4
Ingredients:
- 1 lb. lean beef, boneless & cubed
- 2 tablespoons olive oil
- ½ fennel bulb, sliced
- 3 tablespoons all-purpose flour
- 3 shallots, large & chopped
- ¾ teaspoon black pepper, divided
- 2 thyme sprigs, fresh
- 1 bay leaf
- ½ cup red wine
- 3 cups vegetable stock
- 4 carrots, peeled & sliced into 1-inch pieces
- 4 white potatoes, large & cubed
- 18 small boiling onions, halved
- 1/3 cup flat leaf parsley, fresh and chopped
- 3 portobello mushrooms, chopped

Directions:
1. Take out a shallow bowl and add the flour. Dredge the meat cubes

in it, shaking off the excess flour.
2. Take out a saucepan and add in your oil, heating it over medium heat.
3. Add your beef and cook for five minutes.
4. Add in your fennel and shallots, cooking for seven minutes. Stir in your pepper, bay leaf and thyme. Cook for a minute more.
5. Add your beef to the pan with your stock and wine.
6. Boil it and reduce it to a simmer. Cover, cooking for forty-five minutes.
7. Add in your onions, potatoes, carrots and mushrooms. Cook for another half hour, which should leave your vegetables tender.
8. Remove the thyme sprigs and bay leaf before serving warm. Garnish with parsley.

Nutrition:
Calories: 244, Protein: 21g, Fat: 8g, Carbs: 22.1g, Sodium: 587mg, Cholesterol: 125mg, Potassium: 193mg.

363. Currant Pork Chops

Preparation Time: 10 minutes
Cooking Time: 20 minutes
Servings: 6
Ingredients:
- 2 tablespoons Dijon mustard
- 6 pork loin chops, center cut
- 2 teaspoons olive oil
- 1/3 cup wine vinegar
- ¼ cup black currant jam
- 6 orange slices
- 1/8 teaspoon black pepper

Directions:
1. Start by mixing your mustard and jam in a bowl.
2. Take out a nonstick skillet, and grease it with olive oil before placing it over medium heat. Cook your chops for five minutes per side, and then top with a tablespoon of the jam mixture. Cover, and allow it to cook for two minutes. Transfer them to a serving plate.
3. Pour the wine vinegar into the same pan, and drain the pieces to deglaze the pan, mixing well. Drizzle this over the pork chops.
4. Garnish with pepper and orange slices before serving warm.

Nutrition:
Calories: 265, Protein: 25g, Fat: 6g, Carbs: 11g, Sodium: 120mg,

Cholesterol: 22mg, Potassium: 198mg.

364. Spicy Tomato Shrimp

Preparation Time: 10 minutes
Cooking Time: 25 minutes
Servings: 6
Ingredients:
- ¾ lb. shrimp, uncooked, peeled & deveined
- 2 tablespoons tomato paste
- ½ teaspoon garlic, minced
- ½ teaspoon olive oil
- 1 ½ teaspoons water
- ½ teaspoon oregano, chopped
- ½ teaspoon chipotle chili powder

Directions:
1. Rinse and dry the shrimp before setting them to the side.
2. Take out a bowl and mix your tomato paste, water, chili powder, oil, oregano and garlic. Spread this over your shrimp, and make sure they're coated on both sides.
3. Marinate for about twenty minutes or until you're ready to grill. Preheat a gas grill to medium heat, and then grease the grate with oil. Place it six inches from the heat source. Skewer the shrimp and for four minutes per side. Serve warm.

Nutrition:
Calories: 185, Protein: 16.9g, Fat: 1g, Carbs: 12.4g, Sodium: 394mg, Cholesterol: 15mg, Potassium: 134mg.

365. Beef Stir Fry

Preparation Time: 20 minutes
Cooking Time: 20 minutes
Servings: 4
Ingredients:
- 1 head broccoli chopped into florets
- 1 red bell pepper, sliced thin
- 1 ½ cups brown rice
- 2 scallions, sliced thin
- 2 tablespoons sesame seeds
- ¼ teaspoon black pepper
- 1 lb. flank steak, sliced thin
- 2 tablespoons canola oil
- ¾ cup stir fry sauce

Directions:
1. Start by heating your oil in a large wok over medium-high flame. Add in your steak, seasoning with pepper. Cook for four minutes or until crisp. Remove it from the skillet.

2. Place your broccoli in the skillet and cook for four minutes. Toss occasionally. It should be tender but crisp.
3. Put your steak back in the skillet and pour in your sauce. Allow it to simmer for three minutes.
4. Serve over rice with sesame seeds and scallions.

Nutrition:
Calories: 408, Protein: 31g, Fat: 18g, Carbs: 36g, Sodium: 461mg, Cholesterol: 57mg, Potassium: 83mg.

366. Shrimp & Corn Chowder

Preparation Time: 20 minutes
Cooking Time: 30 minutes
Servings: 6
Ingredients:
- 2 carrots, peeled & sliced
- 1 yellow onion, sliced
- 3 tablespoons olive oil
- 2 celery stalks, diced
- 4 baby red potatoes, diced
- 4 cloves garlic, peeled & minced
- ¼ cup all-purpose flour
- 3 cups vegetable stock, unsalted
- ½ cup milk
- ¾ teaspoon sea salt, fine
- ¼ teaspoon black pepper
- ¼ teaspoon cayenne pepper
- 4 cups corn kernels fresh
- 1 lb. shrimp, peeled & deveined
- 2 scallions sliced thin

Directions:
1. Take out a stockpot and heat your oil using medium flame. Once your oil is hot adding in your carrots, celery, potatoes and onion. Cook for seven minutes. The vegetable should soften. Stir and then add in your garlic. Cook for a minute more.
2. Make a flour roux and increase the heat to medium high. Whisk and bring it to a simmer. Make sure to whisk any lumps out. Whisk in your milk, salt, pepper and cayenne. Allow it to simmer until it thickens. This should take about eight minutes.
3. Add in your shrimp and corn and cook for another five minutes.
4. Divide between bowls to serve warm.

Nutrition:
Calories: 340, Protein: 23g, Fat: 9g, Carbs: 45g, Sodium: 473mg,

Cholesterol: 115mg, Potassium: 76mg.

367. Leek & Cauliflower Soup

Preparation Time: 20 minutes
Cooking Time: 20 minutes
Servings: 6
Ingredients:
- 1 tablespoon olive oil
- 1 leek, trimmed & sliced thin
- 1 yellow onion, peeled & diced
- 1 head cauliflower, chopped into florets
- 3 cloves garlic, minced
- 2 tablespoons thyme, fresh and chopped
- 1 teaspoon smoked paprika
- 1 ¼ teaspoons sea salt, fine
- 1/4teaspoon ground cayenne pepper
- 1 tablespoon heavy cream
- 3 cups vegetable stock, unsalted
- ½ lemon, juiced & zested

Directions:
1. Heat your oil in a stockpot over medium heat, and add in your leek, onion, and cauliflower. Cook for five minutes or until the onion begins to soften. Add in your garlic, thyme, smoked paprika, salt, pepper and cayenne. Pour in your vegetable stock and bring it to a simmer, cooking for fifteen minutes. Your cauliflower should be very tender.
2. Remove from heat and stir in your lemon juice, lemon zest and cream. Use an immersion blender to puree and serve warm.

Nutrition:
Calories: 92, Protein: 5g, Fat: 4g, Carbs: 13g, Sodium: 556mg, Cholesterol: 3mg, Potassium: 133mg.

368. Easy Beef Brisket

Preparation Time: 2 hours
Cooking Time: 1 hour and 10 minutes
Servings: 4
Ingredients:
- 1 teaspoon thyme
- 4 cloves garlic, peeled & smashed
- 1 ½ cups onion, chopped
- 2 ½ lbs. beef brisket, chopped

- 1 tablespoon olive oil
- ¼ teaspoon black pepper
- 14.5 ounces tomatoes & liquid, canned
- ¼ cup red wine vinegar
- 1 cup beef stock, low sodium

Directions:
1. Turn the oven to 350F, and then grease a Dutch oven using a tablespoon of oil. Place it over medium heat.
2. Add in your pepper and brisket. Cook until it browns, and then place your brisket on a plate.
3. Put your onions in the pot and cook until golden brown. Stir in your garlic and thyme, cooking for another full minute before adding in the stock, vinegar and tomatoes.
4. Cook until it comes to a boil and add the brisket again.
5. Reduce to a simmer and cook for three hours in the oven until tender.

Nutrition:
Calories: 299, Protein: 10.2g, Fat: 9g, Carbs: 21.4g, Sodium: 372mg, Cholesterol: 101mg, Potassium: 130mg.

369. Coconut Shrimp

Preparation Time: 10 minutes
Cooking Time: 15 minutes
Servings: 4
Ingredients:
- ¼ cup coconut, sweetened
- ½ teaspoon sea salt, fine
- ¼ cup panko breadcrumbs
- ½ cup coconut milk
- 12 large shrimp, peeled & deveined

Directions:
1. Preheat your oven to 375F, and then take out a baking pan. Grease it with cooking spray before setting it aside.
2. Grind your panko with coconut and salt in a food processor.
3. Add this mixture to a bowl and pour the coconut milk into another bowl.
4. Dip the shrimp in the coconut mixture and then dredge it through the panko mixture. Put the coated shrimp on the baking pan, and then bake for fifteen minutes. Serve warm.

Nutrition:
Calories: 249, Protein: 35g, Fat: 1.7g, Carbs: 1.8g, Sodium: 79mg, Cholesterol: 78mg, Potassium: 132mg.

370. Asian Salmon

Preparation Time: 10 minutes
Cooking Time: 20 minutes
Servings: 2
Ingredients:

- 1 cup fresh fruit, diced
- ¼ teaspoon black pepper
- 2 salmon fillets, 4 ounces each
- ¼ teaspoon sesame oil
- 1 teaspoon soy sauce, low sodium
- 2 cloves garlic, minced
- ½ cup pineapple juice, sugar free

Directions:

1. Start by getting out a bowl and mix your garlic, soy sauce, ginger and pineapple juice together. Place your fish in the dough and make sure it's covered. It marinates for an hour.
2. Flip the fillets after thirty minutes, and then heat the oven to 375F.
3. Take out aluminum squares and grease them with cooking spray. Put the salmon fillet on each square, and drizzle with pepper, diced fruit and sesame oil. Fold the aluminum sheet to seal the fish, and then place them on the baking sheet.
4. Bake for ten minutes per side before serving.

Nutrition:
Calories: 247, Protein: 27g, Fat: 7g, Carbs: 19g, Sodium: 350mg, Cholesterol: 120mg, Potassium: 121mg.

371. Basil Halibut

Preparation Time: 10 minutes
Cooking Time: 20 minutes
Servings: 4
Ingredients:

- 4 halibut fillets, 4 ounces each
- 2 teaspoons olive oil
- 1 tablespoon garlic, minced
- 2 tomatoes, diced
- 2 tablespoons basil, fresh and chopped
- 1 teaspoon oregano, fresh and chopped

Directions:

1. Heat the oven to 350F, and then take out a 9 by 13-inch pan. Grease it down with cooking spray.
2. Toss the basil, olive oil, garlic, oregano and tomato together in

a bowl. Pour this over your fish in the pan.

3. Bake the twelve minutes. Your fish should be flakey.

Nutrition:
Calories: 128, Protein: 21g, Fat: 4g, Carbs: 3g, Sodium: 81mg, Cholesterol: 55mg, Potassium: 109mg.

372. Beef with Mushroom & Broccoli

Preparation Time: 45 minutes
Cooking Time: 12 minutes
Servings: 4
Ingredients:
For Beef Marinade:

- 1 garlic clove, minced
- 1 (2-inch) piece fresh ginger, minced
- Salt and freshly ground black pepper to taste
- 3 tablespoons white wine vinegar
- ¾ cup beef broth
- 1 pound flank steak, trimmed and sliced into thin strips

For Vegetables:

- 2 tablespoons coconut oil, divided
- 2 minced garlic cloves
- 3 cups broccoli Rabe, chopped
- 4-ounce shiitake mushrooms, halved
- 8-ounce Cremini mushrooms, sliced

Directions:

1. For marinade in a substantial bowl, mix all ingredients except beef.
2. Add beef and coat with marinade generously.
3. Refrigerate to marinate for around a quarter-hour.
4. In a substantial skillet, heat oil on medium-high flame.
5. Remove beef from the bowl, reserving the marinade.
6. Add beef and garlic and cook for about 3-4 minutes or till browned.
7. With a slotted spoon, transfer the beef to a bowl.
8. In exactly the same skillet, add reserved marinade, broccoli and mushrooms and cook for approximately 3-4 minutes.
9. Stir in beef and cook for about 3-4 minutes.

Nutrition:

Calories: 128, Protein: 21g, Fat: 4g, Carbs: 3g, Sodium: 81mg, Cholesterol: 55mg, Potassium: 10mg.

373. Beef with Zucchini Noodles

Preparation Time: 15 minutes
Cooking Time: 9 minutes
Servings: 4
Ingredients:

- 1 teaspoon fresh ginger, grated
- 2 medium garlic cloves, minced
- ¼ cup coconut aminos
- 2 tablespoons fresh lime juice
- 1½ pound NY strip steak, trimmed and sliced thinly
- 2 medium zucchinis, spiralized with Blade C
- Salt to taste
- 3 tablespoons essential olive oil
- 2 medium scallions, sliced
- 1 teaspoon red pepper flakes, crushed
- 2 tablespoons fresh cilantro, chopped

Directions:

1. In a big bowl, mix ginger, garlic, coconut aminos and lime juice.
2. Add beef and coat with marinade generously.
3. Refrigerate to marinate for approximately 10 minutes.
4. Place zucchini noodles over a large paper towel and sprinkle with salt.
5. Keep aside for around 10 minutes.
6. In a big skillet, heat oil on medium-high heat.
7. Add scallion and red pepper flakes and sauté for about 1 minute.
8. Add beef with marinade and stir fry for around 3-4 minutes or till browned.
9. Add zucchini and cook for approximately 3-4 minutes.
10. Serve hot with all the topping of cilantro.

Nutrition:
Calories: 128, Protein: 21g, Fat: 4g, Carbs: 3g, Sodium: 81mg, Cholesterol: 55mg, Potassium: 183mg.

374. Spiced Ground Beef

Preparation Time: 10 minutes
Cooking Time: 22 minutes

Servings: 5
Ingredients:
- 2 tablespoons coconut oil
- 2 whole cloves
- 2 whole cardamoms
- 1 (2-inch) piece cinnamon stick
- 2 bay leaves
- 1 teaspoon cumin seeds
- 2 onions, chopped
- Salt to taste
- ½ tablespoon garlic paste
- ½ tablespoon fresh ginger paste
- 1 pound lean ground beef
- 1½ teaspoons fennel seeds powder
- 1 teaspoon ground cumin
- 1½ teaspoons red chili powder
- 1/8 teaspoon ground turmeric
- Freshly ground black pepper to taste
- 1 cup coconut milk
- ¼ cup water
- ¼ cup fresh cilantro, chopped

Directions:
1. In a sizable pan, heat oil on medium heat.
2. Add cloves, cardamoms, cinnamon stick, bay leaves and cumin seeds and sauté for about 20 seconds.
3. Add onion and 2 pinches of salt and sauté for about 3-4 minutes.
4. Add garlic-ginger paste and sauté for about 2 minutes.
5. Add beef and cook for about 4-5 minutes, entering pieces using the spoon.
6. Cover and cook for approximately 5 minutes.
7. Stir in spices and cook, stirring for approximately 2-2½ minutes.
8. Stir in coconut milk and water and cook for about 7-8 minutes.
9. Season with salt and take away from heat.
10. Serve hot using the garnishing of cilantro.

Nutrition:
Calories: 128, Protein: 21g, Fat: 4g, Carbs: 3g, Sodium: 81mg, Cholesterol: 55mg, Potassium: 63mg.

375. Ground Beef with Veggies

Preparation Time: 45 minutes
Cooking Time: 20 minutes
Servings: 4-5
Ingredients:
- 1-2 tablespoons coconut oil
- 1 red onion, sliced
- 2 red jalapeño peppers, seeded and sliced
- 2 minced garlic cloves
- 1 pound lean ground beef
- 1 small head broccoli, chopped
- ½ of head cauliflower, chopped
- 3 carrots, peeled and sliced
- 3 celery ribs, sliced
- Chopped fresh thyme to taste
- Dried sage to taste
- Ground turmeric to taste
- Salt and freshly ground black pepper to taste

Directions:
1. In a large skillet, melt coconut oil on medium heat.
2. Add onion, jalapeño peppers and garlic and sauté for about 5 minutes.
3. Add beef and cook for around 4-5 minutes, entering pieces using the spoon.
4. Add remaining ingredients and cook, stirring occasionally for about 8-10 min.
5. Serve hot.

Nutrition:
Calories: 128, Protein: 21g, Fat: 4g, Carbs: 3g, Sodium: 81mg, Cholesterol: 55mg, Potassium: 70mg.

376. Ground Beef with Greens & Tomatoes

Preparation Time: 15 minutes
Cooking Time: 15 minutes
Servings: 4
Ingredients:
- 1 tbsp. organic olive oil
- ½ of white onion, chopped
- 2 garlic cloves, chopped finely
- 1 jalapeño pepper, chopped finely
- 1 pound lean ground beef
- 1 teaspoon ground coriander
- 1 teaspoon ground cumin
- ½ teaspoon ground turmeric
- ½ teaspoon ground ginger
- ½ teaspoon ground cinnamon
- ½ teaspoon ground fennel seeds
- Salt and freshly ground black pepper to taste
- 8 fresh cherry tomatoes, quartered
- 8 collard greens leaves, stemmed and chopped
- 1 teaspoon fresh lemon juice

Directions:
1. In a big skillet, heat oil on medium heat.
2. Add onion and sauté for approximately 4 minutes.
3. Add garlic and jalapeño pepper and sauté for approximately 1 minute.
4. Add beef and spices and cook for approximately 6 minutes, breaking into pieces while using a spoon.
5. Stir in tomatoes and greens and cook, stirring gently for about 4 minutes.
6. Stir in lemon juice and take away from heat.

Nutrition:
Calories: 128, Protein: 21g, Fat: 4g, Carbs: 3g, Sodium: 81mg, Cholesterol: 55mg, Potassium: 73mg.

377. Curried Beef Meatballs

Preparation Time: 20 minutes
Cooking Time: 22 minutes
Servings: 6
Ingredients:
For Meatballs:
- 1 pound lean ground beef
- 2 organic eggs, beaten
- 3 tablespoons red onion, minced
- ¼ cup fresh basil leaves, chopped
- 1 (1-inch) fresh ginger piece, chopped finely
- 4 garlic cloves, chopped finely
- 3 Thai bird's eye chilies, minced
- 1 teaspoon coconut sugar
- 1 tablespoon red curry paste
- Salt to taste
- 1 tablespoon fish sauce
- 2 tablespoons coconut oil

For Curry:
- 1 red onion, chopped
- Salt to taste
- 4 garlic cloves, minced
- 1 (1-inch) fresh ginger piece, minced
- 2 Thai bird's eye chilies, minced
- 2 tablespoons red curry paste
- 1 (14-ounce) coconut milk
- Salt and freshly ground black pepper to taste
- Lime wedges, for serving

Directions:
1. For meatballs in a large bowl, add all ingredients except oil and mix till well combined.
2. Make small balls from the mixture.
3. In a large skillet, melt coconut oil on medium heat.

4. Add meatballs and cook for about 3-5 minutes or till golden brown on all sides.
5. Transfer the meatballs right into a bowl.
6. In the same skillet, add onion as well as a pinch of salt and sauté for around 5 minutes.
7. Add garlic, ginger and chilies and sauté for about 1 minute.
8. Add curry paste and sauté for around 1 minute.
9. Add coconut milk and meatballs and convey to some gentle simmer.
10. Reduce the warmth to low and simmer, covered for around 10 minutes.
11. Serve using the topping of lime wedges.

Nutrition:
Calories: 128, Protein: 21g, Fat: 4g, Carbs: 3g, Sodium: 81mg, Cholesterol: 55mg, Potassium: 87mg.

378. Grilled Skirt Steak Coconut

Preparation Time: 45 minutes
Cooking Time: 8-9 minutes
Servings: 4
Ingredients:
- 2 teaspoons fresh ginger herb, grated finely
- 2 teaspoons fresh lime zest, grated finely
- ¼ cup coconut sugar
- 2 teaspoons fish sauce
- 2 tablespoons fresh lime juice
- ½ cup coconut milk
- 1 pound beef skirt steak, trimmed and cut into 4-inch slices lengthwise
- Salt to taste

Directions:
1. In a sizable sealable bag, mix all ingredients except steak and salt.
2. Add steak and coat with marinade generously.
3. Seal the bag and refrigerate to marinate for about 4-12 hours.
4. Preheat the grill to high heat. Grease the grill grate.
5. Remove steak from the refrigerator and discard the marinade.
6. With a paper towel, dry the steak and sprinkle with salt evenly.
7. Cook the steak for approximately 3½ minutes.

8. Flip the medial side and cook for around 2½-5 minutes or till the desired doneness.
9. Remove from grill pan and keep side for approximately 5 minutes before slicing. With a clear, crisp knife, cut into desired slices and serve.

Nutrition:
Calories: 128, Protein: 21g, Fat: 4g, Carbs: 3g, Sodium: 81mg, Cholesterol: 55mg, Potassium: 98mg.

379. Lamb with Prunes

Preparation Time: 15 minutes
Cooking Time: 40 minutes
Servings: 6
Ingredients:
- 3 tablespoons coconut oil
- 2 onions, chopped finely
- 1 (1-inch) piece fresh ginger, minced
- 3 garlic cloves, minced
- ½ teaspoon ground turmeric
- 2 ½ pound lamb shoulder, trimmed and cubed into 3-inch size
- Salt and freshly ground black pepper to taste
- ½ teaspoon saffron threads, crumbled
- 1 cinnamon stick
- 3 cups water
- 1 cup runes, pitted and halved

Directions:
1. In a big pan, melt coconut oil on medium heat.
2. Add onions, ginger, garlic cloves and turmeric and sauté for about 3-5 minutes.
3. Sprinkle the lamb with salt and black pepper evenly.
4. In the pan, add lamb and saffron threads and cook for approximately 4-5 minutes.
5. Add cinnamon stick and water and produce to some boil on high heat.
6. Reduce the temperature to low and simmer, covered for around 1½-120 minutes or till the desired doneness of lamb.
7. Stir in prunes and simmer for approximately 20-a half-hour.
8. Remove cinnamon stick and serve hot.

Nutrition:
Calories: 128, Protein: 21g, Fat: 4g, Carbs: 3g, Sodium: 81mg, Cholesterol: 55mg, Potassium: 323mg.

380. Ground Lamb with Peas

Preparation Time: 15 minutes
Cooking Time: 55 minutes
Servings: 4
Ingredients:
- 1 tablespoon coconut oil
- 3 dried red chilies
- 1 (2-inch) cinnamon stick
- 3 green cardamom pods
- ½ teaspoon cumin seeds
- 1 medium red onion, chopped
- 1 (¾-inch) piece fresh ginger, minced
- 4 garlic cloves, minced
- 1½ teaspoons ground coriander
- ½ teaspoon garam masala
- ½ teaspoon ground cumin
- ½ teaspoon ground turmeric
- ¼ teaspoon ground nutmeg
- 2 bay leaves
- 1 pound lean ground lamb
- ½ cup Roma tomatoes, chopped
- 1-1½ cups water
- 1 cup fresh green peas, shelled
- 2 tablespoons plain Greek yogurt, whipped
- ¼ cup fresh cilantro, chopped
- Salt and freshly ground black pepper to taste

Directions:
1. In a Dutch oven, melt coconut oil medium-high heat.
2. Add red chilies, cinnamon stick, cardamom pods and cumin seeds and sauté for around thirty seconds.
3. Add onion and sauté for about 3-4 minutes.
4. Add ginger, garlic cloves and spices and sauté for around thirty seconds.
5. Add lamb and cook for approximately 5 minutes.
6. Add tomatoes and cook approximately 10 minutes.
7. Stir in water and green peas and cook, covered approximately 25-30 minutes.
8. Stir in yogurt, cilantro, salt and black pepper and cook for around 4-5 minutes.
9. Serve hot.

Nutrition:
Calories: 128, Protein: 21g, Fat: 4g, Carbs: 3g, Sodium: 81mg, Cholesterol: 55mg, Potassium: 133mg.

381. Roasted Lamb Chops

Preparation Time: 15 minutes

Cooking Time: 30 minutes
Servings: 4
Ingredients:
For Lamb Marinade:
- 4 garlic cloves, chopped
- 1 (2-inch) piece fresh ginger, chopped
- 2 green chilies, seeded and chopped
- 1 teaspoon fresh lime zest
- 2 teaspoons garam masala
- 1 teaspoon ground coriander
- 1 teaspoon ground cumin
- ½ teaspoon ground cinnamon
- 1 teaspoon coconut oil, melted
- 2 tablespoons fresh lime juice
- 6-7 tablespoons plain Greek yogurt
- 1 (8-bone) rack of lamb, trimmed
- 2 onions, sliced

For Relish:
- ½ of garlic herb, chopped
- 1 (1-inch) piece fresh ginger, chopped
- ¼ cup fresh cilantro, chopped
- ¼ cup fresh mint, chopped
- 1 green chili, seeded and chopped
- 1 teaspoon fresh lime zest
- 1 teaspoon organic honey
- 2 tablespoons fresh apple juice
- 2 tablespoons fresh lime juice

Directions:
1. For chops in a very mixer, add all ingredients except yogurt, chops and onions and pulse till smooth.
2. Transfer the mixture to a large bowl with yogurt and stir to combine well.
3. Add chops and coat with mixture generously.
4. Refrigerate to marinate for approximately twenty-four hours.
5. Preheat the oven to 375 degrees F. Linea roasting pan with foil paper.
6. Place the onion wedges in the bottom of the prepared roasting pan.
7. Arrange rack of lamb over onion wedges.
8. Roast for approximately half an hour.
9. Meanwhile, for the relish in the blender, add all ingredients and pulse until smooth.
10. Serve chops and onions alongside relish.

Nutrition:
Calories: 128, Protein: 21g, Fat: 4g, Carbs: 3g, Sodium: 81mg, Cholesterol: 55mg, Potassium: 118mg.

382. Baked Meatballs & Scallions

Preparation Time: 20 minutes
Cooking Time: 35 minutes
Servings: 4-6
Ingredients:
For Meatballs:
- 1 lemongrass stalk, outer skin peeled and chopped
- 1 (1½-inch) piece fresh ginger, sliced
- 3 garlic cloves, chopped
- 1 cup fresh cilantro leaves, chopped roughly
- ½ cup fresh basil leaves, chopped roughly
- 2 tablespoons plus 1 teaspoon fish sauce
- 2 tablespoons water
- 2 tablespoons fresh lime juice
- ½ pound lean ground pork
- 1 pound lean ground lamb
- 1 carrot, peeled and grated
- 1 organic egg

For Scallions:
- 16 stalks scallions, trimmed
- 2 tablespoons coconut oil, melted
- Salt to taste
- ½ cup water

Directions:
1. Preheat the oven to 375 degrees F. Grease a baking dish.
2. In a blender, add lemongrass, ginger, garlic, fresh herbs, fish sauce, water and lime juice and pulse till chopped finely.
3. Transfer the mixture to a bowl with the remaining ingredients and blend till well combined.
4. Make about 1-inch balls from the mixture.
5. Arrange the balls into the prepared baking dish in a single layer.
6. In another rimmed baking dish, arrange scallion stalks in a single layer.
7. Drizzle with coconut oil and sprinkle with salt.
8. Pour water in the baking dish with foil paper cover it tightly.
9. Bake the scallion for around a half-hour.
10. Bake the meatballs for approximately 30-35 minutes.

11. This stir-fry not only tastes wonderful, but it is also packed with nutritional benefits.

Nutrition:
Calories: 128, Protein: 21g, Fat: 4g, Carbs: 3g, Sodium: 81mg, Cholesterol: 55mg, Potassium: 133mg.

383. Pork Chili

Preparation Time: 45 minutes
Cooking Time: 60 minutes
Servings: 4
Ingredients:
- 2 tablespoons extra-virgin organic olive oil
- 2 pound ground pork
- 1 medium red bell pepper, seeded and chopped
- 1 medium onion, chopped
- 5 garlic cloves, chopped finely
- 1 (2-inch) part of hot pepper, minced
- 1 tablespoon ground cumin
- 1 teaspoon ground turmeric
- 3 tablespoon chili powder
- ½ teaspoon chipotle chili powder
- Salt and freshly ground black pepper to taste
- 1 cup chicken broth
- 1 (28-ounce) can fire-roasted crushed tomatoes
- 2 medium bok choy heads, sliced
- 1 avocado, peeled, pitted and chopped

Directions:
1. In a sizable pan, heat oil on medium flame.
2. Add pork and stir fry for about 5 minutes.
3. Add bell pepper, onion, garlic, hot pepper and spices and stir fry for approximately 5 minutes.
4. Add broth and tomatoes and convey with a boil.
5. Stir in bok choy and cook, covered for approximately twenty minutes.
6. Uncover and cook for approximately 20-half an hour.
7. Serve hot while using avocado topping.

Nutrition:
Calories: 128, Protein: 21g, Fat: 4g, Carbs: 3g, Sodium: 81mg, Cholesterol: 55mg, Potassium: 98mg.

384. Baked Pork & Mushroom Meatballs

Preparation Time: 15 minutes
Cooking Time: 15 minutes
Servings: 6
Ingredients:

- 1 pound lean ground pork
- 1 organic egg white, beaten
- 4 fresh shiitake mushrooms, stemmed and minced
- 1 tablespoon fresh parsley, minced
- 1 tablespoon fresh basil leaves, minced
- 1 tablespoon fresh mint leaves, minced
- 2 teaspoons fresh lemon zest, grated finely
- 1½ teaspoons fresh ginger, grated finely
- Salt and freshly ground black pepper to taste

Directions:

1. Preheat the oven to 425 degrees F. Arrange the rack inside the center of the oven.
2. Line a baking sheet with parchment paper.
3. In a sizable bowl, add all ingredients and mix till well combined.
4. Make small equal-sized balls from the mixture.
5. Arrange the balls onto the prepared baking sheet in a single layer.
6. Bake for approximately 12-quarter-hour or till done completely.

Nutrition:

Calories: 128, Protein: 21g, Fat: 4g, Carbs: 3g, Sodium: 81mg, Cholesterol: 55mg, Potassium: 23mg.

385. Citrus Beef with Bok Choy

Preparation Time: 15 minutes
Cooking Time: 11 minutes
Servings: 4
Ingredients:
For Marinade:

- 2 minced garlic cloves
- 1 (1-inch) piece fresh ginger, grated
- 1/3 cup fresh orange juice
- ½ cup coconut aminos
- 2 teaspoons fish sauce
- 2 teaspoons Sriracha
- 1¼ pound sirloin steak, trimmed and sliced thinly

For Veggies:

- 2 tablespoons coconut oil, divided
- 3-4 wide strips of fresh orange zest
- 1 jalapeño pepper, sliced thinly
- ½ pound string beans, stemmed and halved crosswise
- 1 tablespoon arrowroot powder
- ½ pound bok choy, chopped
- 2 teaspoons sesame seeds

Directions:

1. For marinade in a big bowl, mix garlic, ginger, orange juice, coconut aminos, fish sauce and Sriracha.
2. Add beef and coat with marinade generously.
3. Refrigerate to marinate for around a couple of hours.
4. In a substantial skillet, heat oil on medium-high heat.
5. Add orange zest and sauté for approximately 2 minutes.
6. Remove beef from the bowl, reserving the marinade.
7. In the skillet, add beef and increase the heat to high.
8. Stir fry for about 2-3 minutes or till browned.
9. With a slotted spoon, transfer the beef and orange strips right into a bowl.
10. With a paper towel, wipe out the skillet.
11. In a similar skillet, heat the remaining oil on medium-high heat.
12. Add jalapeño pepper and string beans and stir fry for about 3-4 minutes.
13. Meanwhile, add arrowroot powder in reserved marinade and stir to mix.
14. In the skillet, add marinade mixture, beef and bok choy and cook for about 1-2 minutes.
15. Serve hot with garnishing of sesame seeds.

Nutrition:

Calories: 128, Protein: 21g, Fat: 4g, Carbs: 3g, Sodium: 81mg, Cholesterol: 55mg, Potassium: 33mg.

386. Ground Beef with Cabbage

Preparation Time: 10 minutes
Cooking Time: 45 minutes
Servings: 4
Ingredients:

- 1 tbsp. olive oil
- 1 onion, sliced thinly
- 2 teaspoons fresh ginger, minced
- 4 garlic cloves, minced
- 1 pound lean ground beef
- 1½ tablespoons fish sauce
- 2 tablespoons fresh lime juice
- 1 small head purple cabbage, shredded
- 2 tablespoons peanut butter
- ½ cup fresh cilantro, chopped

Directions:

1. In a large skillet, heat oil on medium heat.
2. Add onion, ginger and garlic and sauté for about 4-5 minutes.
3. Add beef and cook for approximately 7-8 minutes, getting into pieces using the spoon.
4. Drain off the extra liquid in the skillet.
5. Stir in fish sauce and lime juice and cook for approximately 1 minute.
6. Add cabbage and cook approximately 4-5 minutes or till the desired doneness.
7. Stir in peanut butter and cilantro and cook for about 1 minute.
8. Serve hot.

Nutrition:

Calories: 128, Protein: 21g, Fat: 4g, Carbs: 3g, Sodium: 81mg, Cholesterol: 55mg, Potassium: 63mg.

387. Beef & Veggies Chili

Preparation Time: 15 minutes
Cooking Time: 1 hour
Servings: 6-8
Ingredients:

- 2 pounds lean ground beef
- ½ head cauliflower, chopped into large pieces
- 1 onion, chopped
- 6 garlic cloves, minced
- 2 cups pumpkin puree
- 1 teaspoon dried oregano, crushed
- 1 teaspoon dried thyme, crushed
- 1 teaspoon ground cumin
- 1 teaspoon ground turmeric
- 1-2 teaspoons chili powder
- 1 teaspoon paprika
- 1 teaspoon cayenne pepper
- ¼ teaspoon red pepper flakes, crushed
- Salt and freshly ground black pepper to taste
- 1 (26-ounce) can tomatoes, drained

- ½ cup water
- 1 cup beef broth

Directions:

1. Heat a big pan on medium-high flame.
2. Add beef and stir fry for around 5 minutes.
3. Add cauliflower, onion and garlic and stir fry for approximately 5 minutes.
4. Add spices and herbs and stir to mix well.
5. Stir in remaining ingredients and get to a boil.
6. Reduce heat to low and simmer, covered, approximately 30-45 minutes.
7. Serve hot.

Nutrition:

Calories: 128, Protein: 21g, Fat: 4g, Carbs: 3g, Sodium: 81mg, Cholesterol: 55mg, Potassium: 89mg.

388. Beef Meatballs in Tomato Gravy

Preparation Time: 20 minutes
Cooking Time: 37 minutes
Servings: 4
Ingredients:
For Meatballs:

- 1 pound lean ground beef
- 1 organic egg, beaten
- 1 tablespoon fresh ginger, minced
- 1 garlic oil, minced
- 2 tablespoons fresh cilantro, chopped finely
- 2 tablespoons tomato paste
- 1/3 cup almond meal
- 1 tablespoon ground cumin
- Pinch of ground cinnamon
- Salt and freshly ground black pepper to taste
- ¼ cup coconut oil

For Tomato Gravy:

- 2 tablespoons coconut oil
- ½ of small onion, chopped
- 2 garlic cloves, chopped
- 1 teaspoon fresh lemon zest, grated finely
- 2 cups tomatoes, chopped finely
- Pinch of ground cinnamon
- 1 teaspoon red pepper flakes, crushed
- ¾ cup chicken broth
- Salt and freshly ground black pepper to taste
- ¼ cup fresh parsley, chopped

Directions:

1. For meatballs in a sizable bowl, add all ingredients except oil and mix till well combined.
2. Make about 1-inch sized balls from the mixture.
3. In a substantial skillet, melt coconut oil on medium heat.
4. Add meatballs and cook for approximately 3-5 minutes or till golden brown on all sides.
5. Transfer the meatballs to a bowl.
6. For gravy in a big pan, melt coconut oil on medium heat.
7. Add onion and garlic and sauté for approximately 4 minutes.
8. Add lemon zest and sauté for approximately 1 minute.
9. Add tomatoes, cinnamon, red pepper flakes and broth and simmer for approximately 7 minutes.
10. Stir in salt, black pepper and meatballs and reduce the warmth to medium-low.
11. Simmer for approximately twenty minutes.
12. Serve hot with all the garnishing of parsley.

Nutrition:

Calories: 128, Protein: 21g, Fat: 4g, Carbs: 3g, Sodium: 81mg, Cholesterol: 55mg, Potassium: 60mg.

389. Spicy Lamb Curry

Preparation Time: 15 minutes
Cooking Time: 2 hours 45 minutes
Servings: 6-8
Ingredients:
For Spice Mixture:

- 4 teaspoons ground coriander
- 4 teaspoons ground coriander
- 4 teaspoons ground cumin
- ¾ teaspoon ground ginger
- 2 teaspoons ground cinnamon
- ½ teaspoon ground cloves
- ½ teaspoon ground cardamom
- 2 tablespoons sweet paprika
- ½ tablespoon cayenne pepper
- 2 teaspoons chili powder
- 2 teaspoons salt

For Curry:

- 1 tablespoon coconut oil
- 2 pounds boneless lamb, trimmed and cubed into 1-inch size
- Salt and freshly ground black pepper to taste
- 2 cups onions, chopped
- 1¼ cups water

- 1 cup coconut milk

Directions:

1. For spice mixture in a bowl, mix all spices. Keep aside.
2. Season the lamb with salt and black pepper.
3. In a large Dutch oven, heat oil on medium-high heat.
4. Add lamb and stir fry for around 5 minutes.
5. Add onion and cook for approximately 4-5 minutes.
6. Stir in the spice mixture and cook for approximately 1 minute.
7. Add water and coconut milk and provide to some boil on high heat.
8. Reduce the heat to low and simmer, covered for approximately 1-120 minutes or till the desired doneness of lamb.
9. Uncover and simmer for approximately 3-4 minutes.
10. Serve hot.

Nutrition:

Calories: 128, Protein: 21g, Fat: 4g, Carbs: 3g, Sodium: 81mg, Cholesterol: 55mg, Potassium: 65mg.

390. Ground Lamb with Harissa

Preparation Time: 15 minutes
Cooking Time: 1 hour 11 minutes
Servings: 4
Ingredients:

- 1 tablespoon extra-virgin olive oil
- 2 red peppers, seeded and chopped finely
- 1 yellow onion, chopped finely
- 2 garlic cloves, chopped finely
- 1 teaspoon ground cumin
- ½ teaspoon ground turmeric
- ¼ teaspoon ground cinnamon
- ¼ teaspoon ground ginger
- 1½ pound lean ground lamb
- Salt to taste
- 1 (14½-ounce) can diced tomatoes
- 2 tablespoons harissa
- 1 cup water
- Chopped fresh cilantro for garnishing

Directions:

1. In a big pan, heat oil on medium-high flame.
2. Add bell pepper, onion and garlic and sauté for around 5 minutes.

3. Add spices and sauté for around 1 minute.
4. Add lamb and salt and cook for approximately 5 minutes, getting into pieces.
5. Stir in tomatoes, harissa and water and provide with a boil.
6. Reduce the warmth to low and simmer, covered for about 1 hour.
7. Serve hot while using garnishing of harissa.

Nutrition:
Calories: 128, Protein: 21g, Fat: 4g, Carbs: 3g, Sodium: 81mg, Cholesterol: 55mg, Potassium: 297mg.

391. Pan-Seared Lamb Chops

Preparation Time: 10 minutes
Cooking Time: 4-6 minutes
Servings: 4
Ingredients:
- 4 garlic cloves, peeled
- Salt to taste
- 1 teaspoon black mustard seeds, crushed finely
- 2 teaspoons ground cumin
- 1 teaspoon ground ginger
- 1 teaspoon ground coriander
- ½ teaspoon ground cinnamon
- Freshly ground black pepper to taste
- 1 tablespoon coconut oil
- 8 medium lamb chops, trimmed

Directions:
1. Place garlic cloves onto a cutting board and sprinkle with salt.
2. With a knife, crush the garlic until a paste forms.
3. In a bowl, mix garlic paste and spices.
4. With a clear, crisp knife, make 3-4 cuts on both sides in the chops.
5. Rub the chops with garlic mixture generously.
6. In a large skillet, melt butter on medium heat.
7. Add chops and cook for approximately 2-3 minutes per side or till the desired doneness.

Nutrition:
Calories: 128, Protein: 21g, Fat: 4g, Carbs: 3g, Sodium: 81mg, Cholesterol: 55mg, Potassium: 65mg.

392. Lamb & Pineapple Kebabs

Preparation Time: 15 minutes
Cooking Time: 10 minutes
Servings: 4-6
Ingredients:
- 1 large pineapple, cubed
- 1½-inch size, divided
- 1 (½-inch) piece fresh ginger, chopped
- 2 garlic cloves, chopped
- Salt to taste
- 16-24-ounce lamb shoulder steak, trimmed and cubed into 1½-inch size
- Fresh mint leaves coming from a bunch
- Ground cinnamon to taste

Directions:
1. In a blender, add about 1½ servings of pineapple, ginger, garlic and salt and pulse till smooth.
2. Transfer the amalgamation right into a large bowl.
3. Add chops and coat with mixture generously.
4. Refrigerate to marinate for about 1-2 hours.
5. Preheat the grill to medium heat. Grease the grill grate.
6. Thread lam, remaining pineapple and mint leaves onto pre-soaked wooden skewers.
7. Grill the kebabs for approximately 10 min, turning occasionally.

Nutrition:
Calories: 128, Protein: 21g, Fat: 4g, Carbs: 3g, Sodium: 81mg, Cholesterol: 55mg, Potassium: 83mg.

393. Spiced Pork One

Preparation Time: 15 minutes
Cooking Time: 60 minutes 52 minutes
Servings: 4
Ingredients:
- 1 (2-inch) piece fresh ginger, chopped
- 5-10 garlic cloves, chopped
- 1 teaspoon ground cumin
- ½ teaspoon ground turmeric 1 tablespoon hot paprika
- 1 tablespoon red pepper flakes
- Salt to taste
- 2 tablespoons cider vinegar

- 2 pounds pork shoulder, trimmed and cubed into 1½-inch size
- 2 cups domestic hot water, divided
- 1 (1-inch wide) ball tamarind pulp
- ¼ cup olive oil
- 1 teaspoon black mustard seeds, crushed
- 4 green cardamoms
- 5 whole cloves
- 1 (3-inch) cinnamon stick
- 1 cup onion, chopped finely
- 1 large red bell pepper, seeded and chopped

Directions:
1. In a food processor, add ginger, garlic, cumin, turmeric, paprika, red pepper flakes, salt and cider vinegar and pulse till smooth.
2. Transfer the amalgamation to a large bowl.
3. Add pork and coat with mixture generously.
4. Keep aside, covered for around an hour at room temperature.
5. In a bowl, add 1 cup of warm water and tamarind and make aside till water becomes cool.
6. With the hands, crush the tamarind to extract the pulp.
7. Add remaining cup of hot water and mix till well combined.
8. Through a fine sieve, strain the tamarind juice inside a bowl.
9. In a sizable skillet, heat oil on medium-high heat.
10. Add mustard seeds, green cardamoms, cloves and cinnamon stick and sauté for about 4 minutes.
11. Add onion and sauté for approximately 5 minutes.
12. Add pork and stir fry for approximately 6 minutes.
13. Stir in tamarind juice and convey with a boil.
14. Reduce the heat to medium-low and simmer for 1½ hours. 15. Stir in bell pepper and cook for about 7 minutes.

Nutrition:
Calories: 128, Protein: 21g, Fat: 4g, Carbs: 3g, Sodium: 81mg, Cholesterol: 55mg, Potassium: 83mg.

394. Pork chops in Creamy Sauce

Preparation Time: 15 minutes
Cooking Time: 14 minutes
Servings: 4
Ingredients:

- 2 garlic cloves, chopped
- 1 small jalapeño pepper, chopped
- ¼ cup fresh cilantro leaves
- 1½ teaspoons ground turmeric, divided
- 1 tablespoon fish sauce
- 2 tablespoons fresh lime juice
- 1 (13½-ounce) can coconut milk
- 4 (½-inch thick) pork chops
- Salt to taste
- 1 tablespoon coconut oil
- 1 shallot, chopped finely

Directions:

1. In a blender, add garlic, jalapeño pepper, cilantro, 1 teaspoon of ground turmeric, fish sauce, lime juice and coconut milk and pulse till smooth.
2. Sprinkle the pork with salt and remaining turmeric evenly.
3. In a skillet, melt butter on medium-high heat.
4. Add shallots and sauté for approximately 1 minute.
5. Add chops and cook for approximately 2 minutes per side.
6. Transfer the chops inside a bowl.
7. Add coconut mixture and convey to your boil.
8. Reduce heat to medium and simmer, stirring occasionally for approximately 5 minutes.
9. Stir in pork chops and cook for about 3-4 minutes.
10. Serve hot.

Nutrition:

Calories: 128, Protein: 21g, Fat: 4g, Carbs: 3g, Sodium: 81mg, Cholesterol: 55mg, Potassium: 93mg.

Chapter 10. Appetizers

395. Turmeric Endives

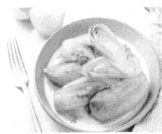

Preparation Time: 10 minutes
Cooking Time: 20 minutes
Servings: 4
Ingredients:
- 2 endives, halved lengthwise
- 2 tablespoons olive oil
- 1 teaspoon rosemary, dried
- ½ teaspoon turmeric powder
- A pinch of black pepper

Directions:
1. Mix the endives with the oil and the other ingredients in a baking pan, toss gently, and bake at 400 degrees F within 20 minutes. Serve as a side dish.

Nutrition:
Calories: 64, Protein: 0.2g, Carbohydrates: 0.8g, Fat: 7.1g, Fiber: 0.6g, Sodium: 3mg, Potassium: 50mg.

396. Parmesan Endives

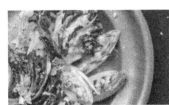

Preparation Time: 10 minutes
Cooking Time: 20 minutes
Servings: 4
Ingredients:
- 4 endives, halved lengthwise
- 1 tablespoon lemon juice
- 1 tablespoon lemon zest, grated
- 2 tablespoons fat-free parmesan, grated
- 2 tablespoons olive oil
- A pinch of black pepper

Directions:

1. In a baking dish, combine the endives with the lemon juice and the other ingredients except for the parmesan and toss. Sprinkle the parmesan on top, bake the endives at 400 degrees F for 20 minutes, and serve.

Nutrition:
Calories: 71, Protein: 0.9g, Carbohydrates: 2.2g, Fat: 7.1g, Fiber: 0.9g, Sodium: 71mg, Potassium: 88mg.

397. Lemon Asparagus

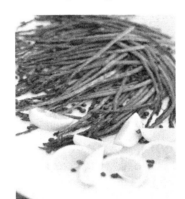

Preparation Time: 10 minutes
Cooking Time: 20 minutes
Servings: 4
Ingredients:
- 1-pound asparagus, trimmed
- 2 tablespoons basil pesto
- 1 tablespoon lemon juice
- A pinch of black pepper
- 3 tablespoons olive oil
- 2 tablespoons cilantro, chopped

Directions:
1. Arrange the asparagus on a lined baking sheet, add the pesto and the other ingredients, toss, bake at 400 degrees F within 20 minutes. Serve as a side dish.

Nutrition:
Calories: 114, Protein: 2.6g, Carbohydrates: 4.5g, Fat: 10.7g, Fiber: 2.4g, Sodium: 3mg, Potassium: 240mg.

398. Lime Carrots

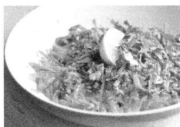

Preparation Time: 10 minutes
Cooking Time: 30 minutes
Servings: 4
Ingredients:
- 1-pound baby carrots, trimmed
- 1 tablespoon sweet paprika
- 1 teaspoon lime juice
- 3 tablespoons olive oil
- A pinch of black pepper
- 1 teaspoon sesame seeds

Directions:
1. Arrange the carrots on a lined baking sheet, add the paprika and the other ingredients except for the sesame seeds, toss, and bake at 400 degrees F within 30 minutes. Divide the carrots between plates, sprinkle sesame seeds on top and serve as a side dish.

Nutrition:
Calories: 139, Protein: 1.1g, Carbohydrates: 10.5g, Fat: 11.2g, Fiber: 4g, Sodium: 89mg, Potassium: 313mg.

399. Garlic Potato Pan

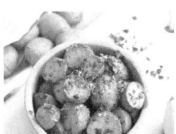

Preparation Time: 10 minutes
Cooking Time: 1 hour
Servings: 8
Ingredients:
- 1-pound gold potatoes, peeled and cut into wedges
- 2 tablespoons olive oil

- 1 red onion, chopped
- 2 garlic cloves, minced
- 2 cups coconut cream
- 1 tablespoon thyme, chopped
- ¼ teaspoon nutmeg, ground
- ½ cup low-fat parmesan, grated

Directions:
1. Heat a pan with the oil over medium heat, put the onion plus the garlic, and sauté for 5 minutes. Add the potatoes and brown them for 5 minutes more.
2. Add the cream and the rest of the ingredients, toss gently, bring to a simmer and cook over medium heat within 40 minutes more. Divide the mix between plates and serve as a side dish.

Nutrition:
Calories: 230, Protein: 3.6g, Carbohydrates: 14.3g, Fat: 19.1g, Fiber: 3.3g, Cholesterol 6mg, Sodium: 105mg, Potassium: 426mg.

400. Balsamic Cabbage

Preparation Time: 10 minutes
Cooking Time: 20 minutes
Servings: 4
Ingredients:
- 1-pound green cabbage, roughly shredded
- 2 tablespoons olive oil
- A pinch of black pepper
- 1 shallot, chopped
- 2 garlic cloves, minced
- 2 tablespoons balsamic vinegar
- 2 teaspoons hot paprika
- 1 teaspoon sesame seeds

Directions:
1. Heat a pan with the oil over medium flame. Add the shallot and the garlic, and sauté for 5 minutes. Add the cabbage and the other ingredients, toss, cook over medium heat for 15 minutes, divide between plates and serve.

Nutrition:
Calories: 100, Protein: 1.8g, Carbohydrates: 8.2g, Fat: 7.5g, Fiber: 3g, Sodium: 22mg, Potassium: 225mg.

401. Chili Broccoli

Preparation Time: 10 minutes
Cooking Time: 30 minutes
Servings: 4
Ingredients:
- 2 tablespoons olive oil
- 1-pound broccoli florets

- 2 garlic cloves, minced
- 2 tablespoons chili sauce
- 1 tablespoon lemon juice
- A pinch of black pepper
- 2 tablespoons cilantro, chopped

Directions:
1. In a baking pan, combine the broccoli with the oil, garlic, and the other, toss a bit, and bake at 400 degrees F for 30 minutes. Divide the mix between plates and serve as a side dish.

Nutrition:
Calories: 103, Protein: 3.4g, Carbohydrates: 8.3g: 7.4g, Fat: Fiber: 3g, Sodium: 229mg, Potassium: 383mg.

402. Hot Brussels Sprouts

Preparation Time: 10 minutes
Cooking Time: 25 minutes
Servings: 4
Ingredients:
- 1 tablespoon olive oil
- 1-pound Brussels sprouts, trimmed and halved
- 2 garlic cloves, minced
- ½ cup low-fat mozzarella, shredded
- A pinch of pepper flakes, crushed

Directions:
1. In a baking dish, combine the sprouts with the oil and the other ingredients except for the cheese and toss. Sprinkle the cheese on top, introduce it in the oven and bake at 400 degrees F for 25 minutes. Divide between plates and serve as a side dish.

Nutrition:
Calories: 111, Protein: 10g, Carbohydrates: 11.6g, Fat: 3.9g, Fiber: 5g, Cholesterol: 4mg, Sodium: 209mg, Potassium: 447mg.

403. Paprika Brussels Sprouts

Preparation Time: 10 minutes
Cooking Time: 25 minutes
Servings: 4
Ingredients:
- 2 tablespoons olive oil
- 1-pound Brussels sprouts, trimmed and halved
- 3 green onions, chopped
- 2 garlic cloves, minced
- 1 tablespoon balsamic vinegar

- 1 tablespoon sweet paprika
- A pinch of black pepper

Directions:
1. In a baking pan, combine the Brussels sprouts with the oil and the other ingredients, toss and bake at 400 degrees F. within 25 minutes. Divide the mix between plates and serve.

Nutrition:
Calories: 121, Protein: 4.4g, Carbohydrates: 12.6g, Fat: 7.6g, Fiber: 5.2g, Sodium: 31mg, Potassium: 521mg.

404. Creamy Cauliflower Mash

Preparation Time: 10 minutes
Cooking Time: 25 minutes
Servings: 4
Ingredients:
- 2 pounds cauliflower florets
- ½ cup of coconut milk
- A pinch of black pepper
- ½ cup low-fat sour cream
- 1 tablespoon cilantro, chopped
- 1 tablespoon chives, chopped

Directions:
1. Put the cauliflower in a pot, add water to cover, bring to a boil over medium heat, and cook for 25 minutes and drain. Mash the cauliflower, add the milk, black pepper, and the cream, whisk well, divide between plates, sprinkle the rest of the ingredients on top, and serve.

Nutrition:
Calories: 188, Protein: 6.1g, Carbohydrates: 15g, Fat: 13.4g, Fiber: 6.4g, Cholesterol: 13mg, Sodium: 88mg, Potassium: 811mg.

405. Avocado, Tomato, and Olives Salad

Preparation Time: 5 minutes
Cooking Time: 0 minutes
Servings: 4
Ingredients:
- 2 tablespoons olive oil
- 2 avocados, cut into wedges
- 1 cup Kalamata olives, pitted and halved
- 1 cup tomatoes, cubed
- 1 tablespoon ginger, grated
- A pinch of black pepper
- 2 cups baby arugula

- 1 tablespoon balsamic vinegar

Directions:
1. In a bowl, combine the avocados with the Kalamata and the other ingredients, toss and serve as a side dish.

Nutrition:
Calories: 320, Protein: 3g, Carbohydrates: 13.9g, Fat: 30.4g, Fiber: 8.7g, Sodium: 305mg, Potassium: 655mg.

406. Radish and Olives Salad

Preparation Time: 5 minutes
Cooking Time: 0 minutes
Servings: 4
Ingredients:
- 2 green onions, sliced
- 1-pound radishes, cubed
- 2 tablespoons balsamic vinegar
- 2 tablespoon olive oil
- 1 teaspoon chili powder
- 1 cup black olives, pitted and halved
- A pinch of black pepper

Directions:
1. Mix radishes with the onions and the other ingredients in a large salad bowl, toss and serve as a side dish.

Nutrition:
Calories: 123, Protein: 1.3g, Carbohydrates: 6.9g, Fat: 10.8g, Fiber: 3.3g, Sodium: 345mg, Potassium: 306mg.

407. Spinach and Endives Salad

Preparation Time: 5 minutes
Cooking Time: 0 minutes
Servings: 4
Ingredients:
- 2 endives, roughly shredded
- 1 tablespoon dill, chopped
- ¼ cup lemon juice
- ¼ cup olive oil
- 2 cups baby spinach
- 2 tomatoes, cubed
- 1 cucumber, sliced
- ½ cups walnuts, chopped

Directions:
1. In a large bowl, combine the endives with the spinach and the other ingredients, toss and serve as a side dish.

Nutrition:
Calories: 238, Protein: 5.7g, Carbohydrates: 8.4g, Fat: 22.3g, Fiber: 3.1g, Sodium: 24mg, Potassium: 506mg.

408. Basil Olives Mix

Preparation Time: 5 minutes
Cooking Time: 0 minutes
Servings: 4
Ingredients:
- 2 tablespoons olive oil
- 1 tablespoon balsamic vinegar
- A pinch of black pepper
- 4 cups corn
- 2 cups black olives, pitted and halved
- 1 red onion, chopped
- ½ cup cherry tomatoes halved
- 1 tablespoon basil, chopped
- 1 tablespoon jalapeno, chopped
- 2 cups romaine lettuce, shredded

Directions:
1. Mix the corn with the olives, lettuce, and the other ingredients in a large bowl, toss well, divide between plates and serve as a side dish.

Nutrition:
Calories: 290, Protein: 6.2g, Carbohydrates: 37.6g, Fat: 16.1g, Fiber: 7.4g, Sodium: 613mg, Potassium: 562mg.

409. Arugula Salad

Preparation Time: 5 minutes
Cooking Time: 0 minutes
Servings: 4
Ingredients:
- ¼ cup pomegranate seeds
- 5 cups baby arugula
- 6 tablespoons green onions, chopped
- 1 tablespoon balsamic vinegar
- 2 tablespoons olive oil
- 3 tablespoons pine nuts
- ½ shallot, chopped

Directions:
1. In a salad bowl, combine the arugula with the pomegranate and the other ingredients, toss and serve.

Nutrition:
Calories: 120, Protein: 1.8g, Carbohydrates: 4.2g, Fat: 11.6g, Fiber: 0.9g, Sodium: 9mg, Potassium: 163mg.

410. Spanish Rice

Preparation Time: 15 minutes

Cooking Time: 1 hour & 35 minutes
Servings: 8
Ingredients:
- 2 cups brown rice
- .25 cup extra virgin olive oil
- 2 cloves garlic, minced
- 1 onion, diced
- 2 tomatoes, diced
- 1 jalapeno, seeded and diced
- 1 tablespoon tomato paste
- .5 cup cilantro, chopped
- 2.5 cups chicken broth, low-sodium

Directions:
1. Heat the oven to Fahrenheit 375F degrees. Puree the tomatoes, onion, plus garlic using a blender or food processor. Measure out two cups of this vegetable puree to use and discard the excess.
2. Into a large oven-safe Dutch pan, heat the extra virgin olive oil over medium heat until hot and shimmering. Add in the jalapeno and rice to toast, cooking while occasionally stirring for two to three minutes.
3. Slowly add the chicken broth to the rice, followed by the vegetable puree and tomato paste. Stir until combined and raise the heat to medium-high until the broth comes to a boil.
4. Cover the Dutch pan with an oven-safe lid, transfer the pot to the preheated oven, and bake within 1 hour and 15 minutes. Remove and stir the cilantro into the rice. Serve.

Nutrition:
Calories: 265, Sodium: 32mg, Potassium: 322mg, Carbs: 40g, Fat: 3g, Protein: 5g.

411. Sweet Potatoes and Apples

Preparation Time: 15 minutes
Cooking Time: 40 minutes
Servings: 4
Ingredients:
- 2 sweet potatoes, sliced into 1" cubes
- 2 apples, cut into 1" cubes
- 3 tablespoons extra virgin olive oil, divided
- 1/4 teaspoon black pepper, ground
- 1 teaspoon cinnamon, ground
- 2 tablespoons maple syrup

Directions:

1. Heat the oven to 425 degrees Fahrenheit and grease a large baking sheet with non-stick cooking spray. Toss the cubed sweet potatoes with two tablespoons of olive oil and black pepper until coated. Roast the potatoes within twenty minutes, stirring them once halfway through the process.

2. Meanwhile, toss the apples with the remaining tablespoon of olive oil, cinnamon, and maple syrup until evenly coated. After the sweet potatoes have cooked for twenty minutes, add the apples to the baking sheet and toss the sweet potatoes and apples.

3. Return to the oven, then roast it for twenty more minutes, once again giving it a good stir halfway through. Once the potatoes and apples are caramelized from the maple syrup, remove them from the oven and serve hot.

Nutrition:

Calories: 100, Carbs: 22g, Fat: 0g, Protein: 2g, Sodium: 38mg, Potassium: 341mg.

412. Roasted Turnips

Preparation Time: 15 minutes
Cooking Time: 30 minutes
Servings: 4
Ingredients:

- 2 cups turnips, peels, and cut into ½" cubes
- 1/4 teaspoon black pepper, ground
- 1/2 teaspoon garlic powder
- 1/2 teaspoon onion powder
- 1 tablespoon extra virgin olive oil

Directions:

1. Heat the oven to 400 degrees Fahrenheit and prepare a large baking sheet, setting it aside. Begin by trimming the top and bottom edges off of the turnips and peeling them if you wish. Slice them into 1/2-inch cubes.

2. Toss the turnips with the extra virgin olive oil and seasonings and then spread them out on the prepared baking sheet. Roast the turnips until tender, stirring them halfway through, about thirty minutes in total.

Nutrition:

Calories: 50, Carbs: 5g, Fat: 4g, Protein: 1g, Sodium: 44mg, Potassium: 134mg.

413. No-Mayo Potato Salad

Preparation Time: 15 minutes
Cooking Time: 20 minutes
Servings: 8
Ingredients:

- 3 pounds red potatoes
- 1/2 cup extra virgin olive oil
- 5 tablespoons white wine vinegar, divided
- 2 teaspoons Dijon mustard
- 1 cup red onion, sliced
- 1/2 teaspoon black pepper, ground
- 2 tablespoons basil, fresh, chopped
- 2 tablespoons dill weed, fresh, chopped
- 2 tablespoons parsley, fresh, chopped

Directions:

1. Add the red potatoes to a large pot and cover them with water until the water level is two inches above the potatoes. Put the pot on high heat, then boil potatoes until they are tender when poked with a fork, about fifteen to twenty minutes. Drain off the water.

2. Let the potatoes cool until they can easily be handled but are still warm, then cut them in half and put them in a large bowl. Stir in three tablespoons of the white wine vinegar, giving the potatoes a good stir so that they can evenly absorb the vinegar.

3. Mix the rest of two tablespoons of vinegar, extra virgin olive oil, Dijon mustard, and black pepper in a small bowl. Add this mixture to the potatoes and give them a good toss to thoroughly coat the potatoes.

4. Toss in the red onion and minced herbs. Serve at room temperature or chilled. Serve immediately or store in the fridge for up to four days.

Nutrition:

Calories: 144, Carbs: 19g, Fat: 7g, Protein: 2g, Sodium: 46m; Potassium: 814mg.

414. Zucchini Tomato Bake

Preparation Time: 15 minutes

Cooking Time: 30 minutes
Servings: 4
Ingredients:

- 10 ounces grape tomatoes, cut in half
- 2 zucchinis
- 5 cloves garlic, minced
- 1 teaspoon Italian herb seasoning
- 1/4 teaspoon black pepper, ground
- 1/3 cup parsley, fresh, chopped
- 1/2 cup parmesan cheese, low-sodium, grated

Directions:

1. Heat the oven to Fahrenheit 350F degrees and coat a large baking sheet with non-stick cooking spray. Mix the tomatoes, zucchini, garlic, Italian herb seasoning, black pepper, and Parmesan cheese in a bowl.

2. Put the mixture out on the baking sheet and roast until the zucchini for thirty minutes. Remove, and garnish with parsley over the top before serving.

Nutrition:

Calories: 35, Carbs: 4g, Fat: 2g, Protein: 2g, Sodium: 30mg, Potassium: 649mg.

415. Creamy Broccoli Cheddar Rice

Preparation Time: 15 minutes
Cooking Time: 40 minutes
Servings: 6
Ingredients:

- 1 cup brown rice
- 2 cups chicken broth, low-sodium
- 1 onion, minced
- 3 tablespoons extra virgin olive oil, divided
- 2 cloves garlic, minced
- 1/2 cup skim milk
- 1/4 teaspoon black pepper, ground
- 1.5 cups broccoli, chopped
- 1 cup cheddar cheese, low-sodium, shredded

Directions:

1. Put one tablespoon of the extra virgin olive oil in a large pot and sauté the onion plus garlic over medium heat within two minutes.

2. Put the chicken broth in a pot and wait for it to come to a boil before adding in the rice.

Simmer the rice over low heat for twenty-five minutes.

3. Stir the skim milk, black pepper, and remaining two tablespoons of olive oil into the rice. Simmer again within five more minutes. Stir in the broccoli and cook the rice for five more minutes until the broccoli is tender. Stir in the rice and serve while warm.

Nutrition:
Calories: 200, Carb: 33g, Fat: 3g, Protein: 10g, Sodium: 50mg, Potassium: 344mg.

416. Smashed Brussels Sprouts

Preparation Time: 15 minutes
Cooking Time: 40 minutes
Servings: 6
Ingredients:
- 2 pounds Brussels sprouts
- 3 cloves garlic, minced
- 3 tablespoons balsamic vinegar
- 1/2 cup extra virgin olive oil
- 1/2 teaspoon black pepper, ground -
- 1 leek washed and thinly sliced
- 1/2 cup parmesan cheese, low-sodium, grated

Directions:
1. Heat the oven to 450 degrees Fahrenheit and prepare two large baking sheets. Trim yellow leaves and stems from Brussels sprouts and steam until tender, twenty to twenty-five minutes.
2. Mix the garlic, black pepper, balsamic vinegar, and extra virgin olive oil in a large bowl. Add the steamed Brussels sprouts and leeks to the bowl and toss until evenly coated.
3. Spread the Brussels sprouts and leaks divided onto the prepared baking sheets.
4. Use a fork or a glass and press down on each of the Brussels sprouts to create flat patties. Put the Parmesan cheese on top and place the smashed sprouts in the oven for fifteen minutes until crispy. Enjoy hot and fresh from the oven.

Nutrition:
Calories: 116, Carbs: 11g, Fat: 5g, Protein: 10g, Sodium: 49mg, Potassium: 642mg.

417. Cilantro Lime Rice

Preparation Time: 15 minutes
Cooking Time: 40 minutes
Servings: 6
Ingredients:
- 1.5 cups brown rice
- 2 tablespoons lime juice
- 1.5 teaspoons lemon juice
- 1/2 teaspoon lime zest
- 1/4 cup cilantro, chopped
- 1 bay leaf
- 1 tablespoon extra virgin olive oil
- Water

Directions:
1. Cook rice and bay leaf in a pot with boiling water. Mix the mixture and allow it to boil for thirty minutes, reducing the heat slightly if need be.
2. Once the rice is tender, drain off the water and return the rice to the pot. Let it sit off of the heat within ten minutes. Remove the bay leaf and use a fork to fluff the rice. Stir the rest of the fixing into the rice and then serve immediately.

Nutrition:
Calories: 94, Carbs: 15g, Fat: 3g, Protein: 2g, Sodium: 184mg, Potassium: 245mg.

418. Corn Salad with Lime Vinaigrette

Preparation Time: 15 minutes
Cooking Time: 7 minutes
Servings: 6
Ingredients:
- 4.5 cups corn kernels, fresh
- 1 tablespoon lemon juice
- 1 red bell pepper, diced
- 1 cup grape tomatoes halved
- 1/4 cup cilantro, chopped
- 1/4 cup green onion, chopped
- 1 jalapeno, diced
- 1/4 red onion, thinly sliced
- 1/2 cup feta cheese
- 2 tablespoons Truvia baking blend
- 2 tablespoons extra virgin olive oil
- 1/2 tablespoon honey
- 3 tablespoons lime juice
- 1/4 teaspoon black pepper, ground
- 1/4 teaspoon cayenne pepper, ground
- 1/4 teaspoon garlic powder

- 1/4 teaspoon onion powder

Directions:
1. To create your lime vinaigrette, add the lime juice, onion powder, garlic powder, black pepper, cayenne pepper, and honey to a bowl. Mix, then slowly add in the extra virgin olive oil while whisking vigorously.
2. Boil a pot of water and add in the lemon juice, Baking Truvia, and corn kernels. Allow the corn to boil for seven minutes until tender. Strain the boiling water and add the corn kernels to a bowl of ice water to stop the cooking process and cool the kernels. Drain off the ice water and reserve the corn.
3. Add the tomatoes, red pepper, jalapeno, green onion, red onion, cilantro, and cooked corn to a large bowl and toss it until the vegetables are well distributed. Add the feta cheese and vinaigrette to the vegetables and then toss until well combined and evenly coated. Serve immediately.

Nutrition:
Calories: 88, Carbs: 23g, Fat: 0g, Protein: 3g, Sodium: 124mg, Potassium: 508mg.

419. Mediterranean Chickpea Salad

Preparation Time: 15 minutes
Cooking Time: 0 minutes
Servings: 6
Ingredients:
- 4 cups chickpeas, cooked
- 2 cups bell pepper, diced
- 1 cup cucumber, chopped
- 1 cup tomato, chopped
- 1 avocado, diced
- 2.5 tablespoons red wine vinegar
- 1 tablespoon lemon juice
- 3 tablespoons extra virgin olive oil
- 1 teaspoon parsley, fresh, chopped
- 1/2 teaspoon oregano, dried
- 1 teaspoon garlic, minced
- 1/4 teaspoon dill weed, dried
- 1/4 teaspoon black pepper, ground

Directions:
1. Add the diced vegetables except for the avocado and the chickpeas to a large bowl and

toss them. In a separate bowl, whisk the seasonings, lemon juice, red wine vinegar, and extra virgin olive oil to create a vinaigrette. Once combined, pour the mixture over the salad and toss to combine.

2. Place the salad in the fridge and allow it to marinate for at least a couple of hours before serving or for up to two days. Immediately before serving the salad, dice the avocado and toss it in.

Nutrition:
Calories: 120, Carbs: 14g, Fat: 5g, Protein: 4g, Sodium: 15mg, Potassium: 696mg.

420. Italian Roasted Cabbage

Preparation Time: 15 minutes
Cooking Time: 15 minutes
Servings: 8
Ingredients:
- 1 cabbage, sliced into 8 wedges
- 1.5 teaspoons black pepper, ground
- 1/3 cup extra virgin olive oil
- 2 teaspoons Italian herb seasoning
- 1/3 cup parmesan cheese, low-sodium, grated

Directions:
1. Heat the oven to Fahrenheit 425 degrees. Prepare a large lined baking sheet with aluminum foil and then spray it with non-stick cooking spray.
2. Slice your cabbage in half, remove the stem, and then cut each half into four wedges so that you are left with eight wedges in total.
3. Arrange the cabbage wedges on the baking sheet and then drizzle half of the extra virgin olive oil over them. Sprinkle half of the seasonings and Parmesan cheese over the top.
4. Place the baking sheet in the hot oven. Allow the cabbage to roast for fifteen minutes, and then flip the wedges. Put the rest of the olive oil over the top and then sprinkle the remaining seasonings and cheese over the top as well.
5. Return the cabbage to the oven and allow it to roast for fifteen more minutes until tender. Serve fresh and hot.

Nutrition:

Calories: 17, Carbs: 4g, Fat: 0g, Protein: 1g, Sodium: 27mg, Potassium: 213mg.

421. Tex-Mex Cole Slaw

Preparation Time: 15 minutes
Cooking Time: 0 minutes
Servings: 12
Ingredients:
- 2 cups black beans, cooked
- 1.5 cups grape tomatoes, sliced in half
- 1.5 cups grilled corn kernels
- 1 jalapeno, seeded and minced
- 1/2 cup cilantro, chopped
- 1 bell pepper, diced
- 16 ounces coleslaw cabbage mix
- 3 tablespoons lime juice
- 1/3 cup light sour cream
- 1 cup olive oil mayonnaise, reduced-fat
- 1 tablespoon chili powder
- 1 teaspoon cumin, ground
- 1 teaspoon onion powder
- 1 teaspoon garlic powder

Directions:
1. Mix the sour cream, mayonnaise, lime juice, garlic powder, onion powder, cumin, and chili powder in a bowl to create the dressing.
2. In a large bowl, toss the vegetables and then add in the prepared dressing and toss again until evenly coated. Chill the mixture in the fridge for thirty minutes to twelve hours before serving.

Nutrition:
Calories: 50, Carbs: 10g, Fat: 1g, Protein: 3g, Sodium: 194mg, Potassium: 345mg.

422. Roasted Okra

Preparation Time: 15 minutes
Cooking Time: 20 minutes
Servings: 4
Ingredients:
- 1 pound okra, fresh
- 2 tablespoons extra virgin olive oil
- 1/4 teaspoon cayenne pepper, ground
- 1 teaspoon paprika
- 1/4 teaspoon garlic powder

Directions:
1. Heat the oven to 450 degrees Fahrenheit and prepare a large baking sheet. Cut the okra into pieces appropriate 1/2-inch in size.

2. Place the okra on the baking pan and top it with the olive oil and seasonings, giving it a good toss until evenly coated. Roast the okra in the heated oven until it is tender and lightly browned and seared. Serve immediately while hot.

Nutrition:
Calories: 65, Carbs: 6g, Fat: 5g, Protein: 2g, Sodium: 9mg, Potassium: 356mg.

423. Brown Sugar Glazed Carrots

Preparation Time: 15 minutes
Cooking Time: 25 minutes
Servings: 6
Ingredients:
- 2 pounds carrots, sliced into 1-inch pieces
- 1/3 cup light olive oil
- 1/4 cup Truvia brown sugar blend
- 1/4 teaspoon black pepper, ground

Directions:
1. Heat the oven to 400 degrees Fahrenheit and prepare a large baking sheet. Toss the carrots with the oil, Truvia, and black pepper until evenly coated and then spread them out on the prepared baking sheet.
2. Place the carrots in the oven and allow them to roast until tender, about twenty to twenty-five minutes. Halfway through the cooking time, give the carrots a good serve. Remove the carrots from the oven and serve them alone or topped with fresh parsley.

Nutrition:
Calories: 110, Carbs: 16g, Fat: 4g, Protein: 1g, Sodium: 105mg, Potassium: 486mg.

424. Oven-Roasted Beets with Honey Ricotta

Preparation Time: 15 minutes
Cooking Time: 40 minutes
Servings: 6
Ingredients:
- 1 pound purple beets
- 1 pound golden beets
- 1/2 cup ricotta cheese, low-fat
- 3 tablespoons extra virgin olive oil

- 1 tablespoon honey
- 1 teaspoon rosemary, fresh, chopped
- 1/4 teaspoon black pepper, ground

Directions:

1. Heat the oven to 375F degrees and prepare a large baking sheet by lining it with kitchen parchment. Slice the beets into 1/2-inch cubes before tossing them with the extra virgin olive oil and black pepper.
2. Put the beets on the prepared baking sheet and allow them to roast until tender, about thirty-five to forty minutes. Halfway through the cooking process, flip the beets over.
3. Meanwhile, in a small bowl, whisk the ricotta with the rosemary and honey. Fridge until ready to serve. Once the beets are done cooking, serve them topped with the ricotta mixture, and enjoy.

Nutrition:

Calories: 195, Carbs: 24g, Fat: 8g, Protein: 8g, Sodium: 139mg, Potassium: 521mg.

425. Easy Carrots Mix

Preparation Time: 10 minutes
Cooking Time: 40 minutes
Servings: 6
Ingredients:

- 15 carrots, halved lengthwise
- 2 tablespoons coconut sugar
- ¼ cup olive oil
- ½ teaspoon rosemary, dried
- ½ teaspoon garlic powder
- A pinch of black pepper

Directions:

1. In a bowl, combine the carrots with the sugar, oil, rosemary, garlic powder, and black pepper, toss well, spread on a lined baking sheet, introduce in the oven and bake at 400 degrees F for 40 minutes. Serve.

Nutrition:

Calories: 60, Carbs: 9g, Fat: 0g, Protein: 2g, Sodium: 0mg, Potassium: 200mg.

426. Tasty Grilled Asparagus

Preparation Time: 10 minutes
Cooking Time: 6 minutes
Servings: 4
Ingredients:

- 2 pounds asparagus, trimmed
- 2 tablespoons olive oil
- A pinch of salt and black pepper

Directions:

1. In a bowl, combine the asparagus with salt, pepper, and oil and toss well. Place the asparagus on a preheated grill over medium-high heat, cook for 3 minutes on each side, then serve.

Nutrition:

Calories: 50, Carbs: 8g, Fat: 1g, Protein: 5g, Sodium: 420mg, Potassium: 186mg.

427. Roasted Carrots

Preparation Time: 10 minutes
Cooking Time: 30 minutes
Servings: 4
Ingredients:

- 2 pounds carrots, quartered
- A pinch of black pepper
- 3 tablespoons olive oil
- 2 tablespoons parsley, chopped

Directions:

1. Arrange the carrots on a lined baking sheet, add black pepper and oil, toss, introduce in the oven, and cook within 30 minutes at 400 degrees F. Add parsley, toss, divide between plates and serve as a side dish.

Nutrition:

Calories: 89, Carbs: 10g, Fat: 6g, Protein: 1g, Sodium: 0mg, Potassium: 187mg.

428. Oven Roasted Asparagus

Preparation Time: 10 minutes
Cooking Time: 25 minutes
Servings: 4
Ingredients:

- 2 pounds asparagus spears, trimmed
- 3 tablespoons olive oil
- A pinch of black pepper
- 2 teaspoons sweet paprika
- 1 teaspoon sesame seeds

Directions:

1. Arrange the asparagus on a lined baking sheet, add oil, black pepper, and paprika. Toss, introduce in the oven and bake within 25 minutes at 400 degrees F. Divide the asparagus between plates, sprinkle sesame

seeds on top, and serve as a side dish.

Nutrition:

Calories: 45, Carbs: 5g, Fat: 2g, Protein: 2g, Sodium: 0mg, Potassium: 109mg.

429. Baked Potato with Thyme

Preparation Time: 10 minutes
Cooking Time: 1 hour and 15 minutes
Servings: 8
Ingredients:

- 6 potatoes, peeled and sliced
- 2 garlic cloves, minced
- 2 tablespoons olive oil
- 1 and ½ cups of coconut cream
- ¼ cup of coconut milk
- 1 tablespoon thyme, chopped
- ¼ teaspoon nutmeg, ground
- A pinch of red pepper flakes
- 1 and ½ cups low-fat cheddar, shredded
- ½ cup low-fat parmesan, grated

Directions:

1. Heat a pan with the oil over medium flame. Add garlic, stir and cook for 1 minute. Add coconut cream, coconut milk, thyme, nutmeg, and pepper flakes, stir, bring to a simmer, adjust to low and cook within 10 minutes.
2. Put one-third of the potatoes in a baking dish. Add 1/3 of the cream, repeat the process with the remaining potatoes and the cream. Sprinkle the cheddar on top, cover with tin foil, introduce in the oven and cook at 375 degrees F for 45 minutes. Uncover the dish, sprinkle the parmesan and bake everything for 20 minutes. Divide between plates, and serve as a side dish.

Nutrition:

Calories: 132, Carbs: 21g, Fat: 4g, Protein: 2g, Sodium: 56mg, Potassium: 106mg.

430. Spicy Brussels Sprouts

Preparation Time: 10 minutes
Cooking Time: 20 minutes
Servings: 6
Ingredients:

- 2 pounds Brussels sprouts, halved
- 2 tablespoons olive oil

- A pinch of black pepper
- 1 tablespoon sesame oil
- 2 garlic cloves, minced
- ½ cup coconut aminos
- 2 teaspoons apple cider vinegar
- 1 tablespoon coconut sugar
- 2 teaspoons chili sauce
- A pinch of red pepper flakes
- Sesame seeds for serving

Directions:
1. Spread the sprouts on a lined baking dish, add the olive oil, sesame oil, black pepper, garlic, aminos, vinegar, coconut sugar, chili sauce, and pepper flakes, toss well, introduce in the oven and bake within 20 minutes at 425 degrees F. Divide the sprouts between plates, sprinkle sesame seeds on top and serve as a side dish.

Nutrition:
Calories: 64, Carbs: 13g, Fat: 0g, Protein: 4g, Sodium: 314mg, Potassium: 156mg.

431. Baked Cauliflower with Chili

Preparation Time: 10 minutes
Cooking Time: 30 minutes
Servings: 4
Ingredients:
- 3 tablespoons olive oil
- 2 tablespoons chili sauce
- Juice of 1 lime
- 3 garlic cloves, minced
- 1 cauliflower head, florets separated
- A pinch of black pepper
- 1 teaspoon cilantro, chopped

Directions:
1. In a bowl, combine the oil with the chili sauce, lime juice, garlic, and black pepper and whisk. Add cauliflower florets, toss, spread on a lined baking sheet, introduce in the oven and bake at 425 degrees F for 30 minutes. Divide the cauliflower between plates, sprinkle cilantro on top, and serve as a side dish.

Nutrition:
Calories: 31, Carbs: 3g, Fat: 0g, Protein: 3g, Sodium: 4mg, Potassium: 86mg.

432. Baked Broccoli

Preparation Time: 10 minutes
Cooking Time: 15 minutes
Servings: 4

Ingredients:
- 1 tablespoon olive oil
- 1 broccoli head, florets separated
- 2 garlic cloves, minced
- ½ cup coconut cream
- ½ cup low-fat mozzarella, shredded
- ¼ cup low-fat parmesan, grated
- A pinch of pepper flakes, crushed

Directions:
1. In a baking dish, combine the broccoli with oil, garlic, cream, pepper flakes, mozzarella, and toss. Sprinkle the parmesan on top, introduce it in the oven and bake at 375 degrees F for 15 minutes. Serve.

Nutrition:
Calories: 90, Carbs: 6g, Fat: 7g, Protein: 3g, Sodium: 30mg, Potassium: 56mg.

433. Slow Cooked Potatoes with Cheddar

Preparation Time: 10 minutes
Cooking Time: 6 hours
Servings: 6
Ingredients:
- Cooking spray
- 2 pounds baby potatoes, quartered
- 3 cups low-fat cheddar cheese, shredded
- 2 garlic cloves, minced
- 8 bacon slices, cooked and chopped
- ¼ cup green onions, chopped
- 1 tablespoon sweet paprika
- A pinch of black pepper

Directions:
1. Grease a slow cooker with the cooking spray, add baby potatoes, cheddar, garlic, bacon, green onions, paprika, and black pepper. Toss, cover, and cook on High for 6 hours. Serve.

Nutrition:
Calories: 112, Carbs: 26g, Fat: 4g, Protein: 8g, Sodium: 234mg, Potassium: 76mg.

434. Squash Salad with Orange

Preparation Time: 10 minutes
Cooking Time: 30 minutes
Servings: 6
Ingredients:
- 1 cup of orange juice

- 3 tablespoons coconut sugar
- 1 and ½ tablespoons mustard
- 1 tablespoon ginger, grated
- 1 and ½ pounds butternut squash, peeled and roughly cubed
- Cooking spray
- A pinch of black pepper
- 1/3 cup olive oil
- 6 cups salad greens
- 1 radicchio, sliced
- ½ cup pistachios, roasted

Directions:
1. Mix the orange juice with the sugar, mustard, ginger, black pepper, squash in a bowl, toss well, spread on a lined baking sheet. Spray everything with cooking oil, and bake for 30 minutes 400 degrees F.
2. In a salad bowl, combine the squash with salad greens, radicchio, pistachios, and oil, toss well, and then serve.

Nutrition:
Calories: 17, Carbs: 2g, Fat: 0g, Protein: 0g, Sodium: 0mg, Potassium: 186mg.

435. Colored Iceberg Salad

Preparation Time: 10 minutes
Cooking Time: 0 minutes
Servings: 4
Ingredients:
- 1 iceberg lettuce head, leaves torn
- 6 bacon slices, cooked and halved
- 2 green onions, sliced
- 3 carrots, shredded
- 6 radishes, sliced
- ¼ cup red vinegar
- ¼ cup olive oil
- 3 garlic cloves, minced
- A pinch of black pepper

Directions:
1. Mix the lettuce leaves with the bacon, green onions, carrots, radishes, vinegar, oil, garlic, and black pepper in a large salad bowl. Toss, divide between plates and serve as a side dish.

Nutrition:
Calories: 15, Carbs: 3g, Fat: 0g, Protein: 1g, Sodium: 15mg, Potassium: 436mg.

436. Fennel Salad with Arugula

Preparation Time: 10 minutes

Cooking Time: 0 minutes
Servings: 4
Ingredients:

- 2 fennel bulbs, trimmed and shaved
- 1 and ¼ cups zucchini, sliced
- 2/3 cup dill, chopped
- ¼ cup lemon juice
- ¼ cup olive oil
- 6 cups arugula
- ½ cups walnuts, chopped
- 1/3 cup low-fat feta cheese, crumbled

Directions:

1. Mix the fennel with the zucchini, dill, lemon juice, arugula, oil, walnuts, and cheese in a large bowl, toss, and then serve.

Nutrition:

Calories: 65, Carbs: 6g, Fat: 5g, Protein: 1g, Sodium: 140mg, Potassium: 21mg.

437. Corn Mix

Preparation Time: 10 minutes
Cooking Time: 0 minutes
Servings: 4
Ingredients:

- ½ cup cider vinegar
- ¼ cup of coconut sugar
- A pinch of black pepper
- 4 cups corn
- ½ cup red onion, chopped
- ½ cup cucumber, sliced
- ½ cup red bell pepper, chopped
- ½ cup cherry tomatoes halved
- 3 tablespoons parsley, chopped
- 1 tablespoon basil, chopped
- 1 tablespoon jalapeno, chopped
- 2 cups baby arugula leaves

Directions:

1. Mix the corn with onion, cucumber, bell pepper, cherry tomatoes, parsley, basil, jalapeno, and arugula in a large bowl. Add vinegar, sugar, and black pepper. Toss well, divide between plates and serve as a side dish.

Nutrition:

Calories: 110, Carbs: 25g, Fat: 0g, Protein: 2g, Sodium: 120mg, Potassium: 86mg.

438. Persimmon Salad

Preparation Time: 10 minutes
Cooking Time: 0 minutes
Servings: 4
Ingredients:

- Seeds from 1 pomegranate
- 2 persimmons, cored and sliced

- 5 cups baby arugula
- 6 tablespoons green onions, chopped
- 4 navel oranges, cut into segments
- ¼ cup white vinegar
- 1/3 cup olive oil
- 3 tablespoons pine nuts
- 1 and ½ teaspoons orange zest, grated
- 2 tablespoons orange juice
- 1 tablespoon coconut sugar
- ½ shallot, chopped
- A pinch of cinnamon powder

Directions:

1. In a salad bowl, combine the pomegranate seeds with persimmons, arugula, green onions, and oranges and toss. In another bowl, combine the vinegar with the oil, pine nuts, orange zest, orange juice, sugar, shallot, and cinnamon, whisk well, add to the salad, toss and serve as a side dish.

Nutrition:

Calories: 310, Carbs: 33g, Fat: 16g, Protein: 7g, Sodium: 320mg, Potassium: 32mg.

439. Avocado Side Salad

Preparation Time: 10 minutes
Cooking Time: 0 minutes
Servings: 4
Ingredients:

- 4 blood oranges, slice into segments
- 2 tablespoons olive oil
- A pinch of red pepper, crushed
- 2 avocados, peeled, cut into wedges
- 1 and ½ cups baby arugula
- ¼ cup almonds, toasted and chopped
- 1 tablespoon lemon juice

Directions:

1. Mix the oranges with the oil, red pepper, avocados, arugula, almonds, and lemon juice in a bowl. Then serve

Nutrition:

Calories: 146, Carbs: 8g, Fat: 7g, Protein: 15g, Sodium: 320mg, Potassium: 65mg.

440. Spiced Broccoli Florets

Preparation Time: 10 minutes
Cooking Time: 3 hours
Servings: 10

Ingredients:

- 6 cups broccoli florets
- 1 and ½ cups low-fat cheddar cheese, shredded
- ½ teaspoon cider vinegar
- ¼ cup yellow onion, chopped
- 10 ounces tomato sauce, Sodium free
- 2 tablespoons olive oil
- A pinch of black pepper

Directions:

1. Grease your slow cooker with the oil, add broccoli, tomato sauce, cider vinegar, onion, and black pepper, cook on High for 2 hours and 30 minutes. Sprinkle the cheese all over. Cover, cook on High for 30 minutes more, divide between plates, and serve as a side dish.

Nutrition:

Calories: 119, Fat: 8.7g, Sodium: 272mg, Carbohydrates: 5.7g, Fiber: 1.9g, Sugars: 2.3g, Protein: 6.2g, Potassium: 76mg.

441. Lima Beans Dish

Preparation Time: 10 minutes
Cooking Time: 5 hours
Servings: 10
Ingredients:

- 1 green bell pepper, chopped
- 1 sweet red pepper, chopped
- 1 and ½ cups tomato sauce, salt-free
- 1 yellow onion, chopped
- ½ cup of water
- 16 ounces canned kidney beans, no-salt-added, drained and rinsed
- 16 ounces canned black-eyed peas, no-salt-added, drained and rinsed
- 15 ounces corn
- 15 ounces canned lima beans, no-salt-added, drained and rinsed
- 15 oz. canned black beans, no-salt-added, drained
- 2 celery ribs, chopped
- 2 bay leaves
- 1 teaspoon ground mustard
- 1 tablespoon cider vinegar

Directions:

1. In your slow cooker, mix the tomato sauce with the onion, celery, red pepper, green bell pepper, water, bay leaves, mustard, vinegar, kidney beans, black-eyed peas, corn, lima beans, and black beans. Cook on Low within 5 hours. Discard bay

leaves, divide the whole mix between plates, and serve.
Nutrition:
Calories: 602, Fat: 4.8g, Sodium: 255mg, Carbohydrates: 117.7g, Fiber: 24.6g, 13.4g, Protein: 33g, Potassium: 56mg.

442. Soy Sauce Green Beans

Preparation Time: 10 minutes
Cooking Time: 2 hours
Servings: 12
Ingredients:
- 3 tablespoons olive oil
- 16 ounces green beans
- ½ teaspoon garlic powder
- ½ cup of coconut sugar
- 1 teaspoon low-sodium soy sauce

Directions:
1. In your slow cooker, mix the green beans with the oil, sugar, soy sauce, and garlic powder, cover, and cook on Low for 2 hours. Toss the beans, divide them between plates, and serve as a side dish.

Nutrition:
Calories: 46, Fat: 3.6g, Sodium: 29mg, Carbohydrates: 3.6g, Fiber: 1.3g, Sugars: 0.6g, Protein: 0.8g, Potassium: 77mg.

443. Butter Corn

Preparation Time: 10 minutes
Cooking Time: 4 hours
Servings: 12
Ingredients:
- 20 ounces fat-free cream cheese
- 10 cups corn
- ½ cup low-fat butter
- ½ cup fat-free milk
- A pinch of black pepper
- 2 tablespoons green onions, chopped

Directions:
1. In your slow cooker, mix the corn with cream cheese, milk, butter, and black pepper, and onions, cook on Low within 4 hours. Toss one more time, divide between plates and serve as a side dish.

Nutrition:
Calories: 279, Fat: 18g, Cholesterol: 52mg, Sodium: 165mg, Carbohydrates: 26g, Fiber: 3.5g, Sugars: 4.8g, Protein: 8.1g, Potassium: 73mg.

444. Stevia Peas with Marjoram

Preparation Time: 10 minutes
Cooking Time: 5 hours
Servings: 12
Ingredients:
- 1-pound carrots, sliced
- 1 yellow onion, chopped
- 16 ounces peas
- 2 tablespoons stevia
- 2 tablespoons olive oil
- 4 garlic cloves, minced
- ¼ cup of water
- 1 teaspoon marjoram, dried
- A pinch of white pepper

Directions:
1. In your slow cooker, mix the carrots with water, onion, oil, stevia, garlic, marjoram, white pepper, peas, toss, cover, and cook on High for 5 hours. Divide between plates and serve as a side dish.

Nutrition:
Calories: 71, Fat: 2.5g, Sodium: 29mg, Carbohydrates: 12.1g, Fiber: 3.1g, Sugars: 4.4g, Protein: 2.5g, Potassium: 85mg.

445. Pilaf with Bella Mushrooms

Preparation Time: 10 minutes
Cooking Time: 3 hours
Servings: 6
Ingredients:
- 1 cup wild rice
- 6 green onions, chopped
- ½ pound baby Bella mushrooms
- 2 cups of water
- 2 tablespoons olive oil
- 2 garlic cloves, minced

Directions:
1. In your slow cooker, mix the rice with garlic, onions, oil, mushrooms and water. Toss, cover, and cook on Low for 3 hours. Stir the pilaf one more time. Divide between plates and serve.

Nutrition:
Calories: 151, Fat: 5.1g, Sodium: 9mg, Carbohydrates: 23.3g, Fiber: 2.6g, Sugars: 1.7g, Protein: 5.2g, Potassium: 43mg.

446. Parsley Fennel

Preparation Time: 10 minutes

Cooking Time: 2 hours and 30 minutes
Servings: 4
Ingredients:
- 2 fennel bulbs, sliced
- Juice and zest of 1 lime
- 2 teaspoons avocado oil
- ½ teaspoon turmeric powder
- 1 tablespoon parsley, chopped
- ¼ cup veggie stock, low-sodium

Directions:
1. In a slow cooker, combine the fennel with the lime juice, zest, and the other ingredients. Cook on Low within 2 hours and 30 minutes. Serve.

Nutrition:
Calories: 47, Fat: 0.6g, Sodium: 71mg, Carbohydrates: 10.8g, Protein: 1.7g, Potassium: 186mg.

447. Sweet Butternut

Preparation Time: 10 minutes
Cooking Time: 4 hours
Servings: 8
Ingredients:
- 1 cup carrots, chopped
- 1 tablespoon olive oil
- 1 yellow onion, chopped
- ½ teaspoon stevia
- 1 garlic clove, minced
- ½ teaspoon curry powder
- 1 butternut squash, cubed
- 2 and ½ cups low-sodium veggie stock
- ½ cup basmati rice
- ¾ cup of coconut milk
- ½ teaspoon cinnamon powder
- ¼ teaspoon ginger, grated

Directions:
1. Heat a pan with the oil over medium-high heat. Add the oil, onion, garlic, stevia, carrots, curry powder, cinnamon, ginger, stir, and cook for 5 minutes and transfer to your slow cooker.
2. Add squash, stock, and coconut milk, stir, cover, and cook on Low for 4 hours. Divide the butternut mix between plates and serve as a side dish.

Nutrition:
Calories: 134, Fat: 7.2g, Sodium: 59mg, Carbohydrates: 16.5g, Fiber: 1.7g, Sugars: 2.7g, Protein: 1.8g, Potassium: 90mg.

448. Mushroom Sausages

Preparation Time: 10 minutes
Cooking Time: 2 hours
Servings: 12
Ingredients:

- 6 celery ribs, chopped
- 1 pound no-sugar, beef sausage, chopped
- 2 tablespoons olive oil
- ½ pound mushrooms, chopped
- ½ cup sunflower seeds, peeled
- 1 cup low-sodium veggie stock
- 1 cup cranberries, dried
- 2 yellow onions, chopped
- 2 garlic cloves, minced
- 1 tablespoon sage, dried
- 1 whole-wheat bread loaf, cubed

Directions:

1. Heat a pan with the oil over medium-high flame. Add beef, stir and brown for a few minutes. Add mushrooms, onion, celery, garlic, and sage, stir, cook for a few more minutes and transfer to your slow cooker.
2. Add stock, cranberries, sunflower seeds, and the bread cubes; cover and cook on High for 2 hours. Stir the whole mix, divide between plates and serve as a side dish.

Nutrition:
Calories: 188, Fat: 13.8g, Sodium: 489mg, Carbohydrates: 8.2g, Fiber: 1.9g, Protein: 7.6g, Potassium: 54mg.

449. Parsley Red Potatoes

Preparation Time: 10 minutes
Cooking Time: 6 hours
Servings: 8
Ingredients:

- 16 baby red potatoes, halved
- 2 cups low-sodium chicken stock
- 1 carrot, sliced
- 1 celery rib, chopped
- ¼ cup yellow onion, chopped
- 1 tablespoon parsley, chopped
- 2 tablespoons olive oil
- A pinch of black pepper
- 1 garlic clove minced

Directions:

1. In your slow cooker, mix the potatoes with the carrot, celery, onion, stock, parsley, garlic, oil, and black pepper, toss, cover, and cook on Low for 6 hours. Serve.

Nutrition:
Calories: 257, Fat: 9.5g, Sodium: 145mg, Carbohydrates: 43.4g, Protein: 4.4g, Potassium: 65mg.

450. Jalapeno Black-Eyed Peas Mix

Preparation Time: 10 minutes
Cooking Time: 5 hours
Servings: 12
Ingredients:

- 17 ounces black-eyed peas
- 1 sweet red pepper, chopped
- ½ cup sausage, chopped
- 1 yellow onion, chopped
- 1 jalapeno, chopped
- 2 garlic cloves minced
- 6 cups of water
- ½ teaspoon cumin, ground
- A pinch of black pepper
- 2 tablespoons cilantro, chopped

Directions:

1. In your slow cooker, mix the peas with the sausage, onion, red pepper, jalapeno, garlic, cumin, black pepper, water, cilantro, cover, and cook low for 5 hours. Serve.

Nutrition:
Calories: 75, Fat: 3.5g, Sodium: 94mg, Carbohydrates: 7.2g, Fiber: 1.7g, Sugars: 0.9g, Protein: 4.3g, Potassium: 65mg.

451. Sour Cream Green Beans

Preparation Time: 10 minutes
Cooking Time: 4 hours
Servings: 8
Ingredients:

- 15 ounces green beans
- 14 ounces corn
- 4 ounces mushrooms, sliced
- 11 ounces cream of mushroom soup, low-fat and Sodium free
- ½ cup low-fat sour cream
- ½ cup almonds, chopped
- ½ cup low-fat cheddar cheese, shredded

Directions:

1. In your slow cooker, mix the green beans with the corn, mushrooms soup, mushrooms, almonds, cheese and sour cream. Toss, cover, and cook on Low for 4 hours. Stir one more time, divide between plates and serve as a side dish.

Nutrition:

Calories: 360, Fat: 12.7g, Sodium: 220mg, Carbohydrates: 58.3g, Fiber: 10g, Sugars: 10.3g, Protein: 14g, Potassium: 45mg.

452. Cumin Brussels Sprouts

Preparation Time: 10 minutes
Cooking Time: 3 hours
Servings: 4
Ingredients:

- 1 cup low-sodium veggie stock
- 1-pound Brussels sprouts, trimmed and halved
- 1 teaspoon rosemary, dried
- 1 teaspoon cumin, ground
- 1 tablespoon mint, chopped

Directions:

1. In your slow cooker, combine the sprouts with the stock and the other ingredients, cook on Low within 3 hours. Serve.

Nutrition:
Calories: 56, Fat: 0.6g, Sodium: 65mg, Carbohydrates: 11.4g, Fiber: 4.5g, Sugars: 2.7g, Protein: 4g, Potassium: 65mg.

453. Peach and Carrots

Preparation Time: 10 minutes
Cooking Time: 6 hours
Servings: 6
Ingredients:

- 2 pounds small carrots, peeled
- ½ cup low-fat butter, melted
- ½ cup canned peach, unsweetened
- 2 tablespoons cornstarch
- 3 tablespoons stevia
- 2 tablespoons water
- ½ teaspoon cinnamon powder
- 1 teaspoon vanilla extract
- A pinch of nutmeg, ground

Directions:

1. In your slow cooker, mix the carrots with the butter, peach, stevia, cinnamon, vanilla, nutmeg, and cornstarch mixed with water, toss, cover, and cook on Low for 6 hours. Toss the carrots one more time, divide between plates and serve as a side dish.

Nutrition:
Calories:139, Fat: 10.7g, Sodium: 199mg, Carbohydrates: 35.4g, Fiber: 4.2g, Sugars: 6.9g, Protein: 3.8g, Potassium: 100mg.

454. Baby Spinach and Grains Mix

Preparation Time: 10 minutes
Cooking Time: 4 hours
Servings: 12
Ingredients:
- 1 butternut squash, peeled and cubed
- 1 cup whole-grain blend, uncooked
- 12 ounces low-sodium veggie stock
- 6 ounces baby spinach
- 1 yellow onion, chopped
- 3 garlic cloves, minced
- ½ cup of water
- 2 teaspoons thyme, chopped
- A pinch of black pepper

Directions:
1. In your slow cooker, mix the squash with whole grain, onion, garlic, water, thyme, black pepper, stock, spinach, cover, and cook on Low for 4 hours. Serve.

Nutrition:
Calories:78, Fat: 0.6g, Sodium: 259mg, Carbohydrates: 16.4g, Fiber: 1.8g, Sugars: 2g, Protein: 2.5g, Potassium: 198mg.

455. Quinoa Curry

Preparation Time: 15 minutes
Cooking Time: 4 hours
Servings: 8
Ingredients:
- 1 chopped sweet potato
- 2 cups green beans
- ½ diced onion (white)
- 1 diced carrot
- 15 oz. chick peas (organic and drained)
- 28 oz. tomatoes (diced)
- 29 oz. coconut milk
- 2 minced cloves of garlic
- ¼ cup quinoa
- 1 tbs. turmeric (ground)
- 1 tbsp. ginger (grated)
- 1 ½ cups water
- 1 tsp. of chili flakes
- 2 tsp. of tamari sauce

Directions:
1. Put all the listed fixing in the slow cooker. Add 1 cup of water. Stir well. Cook on "high" for 4 hrs. Serve with rice.

Nutrition:
Calories: 297, Fat: 18g, Sodium: 364mg, Carbohydrates: 9mg,

Protein: 28g, Potassium: 200mg.

456. Lemon and Cilantro Rice

Preparation Time: 15 minutes
Cooking Time: 6 hours
Servings: 4
Ingredients:
- 3 cups vegetable broth (low sodium)
- 1 ½ cups brown rice (uncooked)
- Juice of 2 lemons
- 2 tbsp. chopped cilantro

Directions:
1. In a slow cooker, place broth and rice. Cook on "low" for 5 hours. Check the rice for doneness with a fork. Add the lemon juice and cilantro before serving.

Nutrition:
Calories: 56, Fats: 0.3g, Sodium: 174mg, Carbohydrates: 12g, Protein: 1g, Potassium: 34mg.

457. Chili Beans

Preparation Time: 15 minutes
Cooking Time: 4 hours
Servings: 5
Ingredients:
- 1 ½ cup chopped bell pepper
- 1 ½ cup sliced mushrooms (white)
- 1 cup chopped onion
- 1 tbsp. olive oil
- 1 tbsp. chili powder
- 2 chopped cloves garlic
- 1 tsp. chopped chipotle chili
- ½ tsp. cumin
- 2 oz. drained black beans
- 1 cup diced tomatoes (no salt)
- 2 tbsp. chopped cilantro

Directions:
1. Put all the fixing above in the slow cooker. Cook on "high" for 4 hours. Serve

Nutrition:
Calories: 343, Fat: 11g, Sodium: 308mg, Carbohydrates: 9mg, Protein: 29g, Potassium: 77mg.

458. Bean Spread

Preparation Time: 15 minutes
Cooking Time: 4 hours
Servings: 20
Ingredients:
- 30 ounces Cannellini beans
- ½ cup broth (chicken or veg)
- 1 tbsp. olive oil

- 3 minced cloves garlic
- ½ tsp. marjoram
- ½ tsp. rosemary
- 1/8 tsp. pepper
- pita chips
- 1 tbsp. olive oil

Directions:
1. Place olive oil, beans, broth, marjoram, garlic, rosemary, and pepper in the slow cooker. Cook on "low" for 4 hours. Mash the mixture and transfer to a bowl. Serve with Pita.

Nutrition:
Calories: 298, Fat: 18g, Sodium: 298mg, Carbohydrates: 30mg, Protein: 19g, Potassium: 87mg.

459. Stir-Fried Steak, Shiitake, and Asparagus

Preparation Time: 15 minutes
Cooking Time: 2 hours & 20 minutes
Servings: 4
Ingredients:
- 1 tbsp. sherry (dry)
- 1 tbsp. vinegar (rice)
- ½ tbsp. soy sauce (low sodium)
- ½ tbsp. cornstarch
- 2 tsp. canola oil
- ¼ tsp. black pepper (ground)
- 1 minced clove garlic
- ½ lb. sliced sirloin steak
- 3 oz. shiitake mushrooms
- ½ tbsp. minced ginger
- 6 oz. sliced asparagus
- 3 oz. peas (sugar snap)
- 2 sliced scallions
- ¼ cup water

Directions:
1. Combine cornstarch, soy sauce, sherry vinegar, broth, and pepper. Place the steaks in 1 teaspoon of hot oil in the slow cooker for 2 minutes. Transfer the steaks to a plate. Sauté ginger and garlic in the remaining oil. Add in the mushrooms, peas, and asparagus.
2. Add water and cook on "low" for 1 hour. Add the scallions and cook again for 30 minutes on low. Change the heat to "high" and add the vinegar. When the sauce has thickened, transfer the steaks to the slow cooker. Stir well and serve immediately.

Nutrition:

Calories: 182, Fats: 7g, Sodium: 157mg, Carbohydrates: 10mg, Protein: 20g, Potassium: 34mg.

460. Chickpeas and Curried Veggies

Preparation Time: 15 minutes
Cooking Time: 4 hours
Servings: 2
Ingredients:

- ½ tbsp. canola oil
- 2 sliced celery ribs
- 1/8 tsp. cayenne pepper
- ¼ cup water
- 2 sliced carrots
- 2 sliced red potatoes (sliced)
- ½ tbsp. curry powder
- ½ cup of coconut milk (light)
- ¼ cup drained chickpeas (low sodium)
- chopped cilantro
- ¼ cup yogurt (low fat)

Directions:

1. Sauté potatoes for 5 minutes in oil. Add the carrots, celery, and onion. Sauté for 5 more mins. Sprinkle on the curry powder and cayenne pepper. Stir well to combine.
2. In a slow cooker, pour water and coconut milk. Add in the potatoes. Cook on "low" for 3 hrs. Add chickpeas and cook for 30 more minutes. Serve in bowls along with the yogurt and cilantro garnish.

Nutrition:

Calories: 271, Fats: 11g, Sodium: 207mg, Carbohydrates: 39g, Protein: 7g, Potassium: 67mg.

461. Brussels Sprouts Casserole

Preparation Time: 15 minutes
Cooking Time: 4 hours & 15 minutes
Servings: 3
Ingredients:

- ¾ lb. Brussels sprouts
- 1 diced slice Pancetta
- 1 minced clove garlic
- 1 tbsp. chopped shallot
- ¼ cup pine nuts (toasted)
- ¼ tsp. black pepper (cracked)
- 4 tbsp. water

Directions:

1. Slice sprouts and place them in the slow cooker along with the

water. Cook on "high" for 1 hr. Drain well. Remove the fat from the pancetta. Sauté the pancetta for 4 minutes. Add the shallots, garlic, and 1/8 cup of pine nuts to the sauté.

2. Now, add the sprouts. Cook for 3 minutes. Transfer the prepared mixture to the slow cooker. Add black pepper. 4 tablespoons of water and cook again on "low" for 2 hours. Serve immediately.

Nutrition:

Calories: 128, Fats: 9g, Sodium: 56mg, Carbohydrates: 5g, Protein: 5g, Potassium: 80mg.

462. Tasty Cauliflower

Preparation Time: 15 minutes
Cooking Time: 6 hours & 15 minutes
Servings: 4
Ingredients:

- 2 minced cloves garlic
- 2 cups cauliflower florets
- 2 tbsp. olive oil
- Pinch of sea salt
- ¼ tsp. pepper flakes (chili)
- Pinch of black pepper (cracked)
- 4 tbsp. water
- Zest of ½ lemon

Directions:

1. In a slow cooker, place cauliflower and oil. Add vinegar. Toss well to coat thoroughly. Put in the rest of the ingredients and toss again. Cook on "low" for 2 hours. Serve immediately.

Nutrition:

Calories: 150, Fats: 14g, Sodium: 69mg, Carbohydrates: 6g, Protein: 2.2g, Potassium: 32mg.

463. Artichoke and Spinach Dip

Preparation Time: 15 minutes
Cooking Time: 2 hours & 10 minutes
Servings: 2
Ingredients:

- 1/8 tsp. basil (dried)
- 14 oz. chopped artichoke hearts
- 1 ½ cups spinach
- ½ minced clove garlic
- ¼ cup sour cream (low fat)
- ¼ cup shredded cheese (parmesan)

- ¼ cup Mozzarella cheese (shredded)
- 1/8 tsp. parsley (dried)
- ½ cup yogurt (Greek)
- pinch of black pepper
- Pinch of Kosher Salt

Directions:

1. Boil spinach in water for 1 minute. Drain the water. Set the spinach aside to cool and then chop. Puree all the ingredients, including spinach, in a blender.
2. Transfer the mixture to the slow cooker. Add cheeses and cook for 1 hour on "low." Serve with sliced vegetables.

Nutrition:

Calories: 263, Fats: 14g, Sodium: 537mg, Carbohydrates: 18g, Protein: 20g, Potassium: 54mg.

464. Apple Salsa

Preparation Time: 15 minutes
Cooking Time: 2 hours
Servings: 3
Ingredients:

- 7 ½ oz. drained black beans
- ¼ cubed apples (granny smith)
- ¼ chopped chili pepper (serrano)
- 1/8 cup chopped onion (red)
- 1 ½ tbsp. chopped cilantro
- ¼ lemon
- ¼ orange
- Pinch of sea salt
- Pinch of black pepper (cracked)

Directions:

1. Mix all the ingredients in the cooker (slow cooker). Cook on "low" for an hour. Transfer to a covered container and allow to cool for 1 hour. Serve.

Nutrition:

Calories: 100, Fats: 0.4g, Sodium: 50mg, Carbohydrates: 20g, Protein: 5g, Potassium: 76mg.

465. Hearty Cashew and Almond Butter

Preparation Time: 5 minutes
Cooking Time: 10 minutes
Servings: 1 and ½ cup
Ingredients:

- 1 cup almonds, blanched
- 1/3 cup cashew nuts
- 2 tablespoons coconut oil
- ½ teaspoon cinnamon

Directions:

1. Preheat your oven to 350 degrees F.
2. Bake almonds and cashews for 12 minutes.
3. Let them cool.
4. Transfer to a food processor and add the remaining ingredients.
5. Add oil and keep blending until smooth.
6. Serve and enjoy!

Nutrition:
Calories: 205, Fat: 19g, Carbohydrates: g, Protein: 2.8g, Sodium: 63mg, Potassium: 123mg.

466. Red Coleslaw

Preparation Time: 10 minutes
Cooking Time: 0 minutes
Servings: 4
Ingredients:
- 1 2/3 pounds red cabbage
- 2 tablespoons ground caraway seeds
- 1 tablespoon whole grain mustard
- 1 1/4 cups mayonnaise, low fat, low sodium
- Salt and black pepper

Directions:
1. Cut the red cabbage into small slices.
2. Take a large-sized bowl and add all the ingredients alongside cabbage.
3. Mix well, season with salt and pepper.
4. Serve and enjoy!

Nutrition:
Calories: 406, Fat: 40.8g, Carbohydrates: 10g, Protein: 2.2g, Sodium: 45mg, Potassium: 165mg.

467. Avocado Mayo Medley

Preparation Time: 5 minutes
Cooking Time: 10 minutes
Servings: 4
Ingredients:
- 1 medium avocado, cut into chunks
- ½ teaspoon ground cayenne pepper
- 2 tablespoons fresh cilantro
- ¼ cup olive oil
- ½ cup mayo, low fat and low sodium

Directions:
1. Take a food processor and add avocado, cayenne pepper, lime juice, salt and cilantro.

2. Mix until smooth.
3. Slowly incorporate olive oil, add 1 tablespoon at a time and keep processing between additions.
4. Store and use as needed!

Nutrition:
Calories: 231, Fat: 20g, Carbohydrates: 5g, Protein: 3g, Sodium: 63mg, Potassium: 13mg.

468. Amazing Garlic Aioli

Preparation Time: 5 minutes
Cooking Time: 10 minutes
Servings: 4
Ingredients:
- ½ cup mayonnaise, low fat and low sodium
- 2 garlic cloves, minced
- Juice of 1 lemon
- 1 tablespoon fresh-flat leaf Italian parsley, chopped
- 1 teaspoon chives, chopped
- Salt and pepper to taste

Directions:
1. Add mayonnaise, garlic, parsley, lemon juice, chives and season with salt and pepper.
2. Blend until combined well.
3. Put in the refrigerator and chill for 30 minutes.
4. Serve and use as needed!

Nutrition:
Calories: 813, Fat: 88g, Carbohydrates: 9g, Protein: 2g, Sodium: 63mg, Potassium: 12mg.

469. Easy Seed Crackers

Preparation Time: 10 minutes
Cooking Time: 60 minutes
Servings: 72 crackers
Ingredients:
- 1 cup boiling water
- 1/3 cup chia seeds
- 1/3 cup sesame seeds
- 1/3 cup pumpkin seeds
- 1/3 cup flaxseeds
- 1/3 cup sunflower seeds
- 1 tablespoon Psyllium powder
- 1 cup almond flour
- 1 teaspoon salt
- ¼ cup coconut oil, melted

Directions:
1. Preheat your oven to 300 degrees F.
2. Line a cookie sheet with parchment paper and keep it on the side.

3. Add listed ingredients (except coconut oil and water) to a food processor and pulse until ground.
4. Transfer to a large mixing bowl and pour melted coconut oil and boiling water, mix.
5. Transfer mix to prepared sheet and spread into a thin layer.
6. Cut dough into crackers and bake for 60 minutes.
7. Cool and serve.
8. Enjoy!

Nutrition:
Total Carbs: 10.6g, Fiber: 3g, Protein: 5g, Fat: 14.6g, Sodium: 103mg, Potassium: 30mg.

470. Hearty Almond Crackers

Preparation Time: 10 minutes
Cooking Time: 20 minutes
Servings: 40 crackers
Ingredients:
- 1 cup almond flour
- ¼ teaspoon baking soda
- 1/8 teaspoon black pepper
- 3 tablespoons sesame seeds
- 1 egg, beaten
- Salt and pepper to taste

Directions:
1. Preheat your oven to 350 degrees F.
2. Line two baking sheets with parchment paper and keep them on the side.
3. Mix the dry ingredients in a large bowl and add egg, mix well and form a dough.
4. Divide dough into two balls.
5. Roll out the dough between two pieces of parchment paper.
6. Cut into crackers and transfer them to a prepared baking sheet.
7. Bake for 15-20 minutes.
8. Repeat until all the dough has been used up.
9. Leave crackers to cool and serve.
10. Enjoy!

Nutrition:
Total Carbs: 8g, Fiber: 2g, Protein: 9g, Fat: 28g, Sodium: 63mg, Potassium: 100mg.

471. Black Bean Salsa

Preparation Time: 10 minutes
Cooking Time: 20 minutes
Servings: 4

Ingredients:

- 1 tablespoon coconut aminos
- ½ teaspoon cumin, ground
- 1 cup canned black beans, no salt
- 1 cup salsa
- 6 cups romaine lettuce, torn
- ½ cup avocado, peeled, pitted and cubed

Directions:

1. Take a bowl and add the beans along with the other ingredients.
2. Toss well and serve.
3. Enjoy!

Nutrition:

Calories: 181, Fat: 5g, Carbohydrates: 14g, Protein: 7g, Sodium: 63mg, Potassium: 78mg.

472. Corn Spread

Preparation Time: 10 minutes
Cooking Time: 10 minutes
Servings: 4
Ingredients:

- 30-ounce canned corn, drained
- 2 green onions, chopped
- ½ cup coconut cream
- 1 jalapeno, chopped
- ½ teaspoon chili powder

Directions:

1. Take a pan and add corn, green onions, jalapeno, and chili powder, stir well.
2. Bring to a simmer over medium heat and cook for 10 minutes.
3. Let it chill and add coconut cream.
4. Stir well.
5. Serve and enjoy!

Nutrition:

Calories: 192, Fat: 5g, Carbohydrates: 11g, Protein: 8g, Sodium: 63mg, Potassium: 54mg.

473. Moroccan Leeks Snack

Preparation Time: 10 minutes
Cooking Time: 20 minutes
Servings: 4
Ingredients:

- 1 bunch radish, sliced
- 3 cups leeks, chopped
- 1 ½ cups olives, pitted and sliced
- Pinch turmeric powder
- 2 tablespoons essential olive oil
- 1 cup cilantro, chopped

Directions:

1. Take a bowl and mix in radishes, leeks, olives and cilantro.
2. Mix well.
3. Season with pepper, oil, turmeric and toss well.
4. Serve and enjoy!

Nutrition:

Calories: 120, Fat: 1g, Carbohydrates: 1g, Protein: 6g, Sodium: 63mg, Potassium: 87mg.

474. The Bell Pepper Fiesta

Preparation Time: 10 minutes
Cooking Time: 20 minutes
Servings: 4
Ingredients:

- 2 tablespoons dill, chopped
- 1 yellow onion, chopped
- 1 pound multi colored peppers, cut, halved, seeded and cut into thin strips
- 3 tablespoons organic olive oil
- 2 ½ tablespoons white wine vinegar
- Black pepper to taste

Directions:

1. Take a bowl and mix in sweet pepper, onion, dill, pepper, oil, vinegar and toss well.
2. Divide between bowls and serve.
3. Enjoy!

Nutrition:

Calories: 120, Fat: 3g, Carbohydrates: 1g, Protein: 6g, Sodium: 63mg, Potassium: 87mg.

475. Spiced Up Pumpkin Seeds Bowls

Preparation Time: 10 minutes
Cooking Time: 20 minutes
Servings: 4
Ingredients:

- ½ tablespoon chili powder
- ½ teaspoon cayenne
- 2 cups pumpkin seeds
- 2 teaspoons lime juice

Directions:

1. Spread pumpkin seeds over a lined baking sheet, add lime juice, cayenne and chili powder.
2. Toss well.
3. Preheat your oven to 275 degrees F.
4. Roast in your oven for 20 minutes and transfer to small bowls.
5. Serve and enjoy!

Nutrition:

Calories: 170, Fat: 3g, Carbohydrates: 10g, Protein: 6g, Sodium: 63mg, Potassium: 88mg.

476. Mozzarella Cauliflower Bars

Preparation Time: 10 minutes
Cooking Time: 40 minutes
Servings: 4
Ingredients:

- 1 cauliflower head, riced
- 12 cup low-fat mozzarella cheese, shredded
- ¼ cup egg whites
- 1 teaspoon Italian dressing, low fat
- Pepper to taste

Directions:

1. Spread cauliflower rice over a lined baking sheet.
2. Preheat your oven to 375 degrees F.
3. Roast for 20 minutes.
4. Transfer to a bowl and spread pepper, cheese, seasoning, egg whites and stir well.
5. Spread in a rectangular pan and press.
6. Transfer to oven and cook for 20 minutes more.
7. Serve and enjoy!

Nutrition:

Calories: 140, Fat: 2g, Carbohydrates: 6g, Protein: 6g, Sodium: 63mg, Potassium: 32mg.

477. Tomato Pesto Crackers

Preparation Time: 10 minutes
Cooking Time: 15 minutes
Servings: 4
Ingredients:

- 1 ¼ cups almond flour
- ½ teaspoon garlic powder
- ½ teaspoon baking powder
- 2 tablespoons sun-dried tomato Pesto
- 3 tablespoons ghee
- ½ teaspoon dried basil
- ¼ teaspoon pepper

Directions:

1. Preheat your oven to 325 degrees F.
2. Take a bowl and add the listed ingredients.
3. Mix well and combine.

4. Take a baking sheet lined with parchment paper and spread the dough.
5. Transfer to oven and bake for 15 minutes.
6. Break into small-sized crackers and serve.
7. Enjoy!

Nutrition:
Calories: 204, Fat: 20g, Carbohydrates: 3g, Protein: 3g, Sodium: 123mg, Potassium: 50mg.

478. Garlic Cottage Cheese Crispy

Preparation Time: 5 minutes
Cooking Time: 2 minutes
Servings: 4
Ingredients:
- 1 cup cottage cheese
- ½ teaspoon garlic powder
- Pinch of pepper
- Pinch of onion powder

Directions:
1. Take a skillet and place it over medium heat.
2. Take a bowl and mix in cheese and spices.
3. Scoop half a teaspoon of the cheese mix and place in the pan.
4. Cook for 1 minute per side.
5. Repeat until done.
6. Enjoy!

Nutrition:
Calories: 70, Fat: 6g, Carbohydrates: 1g, Protein: 6g, Sodium: 63mg, Potassium: 65mg.

479. Tasty Cucumber Bites

Preparation Time: 5 minutes
Cooking Time: 20 minutes
Servings: 4
Ingredients:
- 1 (8 ounce) cream cheese container, low fat
- 1 tablespoon bell pepper, diced
- 1 tablespoon shallots, diced
- 1 tablespoon parsley, chopped
- 2 cucumbers
- Pepper to taste

Directions:
1. Take a bowl and add cream cheese, onion, pepper, parsley.
2. Peel cucumbers and cut them in half.
3. Remove seeds and stuff with cheese mix.

4. Cut into bite-sized portions and enjoy!

Nutrition:
Calories: 85, Fat: 4g, Carbohydrates: 2g, Protein: 3g, Sodium: 34mg, Potassium: 223mg.

480. Juicy Simple Lemon Fat Bombs

Preparation Time: 10 minutes
Cooking Time: 20 minutes
Servings: 3
Ingredients:
- 1 whole lemon
- 4 ounces cream cheese
- 2 ounces butter
- 2 teaspoons natural sweetener

Directions:
1. Take a fine grater and zest your lemon.
2. Squeeze lemon juice into a bowl alongside the zest.
3. Add butter, cream cheese to a bowl and add zest, salt, sweetener and juice.
4. Stir well using a hand mixer until smooth.
5. Spoon mix into molds and freeze for 2 hours.
6. Serve and enjoy!

Nutrition:
Total Carbs: 4g, Fiber: 1g, Protein: 4g, Fat: 43g, Calories: 404, Sodium: 63mg, Potassium: 87mg.

481. Chocolate Coconut Bombs

Preparation Time: 20 minutes
Cooking Time: 20 minutes
Servings: 12
Ingredients:
- ½ cup dark cocoa powder
- ½ tablespoon vanilla extract
- 5 drops stevia
- 1 cup coconut oil, solid
- 1 tablespoon peppermint extract

Directions:
1. Take a high-speed food processor and add all the ingredients.
2. Blend until combined.
3. Take a teaspoon and drop a spoonful onto parchment paper.
4. Refrigerate until solidified and keep refrigerated.

Nutrition:
Total Carbs: 0g, Fiber: 0g, Protein: 0g, Fat: 14g, Calories:

126, Sodium: 124mg, Potassium: 168mg.

482. Terrific Jalapeno Bacon Bombs

Preparation Time: 15 minutes
Cooking Time: 10 minutes
Servings: 2
Ingredients:
- 12 large jalapeno peppers
- 16 bacon strips
- 6 ounces full fat cream cheese
- 2 teaspoon garlic powder
- 1 teaspoon chili powder

Directions:
1. Preheat your oven to 350 degrees F.
2. Place a wire rack over a roasting pan and keep it on the side.
3. Make a slit lengthways across jalapeno pepper and scrape out the seeds, discard them.
4. Place a nonstick skillet over high heat and add half of your bacon strips, cook until crispy.
5. Drain them.
6. Chop the cooked bacon strips and transfer them to a large bowl.
7. Add cream cheese and mix.
8. Season the cream cheese and bacon mixture with garlic and chili powder.
9. Mix well.
10. Stuff the mix into the jalapeno peppers and wrap a raw bacon strip all around.
11. Arrange the stuffed wrapped jalapeno on the prepared wire rack.
12. Roast for 10 minutes.
13. Transfer to a cooling rack and serve!

Nutrition:
Calories: 209, Fat: 9g, Net Carbohydrates: 15g, Protein: 9g, Sodium: 63mg, Potassium: 198mg.

483. Yummy Espresso Fat Bombs

Preparation Time: 20 minutes
Cooking Time: 20 minutes
Servings: 24
Ingredients:
- 5 tablespoons butter, tender
- 3 ounces cream cheese, soft
- 2 ounces espresso
- 4 tablespoons coconut oil

- 2 tablespoons coconut whipping cream
- 2 tablespoons stevia

Directions:
1. Prepare your double boiler and melt all ingredients (except stevia) for 3-4 minutes and mix.
2. Add sweetener and mix using a hand mixer.
3. Spoon mixture into silicone muffin molds and freeze for 4 hours.
4. Remove fat bombs and enjoy!

Nutrition:
   Total Carbs: 1.3g, Fiber: 0.2g, Protein: 0.3g, Fat: 7g, Sodium: 63mg, Potassium: 132mg.

484. Crispy Coconut Bombs

Preparation Time: 10 minutes
Cooking Time: 20 minutes
Servings: 6
Ingredients:
- 14 ½ ounces coconut milk
- ¾ cup coconut oil
- 1 cup unsweetened coconut flakes
- 20 drops stevia

Directions:
1. Microwave your coconut oil for 20 seconds in the microwave.
2. Mix in coconut milk and stevia in the hot oil.
3. Stir in coconut flakes and pour the mixture into molds.
4. Let it chill for 60 minutes in the fridge.
5. Serve and enjoy!

Nutrition:
   Total Carbs: 2g, Fiber: 0.5g, Protein: 1g, Fat: 13g, Calories: 123, Net Carbs: 1g, Sodium: 63mg, Potassium: 145mg.

485. Pumpkin Pie Fat Bombs

Preparation Time: 35 minutes
Cooking Time: 5 minutes
Servings: 12
Ingredients:
- 2 tablespoons coconut oil
- 1/3 cup pumpkin puree
- 1/3 cup almond oil
- ¼ cup almond oil
- 3 ounces sugar-free dark chocolate
- ½ teaspoons pumpkin pie spice mix
- Stevia to taste

Directions:
1. Melt almond oil and dark chocolate over a double boiler.
2. Take this mixture and layer the bottom of 12 muffin cups.
3. Freeze until the crust has set.
4. Meanwhile, take a saucepan and combine the rest of the ingredients.
5. Put the saucepan on low heat.
6. Heat until softened and mix well.
7. Pour this over the initial chocolate mixture.
8. Let it chill for at least 1 hour.

Nutrition:
   Total Carbs: 3g, Fiber: 1g, Protein: 3g, Fat: 13g, Calories: 124, Sodium: 63mg, Potassium: 176mg.

486. Sensational Lemonade Fat Bomb

Preparation Time: 2 hours
Cooking Time: 20 minutes
Servings: 2
Ingredients:
- ½ lemon
- 4 ounces cream cheese
- 2 ounces almond butter
- Salt to taste
- 2 teaspoons natural sweetener

Directions:
1. Take a fine grater and zest lemon.
2. Squeeze lemon juice into a bowl with the zest.
3. Add butter, cream cheese in a bowl and add zest, juice, salt, and sweetener.
4. Mix well using a hand mixer until smooth.
5. Spoon mixture into molds and let them freeze for 2 hours.
6. Serve and enjoy!

Nutrition:
   Calories: 404, Fat: 43g, Carbohydrates: 4g, Protein: 4g, Sodium: 63mg, Potassium: 187mg.

487. Sweet Almond and Coconut Fat Bombs

Preparation Time: 10 minutes
Cooking Time: 20 minutes
Servings: 6
Ingredients:
- ¼ cup melted coconut oil

- 9 ½ tablespoons almond butter
- 90 drops liquid stevia
- 3 tablespoons cocoa
- 9 tablespoons melted butter, salted

Directions:
1. Take a bowl and add all the listed ingredients.
2. Mix them well.
3. Pour 2 tablespoons of the mixture into as many muffin molds as you like.
4. Chill for 20 minutes and pop them out.
5. Serve and enjoy!

Nutrition:
   Total Carbs: 2g, Fiber: 0g, Protein: 2.53g, Fat: 14g, Sodium: 63mg, Potassium: 120mg.

488. Almond and Tomato Balls

Preparation Time: 10 minutes
Cooking Time: 20 minutes
Servings: 6
Ingredients:
- 1/3 cup pistachios, de-shelled
- 10 ounces cream cheese
- 1/3 cup sun-dried tomatoes, diced

Directions:
1. Chop pistachios into small pieces.
2. Add cream cheese, tomatoes to a bowl and mix well.
3. Chill for 15-20 minutes and turn into balls.
4. Roll into pistachios.
5. Serve and enjoy!

Nutrition:
   Carb: 183, Fat: 18g, Carb: 5g, Protein: 5g, Sodium: 63mg, Potassium: 112mg.

489. Mediterranean Pop Corn Bites

Preparation Time: 5 minutes + 20 minutes chill
Cooking Time: 2-3 minutes
Servings: 4
Ingredients:
- 3 cups Medjool dates, chopped
- 12 ounces brewed coffee
- 1 cup pecan, chopped
- ½ cup coconut, shredded
- ½ cup cocoa powder

Directions:
1. Soak dates in warm coffee for 5 minutes.

2. Remove dates from coffee and mash them, making a fine smooth mixture.
3. Stir in remaining ingredients (except cocoa powder) and form small balls out of the mixture.
4. Coat with cocoa powder, serve and enjoy!

Nutrition:
Calories: 265, Fat: 12g, Carbohydrates: 43g, Protein: 3g, Sodium: 145mg, Potassium: 153mg.

490. Hearty Buttery Walnuts

Preparation Time: 10 minutes
Cooking Time: 20 minutes
Servings: 4
Ingredients:
- 4 walnut halves
- ½ tablespoon almond butter

Directions:
1. Spread butter over two walnut halves.
2. Top with other halves.
3. Serve and enjoy!

Nutrition:
Calories: 90, Fat: 10g, Carbohydrates: 0g, Protein: 1g, Sodium: 76mg, Potassium: 176mg.

491. Refreshing Watermelon Sorbet

Preparation Time: 20 minutes + 20 hours chill time
Cooking Time: 20 minutes
Servings: 4
Ingredients:
- 4 cups watermelon, seedless and chunked
- ¼ cup coconut sugar
- 2 tablespoons lime juice

Directions:

1. Add the listed ingredients to a blender and puree.
2. Transfer to a freezer container with a tight-fitting lid.
3. Freeze the mix for about 4-6 hours until you have gelatin-like consistency.
4. Puree the mix once again in batches and return to the container.
5. Chill overnight.
6. Allow the sorbet to stand for 5 minutes before serving and enjoy!

Nutrition:
Calories: 91, Fat: 0g, Carbohydrates: 25g, Protein: 1g , Sodium: 45mg, Potassium: 187mg.

492. Lovely Faux Mac and Cheese

Preparation Time: 15 minutes
Cooking Time: 45 minutes
Servings: 4
Ingredients:
- 5 cups cauliflower florets
- 1 tablespoon Salt and pepper to taste
- 1 cup coconut milk
- ½ cup vegetable broth
- 2 tablespoons coconut flour, sifted
- 1 organic egg, beaten
- 2 cups cheddar cheese

Directions:
1. Preheat your oven to 350 degrees F.
2. Season florets with salt and steam until firm.
3. Place florets in a greased ovenproof dish.
4. Heat coconut milk over medium heat in a skillet, make sure to season the oil with salt and pepper.
5. Stir in broth and add coconut flour to the mix; stir.

6. Cook until the sauce begins to bubble.
7. Remove heat and add beaten egg.
8. Pour the thick sauce over cauliflower and mix in cheese.
9. Bake for 30-45 minutes.
10. Serve and enjoy!

Nutrition:
Calories: 229, Fat: 14g, Carbohydrates: 9g, Protein: 15g, Sodium: 45mg, Potassium: 134mg.

493. Beautiful Banana Custard

Preparation Time: 10 minutes
Cooking Time: 25 minutes
Servings: 3
Ingredients:
- 2 ripe bananas, peeled and mashed finely
- ½ teaspoon of vanilla extract
- 14-ounce unsweetened almond milk
- 3 eggs

Directions:
1. Preheat your oven to 350 degrees F.
2. Grease 8 custard glasses lightly.
3. Arrange the glasses in a large baking dish.
4. Take a large bowl and mix all the ingredients and mix them well until combined nicely.
5. Divide the mixture evenly between the glasses.
6. Pour water into the baking dish.
7. Bake for 25 minutes.
8. Take out and serve.
9. Enjoy!

Nutrition:
Calories: 59, Fat: 2.4g, Carbohydrates: 7g, Protein: 3g, Sodium: 63mg, Potassium: 135mg.

Chapter 11. Pasta and Grain

494. Mackerel Maccheroni

Preparation Time: 10 minutes
Cooking Time: 15 minutes
Servings: 4
Ingredients:
- 12oz Maccheroni
- 1 clove garlic
- 14oz tomato sauce
- 1 sprig chopped parsley
- 2 fresh chili peppers
- 1 teaspoon salt
- 7oz mackerel in oil
- 3 tablespoons extra virgin olive oil

Directions:
1. Start by putting the water to boil in a saucepan. While the water is heating up, take a pan, pour in a little oil and a little garlic and cook over low heat. Once the garlic is cooked, pull it out from the pan.
2. Cut open the chili pepper. Remove the internal seeds and cut into thin strips.
3. Add the cooking water and the chili pepper to the same pan as before. Then, take the mackerel, and after draining the oil and separating it with a fork, put it in the pan with the other ingredients. Lightly sauté it by adding some cooking water.
4. Incorporate all the ingredients, pour tomato puree into the pan. Mix well to even out all the ingredients and then cook on low heat for about 3 minutes.

Let's move on to the pasta:
5. After the water starts boiling, add the salt and the pasta. Drain the maccheroni once they are slightly al dente and add them to the sauce you prepared.
6. Sauté for a few moments in the sauce and after tasting, season with salt and pepper according to your liking.

Nutrition:
Calories: 510, Fat: 15.4g, Carbohydrates: 70g, Protein: 22.9g, Sodium: 63mg, Potassium: 123mg.

495. Maccheroni with Cherry Tomatoes and Anchovies

Preparation Time: 10 minutes
Cooking Time: 15 minutes
Servings: 4
Ingredients:
- 14oz Maccheroni pasta
- 6 salted anchovies
- 4oz cherry tomatoes
- 1 clove garlic
- 3 tablespoons extra virgin olive oil
- Fresh chili peppers to taste
- 3 basil leaves
- Salt to taste

Directions:
1. Start by heating water in a pot and add salt when it is boiling. Meanwhile, prepare the sauce: Take the tomatoes after having washed them and cut them into 4 pieces.
2. Now, take a non-stick pan, sprinkle in a little oil and throw in a clove of garlic. Once cooked, remove it from the pan. Add the clean anchovies to the pan, melting them in the oil.
3. When the anchovies are well dissolved, add the chopped tomato pieces and turn the heat to high until they begin to soften (be careful not to let them soften too much).
4. Add the seeded chilies, cut into small pieces, and season.
5. Transfer the pasta to the pot of boiling water, drain it al dente and let it sauté in the pan for a few moments.

Nutrition:
Calories: 476, Fat: 11g, Carbohydrates: 81.4g, Protein: 12.9g, Sodium: 45mg, Potassium: 73mg.

496. Lemon and Shrimp Risotto

Preparation Time: 10 minutes
Cooking Time: 30 minutes
Servings: 4
Ingredients:
- 1 lemon
- 14oz shelled shrimp
- 1 ¾ cups risotto Rice
- 1 white onion
- 33 fl. oz (1 liter) vegetable broth (even less is fine)
- 2 ½ tablespoons butter
- ½ glass white wine
- Salt to taste
- Black pepper to taste
- Chives to taste

Directions:
1. Start by boiling the shrimps in salted water for 3-4 minutes, drain and set aside.
2. Peel and finely chop an onion, stir fry it with melted butter and once the butter has dried, toast the rice in the pan for a few minutes.
3. Deglaze the rice with half a glass of white wine, then add the juice of 1 lemon. Stir and finish cooking the rice; add a ladle of vegetable stock as needed.
4. Mix well and a few minutes before the end of cooking, add the previously cooked shrimps (keeping some of them aside for garnish) and some black pepper.
5. Once the heat is off, add a knob of butter and stir. The risotto is ready to be served. Decorate with the remaining shrimp and sprinkle with some chives.

Nutrition:
Calories: 510, Fat: 10g, Carbohydrates: 82.4g, Protein: 20.6g, Sodium: 56mg, Potassium: 187mg.

497. Spaghetti with Clams

Preparation Time: 10 minutes
Cooking Time: 40 minutes
Servings: 4
Ingredients:
- 11.5oz of spaghetti
- 2 pounds of clams
- 7oz of tomato sauce, or tomato pulp, for the red version of this dish
- 2 cloves of garlic
- 4 tablespoons extra virgin olive oil
- 1 glass of dry white wine
- 1 tablespoon of finely chopped parsley
- 1 chili pepper

Directions:

1. Start by washing the clams: never "purge" the clams — you should only open them by using heat, otherwise their precious internal liquid is lost along with the sand. Wash the clams quickly with a strainer placed in a salad bowl: this will filter the sand from the shells.
2. Then immediately place the drained clams in a pan with a lid over high heat. Turn them from time to time and, when they are almost all open, remove them from the heat. Clams that remain closed are dead and should be removed. Remove the mollusks from the open ones, leaving some whole to decorate the dishes. Strain the liquid that remains at the bottom of the pan and set aside.
3. Take a large frying pan and add a little oil. Heat a whole bell pepper and one or two cloves of crushed garlic over very low heat until the cloves turn a yellowish color. Add the clams and season with dry white wine.
4. Now add the previously strained clam liquid and some chopped parsley.
5. Strain and immediately pour the spaghetti al dente into the pan, after having cooked it in plenty of salted water. Stir well until the spaghetti absorbs all the liquid from the clams. If a chili pepper has not been used, complete with a light sprinkling of white or black pepper.

Nutrition:
Calories: 167, Fat: 8g, Carbohydrates: 18.63g, Protein: 5g, Sodium: 63mg, Potassium: 156mg.

498. Greek Fish Soup

Preparation Time: 10 minutes
Cooking Time: 60 minutes
Servings: 4
Ingredients:
- Hake or other white fish
- 4 Potatoes
- 4 Spring onions
- 2 Carrots
- 2 stalks of Celery
- 2 tomatoes
- 4 tablespoons extra virgin olive oil
- 2 eggs
- 1 lemon
- 1 cup rice

- Salt to taste
Directions:
1. Choose a fish not exceeding 2.2 pounds in weight, remove its scales, gills and intestines and wash it well. Salt it and set it aside.
2. Wash the potatoes, carrots and onions and put them in the saucepan whole with enough water to soak them and then bring to a boil.
3. Add the celery still tied in bunches so that it does not scatter during cooking. Cut the tomatoes in four parts and add them too, together with the oil and salt.
4. When the vegetables are almost cooked, add more water and the fish. Boil for 20 minutes and remove it from the broth along with the vegetables.
5. Place the fish in a serving dish by adorning it with the vegetables and strain the broth. Put the broth back on the heat, diluting it with a little water. Once it boils, put in the rice and season with salt. When the rice is cooked, pull out the saucepan from the heat.

Prepare the avgolemono sauce:
6. Whisk the eggs well and slowly drizzle the lemon juice. Put some broth in a ladle and slowly pour it into the eggs, mixing constantly.
7. Finally, add the obtained sauce to the soup and mix well.

Nutrition:
Calories: 263, Fat: 17.1g, Carbohydrates: 18.6g, Protein: 9g, Sodium: 89mg, Potassium: 109mg.

499. Venere Rice with Shrimp

Preparation Time: 10 minutes
Cooking Time: 55 minutes
Servings: 3
Ingredients:
- 1 ½ cups of black Venere rice (better if parboiled)
- 5 teaspoons extra virgin olive oil
- 10.5oz shrimp
- 10.5oz zucchini
- 1 Lemon (juice and rind)
- Salt to taste
- Black pepper to taste
- 1 clove garlic
- Tabasco to taste

Directions:
Let's start with the rice:

1. After filling a pot with plenty of water and bringing it to a boil, pour in the rice, add salt and cook for the necessary time (check the cooking instructions on the package).
2. Meanwhile, grate the zucchini with a grater with large holes. In a pan, cook olive oil with the peeled garlic clove. Add the grated zucchini, salt and pepper, and cook for 5 minutes, then remove the garlic clove and set the vegetables aside.

Now clean the shrimp:
3. Remove the shell, cut the tail and divide them in half lengthwise. Remove the intestine (the dark thread in their back). Situate the cleaned shrimps in a bowl and season with olive oil; give it some extra flavor by adding lemon zest, salt and pepper and by adding a few drops of Tabasco if you so choose.
4. Heat the shrimps in a hot pan for a couple of minutes. Once cooked, set aside.
5. Once the Venere rice is ready, strain it in a bowl, add the zucchini mix and stir.

Nutrition:
Calories: 293, Fat: 5g, Carbohydrates: 52g, Protein: 10g, Sodium: 60mg, Potassium: 154mg.

500. Pennette with Salmon and Vodka

Preparation Time: 10 minutes
Cooking Time: 18 minutes
Servings: 4
Ingredients:
- 14oz Pennette Rigate
- 7oz smoked salmon
- 1.2oz shallot
- 40ml vodka
- 5 oz cherry tomatoes
- 7 oz fresh liquid cream (I recommend the vegetable one for a lighter dish)
- Chives to taste
- 3 tablespoons extra virgin olive oil
- Salt to taste
- Black pepper to taste
- Basil to taste (for garnish)

Directions:
1. Wash and cut the tomatoes and the chives. After having peeled

the shallot, chop it with a knife, put it in a saucepan and let it marinate in extra virgin olive oil for a few moments.

2. Meanwhile, cut the salmon into strips and sauté it together with the oil and shallot.
3. Blend everything with the vodka, being careful as there could be a flare (if a flame should rise, don't worry, it will lower as soon as the alcohol has evaporated completely). Add the chopped tomatoes and add a pinch of salt and, if you like, some pepper. Finally, add the cream and chopped chives.
4. While the sauce continues cooking, prepare the pasta. Once the water boils, pour in the Pennette and let them cook until al dente.
5. Strain the pasta, and pour the Pennette into the sauce, letting them cook for a few moments so as allow them to absorb all the flavor. If you like, garnish with a basil leaf.

Nutrition:
Calories: 620, Fat: 21.9g, Carbohydrates: 81.7g, Protein: 24g, Sodium: 63mg, Potassium: 123mg.

501. Seafood Carbonara

Preparation Time: 15 minutes
Cooking Time: 50 minutes
Servings: 3
Ingredients:
- 11.5oz spaghetti
- 3.5oz tuna
- 3.5oz swordfish
- 3.5oz salmon
- 6 Yolks
- 4 tablespoons Parmesan cheese (Parmigiano Reggiano)
- 2 fl. oz (60ml) white wine
- 1 clove garlic
- Extra virgin olive oil to taste
- Salt to taste
- Black pepper to taste

Directions:
1. Prepare boiling water in a pot and add a little salt.
2. Meanwhile, pour 6 egg yolks in a bowl and add the grated parmesan, pepper and salt. Beat with a whisk and dilute with a little cooking water from the pot.
3. Remove any bones from the salmon, the scales from the swordfish, and proceed by

dicing the tuna, salmon and swordfish.

4. Once it boils, toss in the pasta and cook it slightly al dente.
5. Meanwhile, heat a little oil in a large pan, add the whole peeled garlic clove. When hot, throw in the fish cubes and sauté over high heat for about 1 minute. Remove the garlic and add the white wine.
6. Once the alcohol evaporates, take out the fish cubes and lower the heat. As soon as the spaghetti is ready, add them to the pan and sauté for about a minute, stirring constantly and adding the cooking water, as needed.
7. Pour in the egg yolk mixture and the fish cubes. Mix well. Serve.

Nutrition:
Calories: 375, Fat: 17g, Carbohydrates: 41.40g, Protein: 14g, Sodium: 63mg, Potassium: 139mg.

502. Garganelli with Zucchini Pesto and Shrimp

Preparation Time: 10 minutes
Cooking Time: 30 minutes
Servings: 4
Ingredients:
- 14 oz egg-based Garganelli

For the zucchini pesto:
- 7oz zucchini
- 1 cup pine nuts
- 8 tablespoons (0.350z) basil
- 1 teaspoon of table salt
- 9 tablespoons extra virgin olive oil
- 2 tablespoons Parmesan cheese to be grated
- 1oz of Pecorino to be grated

For the sautéed shrimp:
- 8.8oz shrimp
- 1 clove garlic
- 7 teaspoons extra virgin olive oil
- Pinch of salt

Directions:
Start by preparing the pesto:
1. After washing the zucchini, grate them, place them in a colander (to allow them to lose some excess liquid), and lightly salt them. Put the pine nuts, zucchini and basil leaves in the blender. Add the grated

Parmesan, the pecorino and the extra virgin olive oil.

2. Blend everything until the mixture is creamy, stir in a pinch of salt and set aside.

Switch to the shrimp:
3. First of all, pull out the intestine by cutting the shrimp's back with a knife along its entire length and, with the tip of the knife, remove the black thread inside.
4. Cook the clove of garlic in a non-stick pan with extra virgin olive oil. When browned, remove the garlic and add the shrimps. Sauté them for about 5 minutes over medium heat until you see a crispy crust form on the outside.
5. Then, boil a pot of water with a sprinkle of salt and cook the Garganelli. Set a couple of ladles of cooking water aside and drain the pasta al dente.
6. Put the Garganelli in the pan where you cooked the shrimp. Cook together for a minute; add a ladle of cooking water and finally, add the zucchini pesto.
7. Mix everything well to combine the pasta with the sauce.

Nutrition:
Calories: 776, Fat: 46g, Carbohydrates: 68g, Protein: 22.5g, Sodium: 63mg, Potassium: 140mg.

503. Salmon Risotto

Preparation Time: 10 minutes
Cooking Time: 30 minutes
Servings: 4
Ingredients:
- 1 ¾ cup (12.3 oz) of rice
- 8.8oz salmon steaks
- 1 leek
- Extra virgin olive oil to taste
- 1 clove of garlic
- ½ glass white wine
- 3 ½ tablespoons grated Grana Padano
- salt to taste
- Black pepper to taste
- 17 fl. oz (500ml) fish broth
- 1 cup butter

Directions:
1. Start by cleaning the salmon and cutting it into small pieces. Cook 1 tablespoon of oil in a pan with a whole garlic clove and brown the salmon for 2/3

minutes, add salt and set the salmon aside, removing the garlic.

Now, start preparing the risotto:

2. Cut the leek into very small pieces and simmer in a pan over low heat with two tablespoons of oil. Mix in the rice and cook it for a few seconds over medium-high heat, stirring with a wooden spoon.
3. Fill in the white wine and continue cooking, stirring occasionally, trying not to let the rice stick to the pan, and add the stock (vegetable or fish) gradually.
4. Halfway through cooking, add the salmon, butter, and a pinch of salt if necessary. When the rice is well cooked, remove it from heat. Combine with a couple of tablespoons of grated Grana Padano and serve.

Nutrition:
Calories: 521, Fat: 13g, Carbohydrates: 82g, Protein: 19g, Sodium: 104mg, Potassium: 137mg.

504. Pasta with Cherry Tomatoes and Anchovies

Preparation Time: 15 minutes
Cooking Time: 35 minutes
Servings: 4
Ingredients:
- 10.5oz spaghetti
- 1.3-pound cherry tomatoes
- 9oz anchovies (pre-cleaned)
- 2 tablespoons capers
- 1 clove of garlic
- 1 small red onion
- Parsley to taste
- Extra virgin olive oil to taste
- Salt to taste
- Black pepper to taste
- Black olives to taste

Directions:
1. Cut the garlic clove, obtaining thin slices.
2. Cut the cherry tomatoes in two. Peel the onion and slice it thinly.
3. Put a little oil with the sliced garlic and onions in a saucepan. Heat everything over medium flame for 5 minutes; stir occasionally.
4. Once everything has been well flavored, add the cherry tomatoes and a pinch of salt and

pepper. Cook for 15 minutes. In the meantime, put a pot with water on the stove and as soon as it boils, add the salt and the pasta.
5. Once the sauce is almost ready, mix in the anchovies and cook for a couple of minutes. Stir gently.
6. Turn off the heat, chop the parsley and place it in the pan.
7. When cooked, strain the pasta and add it directly to the sauce. Turn the heat back on for a few seconds.

Nutrition:
Calories: 446, Fat: 10g, Carbohydrates: 66.1g, Protein: 22.8g, Sodium: 142mg, Potassium: 159mg.

505. Broccoli and Sausage Orecchiette

Preparation Time: 10 minutes
Cooking Time: 32 minutes
Servings: 4
Ingredients:
- 11.5oz orecchiette
- 10.5 broccoli
- 10.50z sausage
- 40ml white wine
- 1 clove of garlic
- 2 sprigs of thyme
- 7 teaspoons extra virgin olive oil
- Black pepper to taste
- Salt to taste

Directions:
1. Bring the pot full of water and salt to boil. Remove the broccoli florets from the stems and cut them in half or in 4 parts if they are very large. Then place them in the boiling water and cover the pot and cook for 6-7 minutes.
2. Meanwhile, finely chop the thyme and set it aside. Remove the sausage casing and with the help of a fork, crush it gently.
3. Fry the garlic clove with a little olive oil and add the sausage. After a few seconds, add the thyme and a little white wine.
4. Without tossing out the cooking water, remove the cooked broccoli with the help of a slotted spoon and add them to the meat a little at a time. Cook everything for 3-4 minutes. Remove the garlic and add a pinch of black pepper.

5. Allow the water where you cooked the broccoli to reach a boil, then toss in the pasta and let it cook. Once the pasta is cooked, strain it with a slotted spoon, transferring it directly to the broccoli and sausage sauce. Then, mix well, adding black pepper and sautéing everything in the pan for a couple of minutes.

Nutrition:
Calories: 683, Fat: 36g, Carbohydrates: 69.6g, Protein: 20g, Sodium: 63mg, Potassium: 164mg.

506. Radicchio and Smoked Bacon Risotto

Preparation Time: 10 minutes
Cooking Time: 30 minutes
Servings: 3
Ingredients:
- 1 ½ cup of rice
- 14oz radicchio
- 5.3oz smoked bacon
- 34 fl. oz (1l) vegetable broth
- 100ml red wine
- 7 teaspoons extra virgin olive oil
- 1.7oz shallots
- Salt to taste
- Black pepper to taste
- 3 sprigs of thyme

Directions:
1. Let's begin with the preparation of the vegetable broth.
2. Start with the radicchio: cut it in half and remove the central part (the white part). Cut it into strips, rinse well and set it aside. Cut the smoked bacon into tiny strips as well.
3. Finely chop the shallot and put it in a pan with a little oil. Let it simmer over medium heat. Adding a ladle of broth, then add the bacon and let it brown.
4. After about 2 minutes, add the rice and toast it, stirring often. At this point, pour the red wine over high heat.
5. Once all the alcohol has evaporated, continue cooking, adding a ladle of broth at a time. Let the previous one dry before adding another until fully cooked. Add salt and black pepper (it's up to how much you decide to add).
6. At the end of cooking, add the strips of radicchio. Mix them well until they are blended with

the rice, but without cooking them. Add the chopped thyme.

Nutrition:
Calories: 482, Fat: 17.5g, Carbohydrates: 68.1g, Protein: 13g, Sodium: 63mg, Potassium: 172mg.

507. Pasta ala Genovese

Preparation Time: 10 minutes
Cooking Time: 25 minutes
Servings: 3
Ingredients:

- 11.5oz of ziti
- 1 pound of beef
- 3 pounds golden onions
- 2oz celery
- 2oz carrots
- 1 tuft of parsley
- 100ml white wine
- 1 tablespoon Extra virgin olive oil to taste
- 1 tablespoon Salt to taste
- 1 tablespoon Black pepper to taste
- 1 tablespoon Parmesan to taste

Directions:

1. Peel and finely chop the onions and carrots. Then, wash and finely chop the celery (do not throw away the leaves, which must also be chopped and set aside). Next, switch to the meat, clean any excess fat and cut it into 5/6 large pieces. Finally, tie the celery leaves and parsley sprig with kitchen twine to create a fragrant bunch.
2. Add plenty of oil in a large pan. Add the onions, celery, and carrots (which you had previously set aside) and let them cook for a couple of minutes.
3. Then, add the pieces of meat, a pinch of salt and the fragrant bunch. Stir and cook for a few minutes. Next, lower the heat and cover with a lid.
4. Cook for at least 3 hours (do not add water or broth because the onions will release all the liquid needed to prevent the bottom of the pan from drying). Occasionally, check on everything and stir.
5. After 3 hours of cooking, remove the bunch of herbs, increase the heat slightly, add a part of the wine and stir.
6. Cook the meat without a lid for about an hour, stirring often

and adding the wine when the bottom of the pan dries.

7. At this point, take a piece of meat, cut it into slices on a cutting board and set it aside. Chop the ziti and cook them in boiling salted water.
8. Once cooked, drain it and place it back in the pot. Dash a few tablespoons of cooking water and stir. Place on a plate and add a little sauce and crumbled meat (the one set aside in step 7.
9. Add pepper and grated Parmesan to taste.

Nutrition:
Calories: 450, Fat: 8g, Carbohydrates: 80g, Protein: 14.5g, Sodium: 63mg, Potassium: 181mg.

508. Cauliflower Pasta from Naples

Preparation Time: 15 minutes
Cooking Time: 35 minutes
Servings: 3
Ingredients:

- 10.5 oz pasta
- 1 cauliflower
- 100 ml of tomato puree
- 1 clove of garlic
- 1 chili pepper
- 3 tablespoons extra virgin olive oil (or teaspoons)
- Salt to taste
- Pepper to taste

Directions:

1. Clean the cauliflower well, remove the outer leaves and the stalk. Cut it into small florets.
2. Peel the garlic clove, chop it and brown it in a saucepan with the oil and the chili pepper.
3. Add the tomato puree and cauliflower florets and let them brown for a few minutes over medium heat, then cover with a few ladles of water and cook for 15-20 minutes or at least until the cauliflower begins to become creamy.
4. If you see that the bottom of the pan is too dry, add as much water as needed so that the mixture remains liquid.
5. At this point, cover the cauliflower with hot water and, once it comes to a boil, add in the pasta.
6. Season with salt and pepper.

Nutrition:

Calories: 458, Fat: 18g, Carbohydrates: 65g, Protein: 9g, Sodium: 63mg, Potassium: 192mg.

509. Pasta e Fagioli with Orange and Fennel

Preparation Time: 10 minutes
Cooking Time: 30 minutes
Servings: 5
Ingredients:

- 1 tbsp. plus extra for serving extra-virgin olive oil
- 2 ounces, chopped fine Pancetta
- 1, chopped fine onion
- 1 bulb, stalks discarded, bulb halved, cored, and chopped fine fennel
- 1 rib, minced celery
- 2 cloves, minced garlic
- 3, rinsed and minced anchovy fillets
- 1 tbsp. minced fresh oregano
- 2 tsp. grated orange zest
- ½ tsp. fennel seeds
- ¼ tsp. red pepper flakes
- 1 (28-ounce) can diced tomatoes
- 1 rind, plus more for serving Parmesan cheese
- 1 (7-ounce) cans, rinsed Cannellini beans
- 2 ½ cups chicken broth
- 2 ½ cups water
- Salt and pepper
- 1 cup orzo
- ¼ cup minced fresh parsley

Directions:

1. Cook oil in a Dutch oven over medium heat. Add pancetta. Stir-fry for 3 to 5 minutes or until beginning to brown. Stir in celery, fennel, and onion and stir-fry until softened (about 5 to 7 minutes).
2. Stir in pepper flakes, fennel seeds, orange zest, oregano, anchovies, and garlic. Cook for 1 minute. Stir in tomatoes and their juice. Stir in Parmesan rind and beans.
3. Simmer and cook for 10 minutes. Stir in water, broth, and 1 teaspoon of salt. Let it boil on high heat. Stir in pasta and cook until al dente.
4. Remove from heat and discard parmesan rind.
5. Sprinkle parsley and season with salt and pepper to taste.

Pour some olive oil and topped with grated Parmesan. Serve.

Nutrition:
Calories: 502, Fat: 8.8g, Carbohydrates: 72.2g, Protein: 34.9g, Sodium: 63mg, Potassium: 105mg.

510. Spaghetti al Limone

Preparation Time: 10 minutes
Cooking Time: 15 minutes
Servings: 6
Ingredients:

- ½ cup extra-virgin olive oil
- 2 tsp. grated lemon zest
- 1/3 cup lemon juice
- 1 clove, minced to pate garlic
- Salt and pepper
- 2 ounces, grated Parmesan cheese
- 1 pound spaghetti
- 6 tbsp. shredded fresh basil

Directions:

1. In a bowl, whisk garlic, oil, lemon zest, juice, ½ teaspoon of salt and ¼ teaspoon of pepper. Stir in the Parmesan and mix until creamy.
2. Meanwhile, cook the pasta according to package directions. Drain and reserve ½ cup of cooking water. Add the oil mixture and basil to the pasta and toss to combine. Season well and stir in the cooking water as needed. Serve.

Nutrition:
Calories: 398, Fat: 20.7g, Carbohydrates: 42.5g, Protein: 11.9g, Sodium: 63mg, Potassium: 110mg.

511. Spiced Vegetable Couscous

Preparation Time: 10 minutes
Cooking Time: 20 minutes
Servings: 6
Ingredients:

- 1 head, cut into 1-inch florets Cauliflower
- 6 tbsp. plus extra for serving Extra-virgin olive oil
- Salt and pepper
- 1 ½ cups couscous
- 1, cut into ½ inch pieces zucchini
- 1, stemmed, seeded, and cut into ½ inch pieces red bell pepper
- 4 cloves, minced garlic

- 2 tsp. ras el hanout
- 1 tsp. plus lemon wedges for serving grated lemon zest
- 1 ¾ cups chicken broth
- 1 tbsp. minced fresh marjoram

Directions:

1. In a skillet, heat 2 tablespoons of oil over medium heat. Add cauliflowers, ¾ teaspoon of salt, and ½ teaspoon of pepper. Mix. Cook until the florets turn brown and the edges are just translucent.
2. Remove the lid and cook, stirring for 10 minutes, or until the florets turn golden brown. Transfer to a bowl and clean the skillet. Heat 2 tablespoons of oil in the skillet.
3. Add the couscous. Cook and continue stirring for 3 to 5 minutes, or until grains are just beginning to brown. Transfer to a bowl and clean the skillet. Heat the remaining 3 tablespoons of oil in the skillet and add bell pepper, zucchini, and ½ teaspoon of salt. Cook for 8 minutes.
4. Stir in lemon zest, ras el hanout, and garlic. Cook until fragrant (about 30 seconds). Place in the broth and simmer. Stir in the couscous. Pull out from the heat and set aside until tender.
5. Add marjoram and cauliflower; then gently fluff with a fork to incorporate. Drizzle with extra oil and season well. Serve with lemon wedges.

Nutrition:
Calories: 787, Fat: 18.3g, Carbohydrates: 129.6g, Protein: 24.5g, Sodium: 104mg, Potassium: 129mg.

512. Spiced Baked Rice with Fennel

Preparation Time: 10 minutes
Cooking Time: 45 minutes
Servings: 8
Ingredients:

- 1 ½ pounds, peeled and cut into 1-inch pieces sweet potatoes
- ¼ cup extra-virgin olive oil
- salt and pepper
- 1 bulb, chopped fine fennel
- 1, chopped fine small onion
- 1 ½ cups, rinsed long-grain white rice
- 4 cloves, minced garlic
- 2 tsp. ras el hanout

- 2 ¾ cups chicken broth
- ¾ cup, halved large pitted brine-cured green olives
- 2 tbsp. minced fresh cilantro
- Lime wedges

Directions:

1. Put the oven rack to the middle and preheat the oven to 400F. Toss the potatoes with ½ teaspoon of salt and 2 tablespoons of oil.
2. Put the potatoes in a single layer in a rimmed baking sheet and roast for 25 to 30 minutes, or until tender. Stir the potatoes halfway through roasting.
3. Pull out the potatoes and lower the oven temperature to 350F. In a Dutch oven, heat the remaining 2 tablespoons of oil over medium heat.
4. Add onion and fennel; next, cook for 5 to 7 minutes, or until softened. Stir in ras el hanout, garlic, and rice. Stir-fry for 3 minutes.
5. Stir in the olives and broth and let sit for 10 minutes. Add the potatoes to the rice and fluff gently with a fork to combine. Season with salt and pepper to taste. Drizzle with cilantro and serve with lime wedges.

Nutrition:
Calories: 207, Fat: 8.9g, Carbohydrates: 29.4g, Protein: 3.9g, Sodium: 123mg, Potassium: 138mg.

513. Moroccan-Style Couscous with Chickpeas

Preparation Time: 5 minutes
Cooking Time: 18 minutes
Servings: 6
Ingredients:

- ¼ cup, extra for serving extra-virgin olive oil
- 1 ½ cups couscous
- 2 peeled and chopped fine carrots
- 1 chopped fine onion
- 1 tablespoon salt and pepper
- 3 cloves, minced garlic
- 1 tsp. ground coriander
- 1 tsp. ground ginger
- ¼ tsp. ground anise seed
- 1 ¾ cups chicken broth
- 1 (15-ounce) can, rinsed chickpeas
- 1 ½ cups frozen peas
- ½ cup chopped fresh parsley or cilantro

- 4 Lemon wedges

Directions:

1. Heat 2 tablespoons of oil in a skillet over medium heat. Mix in the couscous and cook for 3 to 5 minutes, or until just beginning to brown. Transfer to a bowl and clean the skillet.
2. Heat remaining 2 teaspoons of oil in the skillet and add the onion, carrots, and 1 teaspoon of salt. Cook for 5 to 7 minutes. Stir in anise, ginger, coriander, and garlic. Cook until fragrant (about 30 seconds).
3. Combine the chickpeas and broth and bring to simmer. Stir in the couscous and peas. Cover and remove from the heat. Set aside until the couscous is tender.
4. Add the parsley to the couscous and lint with a fork to combine. Dash with extra oil and season well. Serve with lemon wedges.

Nutrition:
Calories: 649, Fat: 14.2g, Carbohydrates: 102.8g, Protein: 30.1g, Sodium: 63mg, Potassium: 148mg.

514. Vegetarian Paella with Green Beans and Chickpeas

Preparation Time: 10 minutes
Cooking Time: 35 minutes
Servings: 4
Ingredients:

- Pinch of saffron
- 3 cups vegetable broth
- 1 tbsp. olive oil
- 1 large, diced yellow onion
- 4 cloves, sliced garlic
- 1, diced red bell pepper
- ¾ cup, fresh or canned crushed tomatoes
- 2 tbsp. tomato paste
- 1 ½ tsp. hot paprika
- 1 tsp. salt
- ½ tsp. freshly ground black pepper
- 1 ½ cups, trimmed and halved green beans
- 1 (15-ounce) can, drained and rinsed chickpeas
- 1 cup short-grain white rice
- 1, cut into wedges lemon

Directions:

1. Mix the saffron threads with 3 tablespoons of warm water in a small bowl. In a saucepan, simmer the water over medium heat. Reduce the heat and allow to simmer.
2. Cook the oil in a skillet over medium heat. Mix in the onion and stir-fry for 5 minutes. Add the bell pepper and garlic and stir-fry for 7 minutes or until pepper is softened. Stir in the saffron-water mixture, salt, pepper, paprika, tomato paste, and tomatoes.
3. Add the rice, chickpeas, and green beans. Stir in the warm broth and bring to a boil. Lower the heat and simmer uncovered for 20 minutes.
4. Serve hot, garnished with lemon wedges.

Nutrition:
Calories: 709, Fat: 12g, Carbohydrates: 121g, Protein: 33g, Sodium: 63mg, Potassium: 157mg.

515. Garlic Prawns with Tomatoes and Basil

Preparation Time: 10 minutes
Cooking Time: 10 minutes
Servings: 4
Ingredients:

- 2 tbsp. olive oil
- 1 ¼ pounds, peeled and deveined prawns
- 3 cloves, minced garlic
- 1/8 tsp. crushed red pepper flakes
- ¾ cup dry white wine
- 1 ½ cups grape tomatoes
- ¼ cup, plus more for garnish finely chopped fresh basil
- ¾ tsp. salt
- ½ tsp. ground black pepper

Directions:

1. In a skillet, cook oil over medium-high heat. Stir in prawns and cook for 1 minute. Transfer to a plate.
2. Place the red pepper flakes and garlic in the oil in the pan and cook, stirring, for 30 seconds. Stir in the wine and cook until it's reduced by about half.
3. Add the tomatoes and stir-fry until tomatoes begin to break down (about 3 to 4 minutes). Stir in the reserved shrimp, salt, pepper, and basil. Cook for 1 to 2 minutes more.
4. Serve garnished with the remaining basil.

Nutrition:
Calories: 282, Fat: 10g, Carbohydrates: 7g, Protein: 33g, Sodium: 63mg, Potassium: 161mg.

516. Shrimp Paella

Preparation Time: 10 minutes
Cooking Time: 25 minutes
Servings: 4
Ingredients:

- 2 tbsp. olive oil
- 1, diced medium onion
- 1, diced red bell pepper
- 3 cloves, minced garlic
- pinch of saffron
- ¼ tsp. hot paprika
- 1 tsp. salt
- ½ tsp. freshly ground black pepper
- 3 cups, divided chicken broth
- 1 cup short-grain white rice
- 1 pound peeled and deveined large shrimp
- 1 cup, thawed frozen peas

Directions:

1. Heat olive oil in a skillet. Fill in the onion and bell pepper and stir-fry for 6 minutes, or until softened. Add the salt, pepper, paprika, saffron, and garlic and mix. Stir in 2 ½ cups of broth and rice.
2. Allow the mixture to boil, then simmer until the rice is cooked, about 12 minutes. Lay the shrimp and peas over the rice and add the remaining ½ cup broth.
3. Put the lid back on the skillet and cook until all shrimp are just cooked through (about 5 minutes). Serve.

Nutrition:
Calories: 409, Fat: 10g, Carbohydrates: 51g, Protein: 25g, Sodium: 63mg, Potassium: 182mg.

517. Lentil Salad with Olives, Mint, and Feta

Preparation Time: 1 hour
Cooking Time: 1 hour
Servings: 6
Ingredients:

- Salt and pepper
- 1 cup, picked over and rinsed French lentils

- 5 cloves, lightly crushed and peeled garlic
- 1 bay leaf
- 5 tbsp. extra-virgin olive oil
- 3 tbsp. white wine vinegar
- ½ cup chopped pitted Kalamata olives
- ½ cup chopped fresh mint
- 1 large, minced shallot
- 1 ounce, crumbled feta cheese

Directions:
1. Add 4 cups warm water and 1 teaspoon of salt in a bowl. Add the lentils and soak at room temperature for 1 hour. Drain well.
2. Put the oven rack to the middle and heat the oven to 325F. Combine the lentils, 4 cups water, garlic, bay leaf, and ½ teaspoon of salt in a saucepan. Cover and place the saucepan to the oven, and cook for 40 to 60 minutes, or until the lentils are tender.
3. Drain the lentils well, discarding garlic and bay leaf. In a large bowl, scourge oil and vinegar together. Add the shallot, mint, olives, and lentils and toss to combine.
4. Season with salt and pepper to taste. Place nicely in the serving dish and garnish with feta. Serve.

Nutrition:
Calories: 249, Fat: 14.3g, Carbohydrates: 22.1g, Protein: 9.5g, Sodium: 63mg, Potassium: 190mg.

518. Chickpeas with Garlic and Parsley

Preparation Time: 5 minutes
Cooking Time: 20 minutes
Servings: 6
Ingredients:
- ¼ cup extra-virgin olive oil
- 4 cloves, sliced thin garlic
- 1/8 tsp. red pepper flakes
- 1, chopped onion
- salt and pepper
- 2 (15-ounce) cans, rinsed chickpeas
- 1 cup chicken broth
- 2 tbsp. minced fresh parsley
- 2 tsp. lemon juice

Directions:
1. In a skillet, add 3 tablespoons of oil and cook garlic and pepper flakes for 3 minutes. Stir in

onion and ¼ tsp. salt and cook for 5 to 7 minutes.
2. Mix in the chickpeas and broth and bring to a simmer. Lower heat and simmer on low heat for 7 minutes, covered.
3. Uncover and set the heat to high and cook for 3 minutes, or until all liquid has evaporated. Set aside and mix in the lemon juice and parsley.
4. Season with salt and pepper to taste. Drizzle with 1 tablespoon of oil and serve.

Nutrition:
Calories: 611, Fat: 17.6g, Carbohydrates: 89.5g, Protein: 28.7g, Sodium: 53mg, Potassium: 103mg.

519. Stewed Chickpeas with Eggplant and Tomatoes

Preparation Time: 10 minutes
Cooking Time: 1 hour
Servings: 6
Ingredients:
- ¼ cup extra-virgin olive oil
- 2 chopped onions
- 1 chopped fine green bell pepper
- Salt and pepper
- 3 cloves, minced garlic
- 1 tbsp. minced fresh oregano
- 2 bay leaves
- 1 pound, cut into 1-inch pieces eggplant
- 1 can drained with juice reserved, chopped whole peeled tomatoes
- 2(15-ounce) cans, drained with 1 cup liquid reserved chickpeas

Directions:
1. Put the oven rack on the lower-middle part and heat the oven to 400F. Heat oil in the Dutch oven. Add bell pepper, onions, ½ teaspoon of salt, and ¼ teaspoon of pepper. Stir-fry for 5 minutes.
2. Stir in 1 teaspoon of oregano, garlic, and bay leaves and cook for 30 seconds. Stir in tomatoes, eggplant, reserved juice, chickpeas, and reserved liquid and bring to a boil. Transfer the pot to oven and cook, uncovered, for 45 to 60 minutes. Stirring twice.
3. Discard the bay leaves. Stir in the remaining 2 teaspoons of oregano and season with salt and pepper. Serve.

Nutrition:
Calories: 642, Fat: 17.3g, Carbohydrates: 93.8g, Protein: 29.3g, Sodium: 63mg, Potassium: 192mg.

520. Greek Lemon Rice

Preparation Time: 20 minutes
Cooking Time: 45 minutes
Servings: 6
Ingredients:
- 2 cups, uncooked (soaked in cold water for 20 minutes, then drained) long grain rice
- 3 tbsp. extra virgin olive oil
- 1 medium, chopped yellow onion
- 1 clove, minced garlic
- ½ cup orzo pasta
- juice of 2 lemons, plus zest of 1 lemon
- 2 cups low sodium broth
- Pinch salt
- 1 large handful chopped parsley
- 1 tsp. dill weed

Directions:
1. In a saucepan, heat 3 tablespoons of extra virgin olive oil. Add the onions and stir-fry for 3 to 4 minutes. Add the orzo pasta and garlic and toss to mix.
2. Then toss in the rice to coat. Add the broth and lemon juice. Boil and lower the heat. Close and cook for 20 minutes.
3. Remove from the heat. Cover and set aside for 10 minutes. Uncover and stir in the lemon zest, dill weed, and parsley. Serve.

Nutrition:
Calories: 145, Fat: 6.9g, Carbohydrates: 18.3g, Protein: 3.3g, Sodium: 63mg, Potassium: 223mg.

521. Garlic-Herb Rice

Preparation Time: 10 minutes
Cooking Time: 30 minutes
Servings: 4
Ingredients:
- ½ cup, divided extra-virgin olive oil
- 5, minced large garlic cloves
- 2 cups brown jasmine rice
- 4 cups water
- 1 tsp. sea salt
- 1 tsp. black pepper
- 3 tbsp. chopped fresh chives

- 2 tbsp. chopped fresh parsley
- 1 tbsp. chopped fresh basil

Directions:
1. In a saucepan, add ¼-cup of olive oil, garlic, and rice. Stir and heat over medium heat. Stir in the water, sea salt, and black pepper. Next, mix again.
2. Boil and lower the heat. Simmer, uncovered, stirring occasionally.
3. When the water is almost absorbed, mix the remaining ¼-cup of olive oil, along with the basil, parsley, and chives.
4. Stir until the herbs are incorporated and all the water is absorbed.

Nutrition:
Calories: 304, Fat: 25.8g, Carb: 19.3g, Protein: 2g, Sodium: 53mg, Potassium: 154mg.

522. Mediterranean Rice Salad

Preparation Time: 10 minutes
Cooking Time: 25 minutes
Servings: 4
Ingredients:
- ½ cup, divided extra virgin olive oil
- 1 cup long-grain brown rice
- 2 cups water
- ¼ cup fresh lemon juice
- 1, minced garlic clove
- 1 tsp. minced fresh rosemary
- 1 tsp. minced fresh mint
- 3, chopped Belgian endives
- 3, chopped red bell pepper
- 1, chopped hothouse cucumber
- ½ cup chopped whole green onion
- ½ cup chopped Kalamata olives
- ¼ tsp. red pepper flakes
- ¾ cup crumbled feta cheese
- Sea salt and black pepper

Directions:
1. Heat ¼-cup of olive oil, rice, and a pinch of salt in a saucepan over low heat. Stir to coat the rice. Add the water and let simmer until the water is absorbed. Stirring occasionally. Fill in the rice into a big bowl and cool.
2. Scourge remaining ¼ cup of olive oil, red pepper flakes, olives, green onion, cucumber, bell pepper, endives, mint, rosemary, garlic, and lemon juice.
3. Place the rice into the mixture and toss to combine. Gently mix in the feta cheese.

4. Adjust the seasoning. Serve.

Nutrition:
Calories: 415, Fat: 34g, Carbohydrates: 28.3g, Protein: 7g, Sodium: 83mg, Potassium: 87mg.

523. Fresh Bean and Tuna Salad

Preparation Time: 5 minutes
Cooking Time: 20 minutes
Servings: 6
Ingredients:
- 2 cups shelled (shucked) fresh beans
- 2 bay leaves
- 3 tbsp. extra-virgin olive oil
- 1 tbsp. red wine vinegar
- Salt and black pepper
- 1 (6-ounce) can, packed in olive oil Best-quality tuna
- 1 tbsp. soaked and dried salted capers
- 2 tbsp. finely minced flat-leaf parsley
- 1, sliced red onion

Directions:
1. Boil lightly salted water in a pot. Add the beans and bay leaves; next, cook for 15 to 20 minutes, or until the beans are tender but still firm. Drain, discard aromatics and transfer to a bowl.
2. Immediately dress the beans with vinegar and oil. Add the salt and black pepper. Mix well and adjust seasoning. Drain the tuna and flake the tuna flesh into the bean salad. Add the parsley and capers. Toss to mix and scatter the red onion slices over the top. Serve.

Nutrition:
Calories: 85, Fat: 7.1g, Carbohydrates: 4.7g, Protein: 1.8g, Sodium: 60mg, Potassium: 77mg.

524. Delicious Chicken Pasta

Preparation Time: 10 minutes
Cooking Time: 17 minutes
Servings: 4
Ingredients:
- 3 chicken breasts, skinless, boneless, cut into pieces
- 9 oz whole-grain pasta
- 1/2 cup olives, sliced
- 1/2 cup sun-dried tomatoes
- 1 tbsp roasted red peppers, chopped

- 14 oz can tomato, diced
- 2 cups marinara sauce
- 1 cup chicken broth
- Pepper
- Salt

Directions:
1. Stir in all ingredients except whole-grain pasta into the Instant Pot.
2. Close the lid and cook on High for 12 minutes.
3. Once done, allow to release pressure naturally. Remove lid.
4. Add pasta and stir well. Seal pot again and select manual and set timer for 5 minutes.
5. When finished, release the pressure for 5 minutes and then release the remainder using the quick release. Remove the lid. Stir well and serve.

Nutrition:
Calories: 615, Fat: 15.4g, Carbohydrates: 71g, Protein: 48g, Sodium: 56mg, Potassium: 87mg.

525. Flavors Taco Rice Bowl

Preparation Time: 10 minutes
Cooking Time: 14 minutes
Servings: 8
Ingredients:
- 1 lb. ground beef
- 8 oz cheddar cheese, shredded
- 14 oz can red beans
- 2 oz taco seasoning
- 16 oz salsa
- 2 cups of water
- 2 cups brown rice
- Pepper
- Salt

Directions:
1. Set Instant Pot on sauté mode.
2. Add meat to the pot and sauté until brown.
3. Add water, beans, rice, taco seasoning, pepper, and salt and stir well.
4. Top with salsa. Close then cook on High for 14 minutes.
5. Once done, release pressure using quick release. Remove lid.
6. Sprinkle cheddar cheese and stir until cheese is melted.
7. Serve and enjoy.

Nutrition:
Calories: 464, Fat: 15.3g, Carbohydrates: 48.9g, Protein: 32.2g, Sodium: 54mg, Potassium: 78mg.

526. Flavorful Mac & Cheese

Preparation Time: 10 minutes
Cooking Time: 10 minutes
Servings: 6
Ingredients:

- 16 oz whole-grain elbow pasta
- 4 cups of water
- 1 cup can tomato, diced
- 1 tsp garlic, chopped
- 2 tbsp olive oil
- 1/4 cup green onions, chopped
- 1/2 cup parmesan cheese, grated
- 1/2 cup mozzarella cheese, grated
- 1 cup cheddar cheese, grated
- 1/4 cup passata
- 1 cup unsweetened almond milk
- 1 cup marinated artichoke, diced
- 1/2 cup sun-dried tomatoes, sliced
- 1/2 cup olives, sliced
- 1 tsp salt

Directions:

1. Add pasta, water, tomatoes, garlic, oil, and salt into the Instant Pot and stir well. Cover the lid and cook on High.
2. Once done, release pressure for few minutes and then release the remaining using quick discharge. Remove lid.
3. Set pot on sauté mode. Add green onion, parmesan cheese, mozzarella cheese, cheddar cheese, passata, almond milk, artichoke, sun-dried tomatoes, and olive. Mix well.
4. Stir well and cook until cheese is melted.
5. Serve and enjoy.

Nutrition:

Calories: 519, Fat: 17.1g, Carbohydrates: 66.5g, Protein: 25g, Sodium: 63mg, Potassium: 45mg.

527. Cucumber Olive Rice

Preparation Time: 10 minutes
Cooking Time: 10 minutes
Servings: 8
Ingredients:

- 2 cups rice, rinsed
- 1/2 cup olives, pitted
- 1 cup cucumber, chopped
- 1 tbsp red wine vinegar
- 1 tsp lemon zest, grated
- 1 tbsp fresh lemon juice
- 2 tbsp olive oil
- 2 cups vegetable broth
- 1/2 tsp dried oregano

- 1 red bell pepper, chopped
- 1/2 cup onion, chopped
- 1 tbsp olive oil
- Pepper
- Salt

Directions:

1. Add oil into the inner pot of the Instant Pot and select the pot on sauté mode. Add onion and sauté for 3 minutes. Add bell pepper and oregano and sauté for 1 minute.
2. Add rice and broth and stir well. Secure the lid and cook at high for 6 minutes. Once done, allow pressure release for 10 minutes; then release remaining using quick release. Remove lid.
3. Add remaining ingredients and stir everything well to mix. Serve immediately and enjoy it.

Nutrition:

Calories: 229, Fat: 5.1g, Carbohydrates: 40.2g, Protein: 4.9g, Sodium: 56mg, Potassium: 65mg.

528. Flavors Herb Risotto

Preparation Time: 10 minutes
Cooking Time: 15 minutes
Servings: 4
Ingredients:

- 2 cups of rice
- 2 tbsp parmesan cheese, grated
- 2 oz heavy cream
- 1 tbsp fresh oregano, chopped
- 1 tbsp fresh basil, chopped
- 1/2 tbsp sage, chopped
- 1 onion, chopped
- 2 tbsp olive oil
- 1 tsp garlic, minced
- 4 cups vegetable stock
- 1 tsp Pepper
- 1 tsp Salt

Directions:

1. Add oil into the inner vessel of the Instant Pot and click the pot on sauté mode. Add garlic and onion to the inner pan of the Instant Pot and press the pot on sauté mode. Add garlic and onion and sauté for 2-3 minutes.
2. Add remaining ingredients except for parmesan cheese and heavy cream and stir well. Seal lid and cook on High for 12 minutes.
3. Once done, discharge the pressure for 10 minutes, then release the remaining using quick release. Remove lid. Stir in cream and cheese and serve.

Nutrition:

Calories: 514, Fat: 17.6g, Carbohydrates: 79.4g, Protein: 8.8g, Sodium: 76mg, Potassium: 78mg.

529. Delicious Pasta Primavera

Preparation Time: 10 minutes
Cooking Time: 4 minutes
Servings: 4
Ingredients:

- 8 oz whole wheat penne pasta
- 1 tbsp fresh lemon juice
- 2 tbsp fresh parsley, chopped
- 1/4 cup almonds slivered
- 1/4 cup parmesan cheese, grated
- 14 oz can tomato, diced
- 1/2 cup prunes
- 1/2 cup zucchini, chopped
- 1/2 cup asparagus
- 1/2 cup carrots, chopped
- 1/2 cup broccoli, chopped
- 1 3/4 cups vegetable stock
- Pepper
- Salt

Directions:

1. Add stock, parsley, tomatoes, prunes, zucchini, asparagus, carrots, and broccoli into the Instant Pot and stir well. Close and cook on High for 4 minutes. Once done, release pressure using quick release. Take out the lid. Stir remaining ingredients well and serve.

Nutrition:

Calories: 303, Fat: 2.6g, Carbohydrates: 63.5g, Protein: 12.8g, Sodium: 23mg, Potassium: 54mg.

530. Roasted Pepper Pasta

Preparation Time: 10 minutes
Cooking Time: 13 minutes
Servings: 6
Ingredients:

- 1 lb. whole wheat penne pasta
- 1 tbsp Italian seasoning
- 4 cups vegetable broth
- 1 tbsp garlic, minced
- 1/2 onion, chopped
- 14 oz jar roasted red peppers
- 1 cup feta cheese, crumbled
- 1 tbsp olive oil
- Pepper
- Salt

Directions:

1. Add roasted pepper into the blender and blend until smooth. Add oil into the inner pot of the Instant Pot and set the jug on sauté mode. Add garlic and onion to the inner cup of the Instant Pot and set the pot on sauté. Cook for 2-3 minutes.
2. Add blended roasted pepper and sauté for 2 minutes.
3. Add remaining ingredients except for feta cheese and stir well. Seal it tight and cook on High for 8 minutes. When done, release pressure naturally for 5 minutes, then release the remaining using quick release. Remove lid. Top with feta cheese and serve.

Nutrition:
Calories: 459, Fat: 10.6g, Carbohydrates: 68.1g, Protein: 21.3g, Sodium: 65mg, Potassium: 54mg.

531. Cheese Basil Tomato Rice
Preparation Time: 10 minutes
Cooking Time: 26 minutes
Servings: 8
Ingredients:
- 1 1/2 cups brown rice
- 1 cup parmesan cheese, grated
- 1/4 cup fresh basil, chopped
- 2 cups grape tomatoes, halved
- 8 oz can tomato sauce
- 1 3/4 cup vegetable broth
- 1 tbsp garlic, minced
- 1/2 cup onion, diced
- 1 tbsp olive oil
- Pepper
- Salt

Directions:
1. Add oil into the inner basin of the Instant Pot and select the pot on sauté. Put garlic and onion in the inner vessel of the Instant Pot and set it on sauté manner. Mix in garlic and onion and sauté for 4 minutes. Add rice, tomato sauce, broth, pepper, and salt and stir well.
2. Seal it and cook on High for 22 minutes.
3. Once done, let it release pressure for 10 minutes, then release the remaining using quick release. Remove cap. Stir in remaining ingredients and mix. Serve and enjoy.

Nutrition:
Calories: 208, Fat: 5.6g, Carbohydrates: 32.1g, Protein: 8.3g, Sodium: 63mg, Potassium: 58mg.

532. Mac & Cheese
Preparation Time: 10 minutes
Cooking Time: 4 minutes
Servings: 8
Ingredients:
- 1 lb. whole grain pasta
- 1/2 cup parmesan cheese, grated
- 4 cups cheddar cheese, shredded
- 1 cup milk
- 1/4 tsp garlic powder
- 1/2 tsp ground mustard
- 2 tbsp olive oil
- 4 cups of water
- Pepper
- Salt

Directions:
1. Add pasta, garlic powder, mustard, oil, water, pepper, and salt into the Instant Pot. Seal tight and cook on High for 4 minutes. When done, release pressure using quick release. Open lid. Put remaining ingredients and stir well and serve.

Nutrition:

Calories: 509, Fat: 25.7g, Carbohydrates: 43.8g, Protein: 27.3g, Sodium: 54mg, Potassium: 87mg.

533. Tuna Pasta
Preparation Time: 10 minutes
Cooking Time: 8 minutes
Servings: 6
Ingredients:
- 10 oz can tuna, drained
- 15 oz whole wheat rotini pasta
- 4 oz mozzarella cheese, cubed
- 1/2 cup parmesan cheese, grated
- 1 tsp dried basil
- 14 oz can tomato
- 4 cups vegetable broth
- 1 tbsp garlic, minced
- 8 oz mushrooms, sliced
- 2 zucchinis, sliced
- 1 onion, chopped
- 2 tbsp olive oil
- Pepper
- Salt

Directions:
1. Pour oil into the inner pot of the Instant Pot and press the pot on sauté. Add mushrooms, zucchini, and onion and sauté until onion is softened. Add garlic and sauté for a minute.
2. Add pasta, basil, tuna, tomatoes, and broth and stir well. Secure and cook on High for 4 minutes. When completed, release pressure for 5 minutes, then release the remaining using quick release. Remove lid. Add remaining ingredients and stir well and serve.

Nutrition:
Calories: 346, Fat: 11.9g, Carbohydrates: 31.3g, Protein: 6.3g, Sodium: 20mg, Potassium: 59mg.

Chapter 12. Salad

534. Watermelon Salad

Preparation Time: 18 minutes
Cooking Time: 0 minutes
Servings: 6
Ingredients:
- ¼ teaspoon sea salt
- ¼ teaspoon black pepper
- 1 tablespoon balsamic vinegar
- 1 cantaloupe, quartered & seeded
- 12 watermelon, small & seedless
- 2 cups mozzarella balls, fresh
- 1/3 cup basil, fresh and torn
- 2 tablespoons olive oil

Directions:
1. Scoop out balls of cantaloupe and put them in a colander over a bowl.
2. With a melon baller, slice the watermelon.
3. Allow your fruit to drain for ten minutes, and then refrigerate the juice.
4. Wipe the bowl dry, and then place your fruit in it.
5. Stir in basil, oil, vinegar, mozzarella and tomatoes before seasoning.
6. Mix well and serve.

Nutrition:
Calories: 218, Protein: 10g, Fat: 13g, Sodium: 59mg, Potassium: 43mg.

535. Orange Celery Salad

Preparation Time: 16 minutes
Cooking Time: 0 minutes
Servings: 6
Ingredients:
- 1 tablespoon lemon juice, fresh
- ¼ teaspoon sea salt, fine
- ¼ teaspoon black pepper
- 1 tablespoon olive brine
- 1 tablespoon olive oil
- ¼ cup red onion, sliced
- ½ cup green olives
- 2 oranges, peeled & sliced
- 3 celery stalks, sliced diagonally in ½ inch slices

Directions:
1. Put your oranges, olives, onion and celery in a shallow bowl.
2. Stir oil, olive brine and lemon juice, pour this over your salad.

---

3. Season with salt and pepper before serving.

Nutrition:
Calories: 65, Protein: 2g, Fat: 0.2g, Sodium: 43mg, Potassium: 123mg.

536. Roasted Broccoli Salad

Preparation Time: 9 minutes
Cooking Time: 17 minutes
Servings: 4
Ingredients:
- 1 lb. broccoli
- 3 tablespoons olive oil, divided
- 1-pint cherry tomatoes
- 1 ½ teaspoons honey
- 3 cups cubed bread, whole grain
- 1 tablespoon balsamic vinegar
- ½ teaspoon black pepper
- ¼ teaspoon sea salt, fine
- grated parmesan for serving

Directions:
1. Set the oven to 450F, and then place the rimmed baking sheet.
2. Drizzle your broccoli with a tablespoon of oil and toss to coat.
3. Take out from the oven and spoon the broccoli. Leave oil at the bottom of the bowl and add in your tomatoes, toss to coat, then mix tomatoes with a tablespoon of honey. Place on the same baking sheet.
4. Roast for fifteen minutes and stir halfway through your cooking time.
5. Add in your bread, and then roast for three more minutes.
6. Whisk two tablespoons of oil, vinegar, and remaining honey. Season. Pour this over your broccoli mix to serve.

Nutrition:
Calories: 226, Protein: 7g, Fat: 12g, Sodium: 23mg, Potassium: 54mg.

537. Tomato Salad

Preparation Time: 22 minutes
Cooking Time: 0 minutes
Servings: 4
Ingredients:
- 1 cucumber, sliced
- ¼ cup sun-dried tomatoes, chopped

- 1 lb. tomatoes, cubed
- ½ cup black olives
- 1 red onion, sliced
- 1 tablespoon balsamic vinegar
- ¼ cup parsley, fresh and chopped
- 2 tablespoons olive oil

Directions:
1. Take out a bowl and combine all of your vegetables. To make your dressing, mix all your seasoning, olive oil and vinegar.
2. Toss with your salad and serve fresh.

Nutrition:
Calories: 126, Protein: 2.1g, Fat: 9.2g, Sodium: 86mg, Potassium: 90mg.

538. Feta Beet Salad

Preparation Time: 16 minutes
Cooking Time: 0 minutes
Servings: 4
Ingredients:
- 6 Red beets, cooked and peeled
- 3 ounces feta cheese, cubed
- 2 tablespoons olive oil
- 2 tablespoons balsamic vinegar

Directions:
1. Combine everything, and then serve.

Nutrition:
Calories: 230, Protein: 7.3g, Fat: 12g, Sodium: 53mg, Potassium: 76mg.

539. Cauliflower & Tomato Salad

Preparation Time: 17 minutes
Cooking Time: 0 minutes
Servings: 4
Ingredients:
- 1 head cauliflower, chopped
- 2 tablespoons parsley, fresh and chopped
- 2 cups cherry tomatoes, halved
- 2 tablespoons lemon juice, fresh
- 2 tablespoons pine nuts

Directions:
1. Incorporate lemon juice, cherry tomatoes, cauliflower and parsley and season well. Sprinkle the pine nuts, and mix.

Nutrition:

Calories: 64, Protein: 2.8g, Fat: 3.3g, Sodium: 77mg, Potassium: 43mg.

540. Tahini Spinach

Preparation Time: 11 minutes
Cooking Time: 6 minutes
Servings: 3
Ingredients:
- 10 spinach, chopped
- ½ cup water
- 1 tablespoon tahini
- 2 cloves garlic, minced
- ¼ teaspoon cumin
- ¼ teaspoon paprika
- ¼ teaspoon cayenne pepper
- 1/3 cup red wine vinegar

Directions:
1. Add your spinach and water to the saucepan, and then boil it on high heat. Once boiling, reduce to low, and cover. Allow it to cook on simmer for five minutes.
2. Add in your garlic, cumin, cayenne, red wine vinegar, paprika and tahini. Whisk well, and season with salt and pepper.
3. Drain your spinach and top with tahini sauce to serve.

Nutrition:
Calories: 69, Protein: 5g, Fat: 3g, Sodium: 42mg, Potassium: 98mg.

541. Pilaf with Cream Cheese

Preparation Time: 11 minutes
Cooking Time: 34 minutes
Servings: 6
Ingredients:
- 2 cups yellow long grain rice, parboiled
- 1 cup onion
- 4 green onions
- 3 tablespoons butter
- 3 tablespoons vegetable broth
- 2 teaspoons cayenne pepper
- 1 teaspoon paprika
- ½ teaspoon cloves, minced
- 2 tablespoons mint leaves
- 1 bunch fresh mint leaves to garnish
- 1 tablespoon olive oil

Cheese Cream:
- 3 tablespoons olive oil
- sea salt and black pepper to taste

- 9 ounces cream cheese

Directions:
1. Start by heating your oven to 360F, and then take out a pan. Heat your butter and olive oil together and cook your onions and spring onions for two minutes.
2. Add in your salt, pepper, paprika, cloves, vegetable broth, rice and remaining seasoning.
3. Sauté for three minutes.
4. Wrap with foil and bake for another half hour. Allow it to cool.
5. Mix in the cream cheese, cheese, olive oil, salt and pepper. Serve your pilaf garnished with fresh mint leaves.

Nutrition:
Calories: 364, Protein: 5g, Fat: 30g, Sodium: 123mg, Potassium: 34mg.

542. Easy Spaghetti Squash

Preparation Time: 13 minutes
Cooking Time: 45 minutes
Servings: 6
Ingredients:
- 2 spring onions, chopped fine
- 3 cloves garlic, minced
- 1 zucchini, diced
- 1 red bell pepper, diced
- 1 tablespoon Italian seasoning
- 1 tomato, small & chopped fine
- 1 tablespoon parsley, fresh and chopped
- pinch lemon pepper
- dash sea salt, fine
- 4 ounces feta cheese, crumbled
- 3 Italian sausage links, casing removed
- 2 tablespoons olive oil
- 1 spaghetti sauce, halved lengthwise

Directions:
1. Prep oven to 350F and take out a large baking sheet. Coat it with cooking spray, and then put your squash on it with the cut side down.
2. Bake at 350F during forty-five minutes. It should be tender.
3. Turn the squash over and bake for five more minutes. Scrape the strands into a larger bowl.
4. Cook tablespoon of olive oil in a skillet, and then add in your Italian sausage. Cook at eight minutes before removing it and placing it in a bowl.

5. Pour an additional tablespoon of olive oil into the skillet and cook your garlic and onions until softened. This will take five minutes. Throw in your Italian seasoning, red peppers and zucchini. Cook for another five minutes. Your vegetables should be softened.
6. Mix in your feta cheese and squash, cooking until the cheese has melted.
7. Stir in your sausage, and then season with lemon pepper and salt. Serve with parsley and tomato.

Nutrition:
Calories: 423, Protein: 18g, Fat: 30g, Sodium: 65mg, Potassium: 87mg.

543. Roasted Eggplant Salad

Preparation Time: 14 minutes
Cooking Time: 36 minutes
Servings: 6
Ingredients:
- 1 red onion, sliced
- 2 tablespoons parsley
- 1 teaspoon thyme
- 2 cups cherry tomatoes
- 1 teaspoon oregano
- 3 tablespoons olive oil
- 1 teaspoon basil
- 3 eggplants, peeled and cubed

Directions:
1. Start by heating your oven to 350F.
2. Season your eggplant with basil, salt, pepper, oregano, thyme and olive oil.
3. Arrange it on a baking tray and bake for a half hour.
4. Toss with your remaining ingredients before serving.

Nutrition:
Calories: 148, Protein: 3.5g, Fat: 7.7g, Sodium: 12mg, Potassium: 45mg.

544. Penne with Tahini Sauce

Preparation Time: 16 minutes
Cooking Time: 22 minutes
Servings: 8
Ingredients:
- 1/3 cup water
- 1 cup yogurt, plain
- 1/8 cup lemon juice
- 3 tablespoons tahini
- 3 cloves garlic

- 1 onion, chopped
- ¼ cup olive oil
- 2 portobello mushrooms, large & sliced
- ½ red bell pepper, diced
- 16 ounces penne pasta
- ½ cup parsley, fresh and chopped

Directions:
1. Start by taking out a pot and bringing a pot of salted water to a boil. Cook the pasta al dente according to package directions.
2. Mix the lemon juice and tahini, and place them in a food processor. Process with garlic, water and yogurt.
3. Place a pan over medium fire. Heat your oil and cook your onions until soft.
4. Add in your mushroom and continue to cook until softened.
5. Add in your bell pepper and cook until crispy.
6. Drain your pasta, and then toss with your tahini sauce, top with parsley and pepper and serve with vegetables.

Nutrition:
Calories: 332, Proteins 11g, Fat: 12g, Sodium: 67mg, Potassium: 98mg.

545. Roasted Veggies
Preparation Time: 14 minutes
Cooking Time: 26 minutes
Servings: 12
Ingredients:
- 6 cloves garlic
- 6 tablespoons olive oil
- 1 fennel bulb, diced
- 1 zucchini, diced
- 2 red bell peppers, diced
- 6 potatoes, large and diced
- 2 teaspoons sea salt
- ½ cup balsamic vinegar
- ¼ cup rosemary, chopped and fresh
- 2 teaspoons vegetable bouillon powder

Directions:
1. Start by heating your oven to 400F.
2. Take out a baking dish and place your potatoes, zucchini, garlic and fennel on a baking dish, drizzling with olive oil. Sprinkle with salt, bouillon powder, and rosemary. Mix well, and then bake at 450F for thirty to forty minutes. Mix your vinegar into the vegetables before serving.

Nutrition:
Calories: 675, Protein: 13g, Fat: 21g, Sodium: 42mg, Potassium: 67mg.

546. Zucchini Pasta
Preparation Time: 9 minutes
Cooking Time: 32 minutes
Servings: 4
Ingredients:
- 3 tablespoons olive oil
- 2 cloves garlic, minced
- 3 zucchinis, large and diced
- sea salt and black pepper to taste
- ½ cup milk, 2%
- ¼ teaspoon nutmeg
- 1 tablespoon lemon juice, fresh
- ½ cup parmesan, grated
- 8 ounces uncooked farfalle pasta

Directions:
1. Take out a skillet, place it over medium flame, and heat the oil. Stir in your garlic and cook for a minute. Stir often so that it doesn't burn. Add in your salt, pepper and zucchini. Stir well and cook covered for fifteen minutes. During this time, you should stir the mixture twice.
2. Take out a microwave safe bowl and heat the milk for thirty seconds. Stir in your nutmeg, and then pour it into the skillet. Cook uncovered for five minutes. Stir occasionally to keep from burning.
3. Take out a stockpot and cook your pasta per package instructions. Drain the pasta, and then save two tablespoons of pasta water.
4. Stir everything together and add in the cheese and lemon juice and pasta water.

Nutrition:
Calories: 410, Protein: 15g, Fat: 17g, Sodium: 50mg, Potassium: 43mg.

547. Asparagus Pasta
Preparation Time: 8 minutes
Cooking Time: 33 minutes
Servings: 6
Ingredients:
- 8 ounces farfalle pasta, uncooked
- 1 ½ cups asparagus
- 1-pint grape tomatoes, halved
- 2 tablespoons olive oil

- 2 cups mozzarella, fresh and drained
- 1/3 cup basil leaves, fresh and torn
- 2 tablespoons balsamic vinegar

Directions:
1. Start by heating the oven to 400F, and then take out a stockpot. Cook your pasta per package instructions, and reserve ¼ cup of pasta water.
2. Take out a bowl and toss the tomatoes, oil, asparagus, and season with salt and pepper. Spread this mixture on a baking sheet and bake for fifteen minutes. Stir twice this time.
3. Remove your vegetables from the oven, and then add the cooked pasta to your baking sheet. Mix with a few tablespoons of pasta water so that your sauce becomes smoother.
4. Mix in your basil and mozzarella, drizzling with balsamic vinegar. Serve warm.

Nutrition:
Calories: 307, Protein: 18g, Fat: 14g, Sodium: 39mg, Potassium: 54mg.

548. Feta & Spinach Pita Bake
Preparation Time: 11 minutes
Cooking Time: 36 minutes
Servings: 6
Ingredients:
- 2 Roma tomatoes
- 6 whole wheat pita bread
- 1 jar sun-dried tomato pesto
- 4 mushrooms, fresh and sliced
- 1 bunch spinach
- 2 tablespoons parmesan cheese
- 3 tablespoons olive oil
- ½ cup feta cheese

Directions:
1. Start by heating the oven to 350F and get to your pita bread. Spread the tomato pesto on the side of each one. Put them in a baking pan with the tomato side up.
2. Top with tomatoes, spinach, mushrooms, parmesan and feta. Pour in olive oil and season with pepper.
3. Bake for twelve minutes, and then serve cut into quarters.

Nutrition:
Calories: 350, Protein: 12g, Fat: 17g, Sodium: 32mg, Potassium: 87mg.

549. Spelled Salad

Preparation Time: 15 minutes
Cooking Time: 30 minutes
Servings: 4
Ingredients:
Salad:
- 2 ½ cups of vegetable broth
- ¾ cup of crumbled feta cheese
- 1 can chickpeas, drained
- 1 cucumber, chopped
- 1 ½ cup pearl spelled
- 1 tablespoon of olive oil
- ½ sliced onion
- 2 cups of baby spinach, chopped
- 1 pint of cherry tomatoes
- 1 ¼ cups of water

Dressing:
- 2 tablespoons of lemon juice
- 1 tablespoon of honey
- ¼ cup olive oil
- ¼ tsp oregano
- 1 pinch of red pepper flakes
- ¼ teaspoon of salt
- 1 tablespoon of red wine vinegar

Directions:
1. Heat the oil in a skillet. Add the spelled and cook for a minute. Be sure to stir it regularly during cooking. Fill in water and broth, then bring to a boil. Reduce the heat and simmer until the spelled is tender, about 30 minutes. Drain the water and transfer the spelled to a bowl.
2. Add the spinach and mix. Let cool for about 20 minutes. Add the cucumber, onions, tomatoes, peppers, chickpeas and feta. Mix well to get a good mixture. Step back and prepare the dressing.
3. Mix all the dressing ingredients and mix well until smooth. Pour it into the bowl and mix it well. Season well to taste.

Nutrition:
Calories: 365, Fat: 10g, Carbohydrates: 43g, Protein: 13g, Sodium: 78mg, Potassium: 06mg.

550. Chickpea and Zucchini Salad

Preparation Time: 10 minutes
Cooking Time: 0 minutes
Servings: 3
Ingredients:
- ¼ cup balsamic vinegar
- 1/3 cup chopped basil leaves
- 1 tablespoon of capers, drained and chopped
- ½ cup crumbled feta cheese

- 1 can chickpeas, drained
- 1 garlic clove, chopped
- ½ cup Kalamata olives, chopped
- 1/3 cup of olive oil
- ½ cup sweet onion, chopped
- ½ tsp oregano
- 1 pinch of red pepper flakes, crushed
- ¾ cup red bell pepper, chopped
- 1 tablespoon chopped rosemary
- 2 cups of zucchini, diced
- salt and pepper to taste

Directions:
1. Combine the vegetables in a bowl and cover well.
2. Serve at room temperature. But for best results, refrigerate the bowl for a few hours before serving to allow the flavors to blend.

Nutrition:
Calories: 258, Fat: 12g, Carbohydrates: 19g, Protein: 5.6g, Sodium: 54mg, Potassium: 29mg.

551. Provencal Artichoke Salad

Preparation Time: 15 minutes
Cooking Time: 5 minutes
Servings: 3
Ingredients:
- 9 oz artichoke hearts
- 1 teaspoon of chopped basil
- 2 garlic cloves, chopped
- 1 lemon zest
- 1 tablespoon olives, chopped
- 1 tablespoon of olive oil
- ½ chopped onion
- 1 pinch, ½ teaspoon of salt
- 2 tomatoes, chopped
- 3 tablespoons of water
- ½ glass of white wine
- salt and pepper to taste

Directions:
1. Heat the oil in a skillet. Sauté the onion and garlic. Cook until the onions are translucent and season with a pinch of salt. Pour in the white wine and simmer until the wine is reduced by half.
2. Add the chopped tomatoes, artichoke hearts and water. Simmer and add the lemon zest and about ½ teaspoon of salt. Cover and cook for about 6 minutes.
3. Add the olives and basil. Season well and enjoy!

Nutrition:
Calories: 147, Fat: 13g, Carbohydrates: 18g, Protein: 4g,

Sodium: 49mg, Potassium: 67mg.

552. Bulgarian Salad

Preparation Time: 10 minutes
Cooking Time: 20 minutes
Servings: 2
Ingredients:
- 2 cups of bulgur
- 1 tablespoon of butter
- 1 cucumber, cut into pieces
- ¼ cup dill
- ¼ cup black olives, cut in half
- 1 tablespoon, 2 teaspoons of olive oil
- 4 cups of water
- 2 teaspoons of red wine vinegar
- salt to taste

Directions:
1. In a saucepan, toast the bulgur on a mixture of butter and olive oil. Leave to cook until the bulgur is golden brown and begins to crack.
2. Add water and season with salt. Wrap everything and simmer for about 20 minutes or until the bulgur is tender.
3. In a bowl, mix the cucumber pieces with the olive oil, dill, red wine vinegar and black olives. Mix everything well.
4. Combine cucumber and bulgur.

Nutrition:
Calories: 386, Fat: 14g, Carbohydrates: 55g, Protein: 9g, Sodium: 34mg, Potassium: 95mg.

553. Falafel Salad Bowl

Preparation Time: 15 minutes
Cooking Time: 5 minutes
Servings: 2
Ingredients:
- 1 tablespoon of chili garlic sauce
- 1 tablespoon of garlic and dill sauce
- 1 pack of vegetarian falafels
- 1 box of hummus
- 2 tablespoons of lemon juice
- 1 tablespoon of pitted kalamata olives
- 1 tablespoon of extra virgin olive oil
- ¼ cup onion, diced
- 2 cups of chopped parsley
- 2 cups of crisp pita
- 1 pinch of salt
- 1 tablespoon of tahini sauce

- ½ cup diced tomato

Directions:
1. Cook the prepared falafels. Put it aside. Prepare the salad. Mix the parsley, onion, tomato, lemon juice, olive oil and salt. Throw it all out and put everything aside.
2. Transfer everything to the serving bowls. Add the parsley and cover with hummus and falafel. Sprinkle bowl with tahini sauce, chili garlic sauce and dill sauce. Upon serving, add the lemon juice and mix the salad well. Serve with pita bread on the side.

Nutrition:
Calories: 561, Fat: 11g, Carbohydrates: 60.1g, Protein: 18.5g, Sodium: 43mg, Potassium: 96mg.

554. Easy Greek Salad

Preparation Time: 15 minutes
Cooking Time: 0 minutes
Servings: 2
Ingredients:
- 4 oz Greek feta cheese, cubed
- 5 cucumbers, cut lengthwise
- 1 teaspoon of honey
- 1 lemon, chewed and grated
- 1 cup kalamata olives, pitted and halved
- ¼ cup extra virgin olive oil
- 1 onion, sliced
- 1 teaspoon of oregano
- 1 pinch of fresh oregano (for garnish)
- 12 tomatoes, quartered
- ¼ cup red wine vinegar
- salt and pepper to taste

Directions:
1. In a bowl, soak the onions in salted water for 15 minutes. In a large bowl, combine the honey, lemon juice, lemon peel, oregano, salt and pepper.
2. Mix everything. Gradually add the olive oil, beating as you do until the oil emulsifies. Add the olives and tomatoes. Put it right. Add the cucumbers
3. Drain the onions soaked in salted water and add them to the salad mixture. Top the salad with fresh oregano and feta. Dash with olive oil and season with pepper to taste.

Nutrition:
Calories: 292, Fat: 17g, Carbohydrates: 12g, Protein: 6g,

Sodium: 49mg, Potassium: 60mg.

555. Arugula Salad with Figs and Walnuts

Preparation Time: 15 minutes
Cooking Time: 10 minutes
Servings: 2
Ingredients:
- 5 oz arugula
- 1 carrot, scraped
- 1/8 teaspoon of cayenne pepper
- 3 oz of goat cheese, crumbled
- 1 can salt-free chickpeas, drained
- ½ cup dried figs, cut into wedges
- 1 teaspoon of honey
- 3 tablespoons of olive oil
- 2 teaspoons of balsamic vinegar
- ½ walnuts cut in half
- salt to taste

Directions:
1. Preheat the oven to 175 degrees. In a baking dish, combine the nuts, 1 tablespoon of olive oil, cayenne pepper and 1/8 teaspoon of salt. Transfer the baking sheet to the oven and bake it until the nuts are golden. Set it aside when you are done.
2. In a bowl, incorporate the honey, balsamic vinegar, 2 tablespoons of oil and ¾ teaspoon of salt.
3. In a large bowl, combine the arugula, carrot and figs. Add nuts and goat cheese and drizzle with balsamic honey vinaigrette. Make sure you cover everything.

Nutrition:
Calories: 403, Fat: 9g, Carbohydrates: 35g, Protein: 13g, Sodium: 92mg, Potassium: 38mg.

556. Cauliflower Salad with Tahini Vinaigrette

Preparation Time: 15 minutes
Cooking Time: 5 minutes
Servings: 2
Ingredients:
- 1 ½ lb. of cauliflower
- ¼ cup of dried cherries
- 3 tablespoons of lemon juice
- 1 tablespoon of fresh mint, chopped

- 1 teaspoon of olive oil
- ½ cup chopped parsley
- 3 tablespoons of roasted salted pistachios, chopped
- ½ teaspoon of salt
- ¼ cup of shallot, chopped
- 2 tablespoons of tahini

Directions:
1. Grate the cauliflower in a microwave-safe container. Add olive oil and ¼ salt. Be sure to cover and season the cauliflower evenly. Wrap the bowl with plastic wrap and heat it in the microwave for about 3 minutes.
2. Put the rice with the cauliflower on a baking sheet and let cool for about 10 minutes. Add the lemon juice and the shallots. Let it rest to allow the cauliflower to absorb the flavor.
3. Add the mixture of tahini, cherries, parsley, mint and salt. Mix everything well. Sprinkle with roasted pistachios before serving.

Nutrition:
Calories: 165, Fat: 10g, Carbohydrates: 20g, Protein: 6g, Sodium: 40mg, Potassium: 84mg.

557. Mediterranean Potato Salad

Preparation Time: 15 minutes
Cooking Time: 10 minutes
Servings: 2
Ingredients:
- 1 bunch of basil leaves, torn
- 1 garlic clove, crushed
- 1 tablespoon of olive oil
- 1 onion, sliced
- 1 teaspoon of oregano
- 100 g of roasted red pepper. Slices
- 300g potatoes, cut in half
- 1 can of cherry tomatoes
- salt and pepper to taste

Directions:
1. Sauté the onions in a saucepan. Add oregano and garlic. Then cooks everything for one minute. Add the pepper and tomatoes. Season well, and simmer for about 10 minutes. Put that aside.
2. In a saucepan, boil the potatoes in salted water. Cook until tender, about 15 minutes. Drain well. Mix the potatoes with the sauce and add the basil and olives. Finally, throw everything away before serving.

Nutrition:
Calories: 111, Fat: 9g, Carbohydrates: 16g, Protein: 3g, Sodium: 59mg, Potassium: 75mg.

558. Quinoa and Pistachio Salad

Preparation Time: 10 minutes
Cooking Time: 15 minutes
Servings: 2
Ingredients:
- ¼ teaspoon of cumin
- ½ cup of dried currants
- 1 teaspoon grated lemon zest
- 2 tablespoons of lemon juice
- ½ cup green onions, chopped
- 1 tablespoon of chopped mint
- 2 tablespoons of extra virgin olive oil
- ¼ cup chopped parsley
- ¼ teaspoon ground pepper
- 1/3 cup pistachios, chopped
- 1 ¼ cups uncooked quinoa
- 1 2/3 cup of water

Directions:
1. In a saucepan, combine 1 2/3 cups of water, raisins and quinoa. Cook everything until boiling and then reduce the heat. Simmer everything for about 10 minutes and let the quinoa become frothy.
2. Set it aside for about 5 minutes. In a container, transfer the quinoa mixture. Add the nuts, mint, onions and parsley. Mix everything. In a separate bowl, incorporate the lemon zest, lemon juice, currants, cumin and oil. Beat them together. Mix the dry and wet ingredients.

Nutrition:
Calories: 248, Fat: 8g, Carbohydrates: 35g, Protein: 7g, Sodium: 63mg, Potassium: 94mg.

559. Cucumber Chicken Salad with Spicy Peanut Dressing

Preparation Time: 15 minutes
Cooking Time: 0 minutes
Servings: 2
Ingredients:
- 1/2 cup peanut butter

- 1 tablespoon sambal oelek (chili paste)
- 1 tablespoon low-sodium soy sauce
- 1 teaspoon grilled sesame oil
- 4 tablespoons of water, or more if necessary
- 1 cucumber with peeled and cut into thin strips
- 1 cooked chicken fillet, grated into thin strips
- 2 tablespoons chopped peanuts

Directions:
1. Combine peanut butter, soy sauce, sesame oil, sambal oelek, and water in a bowl. Place the cucumber slices on a dish. Garnish with grated chicken and sprinkle with sauce. Sprinkle the chopped peanuts.

Nutrition:
Calories: 720, Fat: 54g, Carbohydrates: 8.9g, Protein: 45.9g, Sodium: 54mg, Potassium: 95mg.

560. German Hot Potato Salad

Preparation Time: 10 minutes
Cooking Time: 30 minutes
Servings: 12
Ingredients:
- 9 peeled potatoes
- 6 slices of bacon
- 1/8 teaspoon ground black pepper
- 1/2 teaspoon celery seed
- 2 tablespoons white sugar
- 2 teaspoons salt
- 3/4 cup water
- 1/3 cup distilled white vinegar
- 2 tablespoons all-purpose flour
- 3/4 cup chopped onions

Directions:
1. Boil salted water in a large pot. Put in the potatoes and cook until soft but still firm, about 30 minutes. Drain, let cool and cut finely. Over medium heat, cook bacon in a pan. Drain, crumble and set aside. Save the cooking juices. Cook onions in bacon grease until golden brown.
2. Combine flour, sugar, salt, celery seed, and pepper in a small bowl. Add sautéed onions and cook, stirring until bubbling, and remove from heat. Stir in the water and vinegar, then bring back to the fire and bring to a boil, stirring constantly. Boil and stir. Slowly add bacon and potato slices to

the vinegar/water mixture, stirring gently until the potatoes are warmed up.

Nutrition:
Calories: 205, Fat: 6.5g, Carbohydrates: 32.9g, Protein: 4.3g, Sodium: 54mg, Potassium: 40mg.

561. Chicken Fiesta Salad

Preparation Time: 20 minutes
Cooking Time: 20 minutes
Servings: 4
Ingredients:
- 2 halves of chicken fillet without skin or bones
- 1 packet of herbs for fajitas, divided
- 1 tablespoon vegetable oil
- 1 can black beans, rinsed and drained
- 1 box of Mexican-style corn
- 1/2 cup of salsa
- 1 packet of green salad
- 1 onion, minced
- 1 tomato, quartered

Directions:
1. Rub the chicken evenly with 1/2 of the herbs for fajitas. Cook the oil in a frying pan over medium heat and cook the chicken for 8 minutes on the side by side or until the juice is clear; put aside.
2. Combine beans, corn, salsa, and other 1/2 fajita spices in a large pan. Heat over medium heat until lukewarm. Prepare the salad by mixing green vegetables, onion, and tomato. Cover the chicken salad and dress the beans and corn mixture.

Nutrition:
Calories: 311, Fat: 6.4g, Carbohydrates: 42.2g, Protein: 23g, Sodium: 47mg, Potassium: 96mg.

562. Corn & Black Bean Salad

Preparation Time: 10 minutes
Cooking Time: 0 minutes
Servings: 4
Ingredients:
- 2 tablespoons vegetable oil
- 1/4 cup balsamic vinegar
- 1/2 teaspoon of salt
- 1/2 teaspoon of white sugar
- 1/2 teaspoon ground cumin
- 1/2 teaspoon ground black pepper

- 1/2 teaspoon chili powder
- 3 tablespoons chopped fresh coriander
- 1 can black beans (15 oz)
- 1 can of sweetened corn (8.75 oz) drained

Directions:
1. Combine balsamic vinegar, oil, salt, sugar, black pepper, cumin and chili powder in a small bowl. Combine black corn and beans in a medium bowl.
2. Mix with vinegar and oil vinaigrette and garnish with coriander. Cover and refrigerate overnight.

Nutrition:
Calories: 214, Fat: 8.4g, Carbohydrates: 28.6g, Protein: 7.5g, Sodium: 57mg, Potassium: 60mg.

563. Awesome Pasta Salad

Preparation Time: 30 minutes
Cooking Time: 10 minutes
Servings: 16
Ingredients:
- 1 (16-oz) fusilli pasta package
- 3 cups of cherry tomatoes
- 1/2 pound of provolone, diced
- 1/2 pound of sausage, diced
- 1/4 pound of pepperoni, cut in half
- 1 large green pepper
- 1 can of black olives, drained
- 1 jar of chilis, drained
- 1 bottle (8 oz) Italian vinaigrette

Directions:
1. Bring lightly salted water to a boil in a saucepan. Add pasta and cook for 8 to 10 minutes or until al dente. Drain and rinse with cold water.
2. Combine pasta with tomatoes, cheese, salami, pepperoni, green pepper, olives, and peppers in a large bowl. Pour the vinaigrette and mix well.

Nutrition:
Calories: 310, Fat: 17.7g, Carbohydrates: 25.9g, Protein: 12.9g, Sodium: 86mg, Potassium: 53mg.

564. Tuna Salad

Preparation Time: 20 minutes
Cooking Time: 0 minutes
Servings: 4
Ingredients:
- 1 (19 ounce) can of garbanzo beans
- 2 tablespoons mayonnaise

- 2 teaspoons of spicy brown mustard
- 1 tablespoon sweet pickle
- Salt and pepper to taste
- 2 chopped green onions

Directions:
1. Combine green beans, mayonnaise, mustard, sauce, chopped green onions, salt and pepper in a medium bowl. Mix well.

Nutrition:
Calories: 220, Fat: 7.2g, Carbohydrates: 32.7g, Protein: 7g, Sodium: 53mg, Potassium: 95mg.

565. Southern Potato Salad

Preparation Time: 15 minutes
Cooking Time: 15 minutes
Servings: 4
Ingredients:
- 4 potatoes
- 4 eggs
- 1/2 stalk of celery, finely chopped
- 1/4 cup sweet taste
- 1 clove of garlic minced
- 2 tablespoons mustard
- 1/2 cup mayonnaise
- salt and pepper to taste

Directions:
1. Boil water in a saucepan and place the potatoes; cook them until they are soft but still firm, about 15 minutes; drain and chop them. Place the eggs in a saucepan and cover with cold water.
2. Bring the water to a boil; cover, remove from the heat and let the eggs soak in hot water for 10 minutes. Remove the shells and chop them.
3. Combine potatoes, eggs, celery, sweet sauce, garlic, mustard, mayonnaise, salt, and pepper in a large bowl. Mix and serve hot.

Nutrition:
Calories: 460, Fat: 27.4g, Carbohydrates: 44.6g, Protein: 11.3g, Sodium: 74mg, Potassium: 99mg.

566. Seven-Layer Salad

Preparation Time: 15 minutes
Cooking Time: 5 minutes
Servings: 10
Ingredients:
- 1-pound bacon

- 1 head iceberg lettuce
- 1 red onion, minced
- 1 pack of 10 frozen peas, thawed
- 10 oz grated cheddar cheese
- 1 cup chopped cauliflower
- 1 1/4 cup mayonnaise
- 2 tablespoons white sugar
- 2/3 cup grated Parmesan cheese

Directions:
1. Put the bacon in a huge, shallow frying pan. Bake over medium heat until smooth. Crumble and set aside. Place the chopped lettuce in a large bowl and cover it with a layer of onion, peas, grated cheese, cauliflower, and bacon.
2. Prepare the vinaigrette by mixing the mayonnaise, sugar, and parmesan cheese. Pour over the salad and cool to cool.

Nutrition:
Calories: 387, Fat: 32.7g, Carbohydrates: 9.9g, Protein: 14.5g, Sodium: 67mg, Potassium: 78mg.

567. Kale, Quinoa & Avocado Salad

Preparation Time: 5 minutes
Cooking Time: 25 minutes
Servings: 4
Ingredients:
- 2/3 cup of quinoa
- 1 1/3 cup of water
- 1 bunch of kale, torn into bite-sized pieces
- 1/2 avocado - peeled, diced and pitted
- 1/2 cup chopped cucumber
- 1/3 cup chopped red pepper
- 2 tablespoons chopped red onion
- 1 tablespoon of feta crumbled

Directions:
1. Boil the quinoa and 1 1/3 cup of water in a pan. Adjust heat and simmer until quinoa is tender and water is absorbed for about 15 to 20 minutes. Set aside to cool.
2. Place the cabbage in a steam basket over more than an inch of boiling water in a pan. Seal the pan with a lid and steam until hot, about 45 seconds; transfer to a large plate. Garnish with cabbage, quinoa, avocado, cucumber, pepper, red onion, and feta cheese.
3. Combine olive oil, lemon juice, Dijon mustard, sea salt, and

black pepper in a bowl until the oil is emulsified in the dressing, pour over the salad.

Nutrition:

Calories: 342, Fat: 20.3g, Carbohydrates: 35.4g, Protein: 8.9g, Sodium: 32mg, Potassium: 05mg.

568. Chicken Salad

Preparation Time: 20 minutes
Cooking Time: 0 minutes
Servings: 9
Ingredients:

- 1/2 cup mayonnaise
- 1/2 teaspoon of salt
- 3/4 teaspoon of poultry herbs
- 1 tablespoon lemon juice
- 3 cups cooked chicken breast, diced
- 1/4 teaspoon ground black pepper
- 1/4 teaspoon garlic powder
- 1/4 teaspoon onion powder
- 1/2 cup finely chopped celery
- 1 (8 oz) box of water chestnuts, drained and chopped
- 1/2 cup chopped green onions
- 1 1/2 cups green grapes cut in half
- 1 1/2 cups diced Swiss cheese

Directions:

1. Combine mayonnaise, salt, chicken spices, onion powder, garlic powder, pepper, and lemon juice in a medium bowl.
2. Combine chicken, celery, green onions, water chestnuts, Swiss cheese, and raisins in a big bowl. Stir in the mayonnaise mixture and coat. Cool until ready to serve.

Nutrition:

Calories: 293, Fat: 19.5g, Carbohydrates: 10.3g, Protein: 19.4g, Sodium: 45mg, Potassium: 96mg.

569. Cobb Salad

Preparation Time: 5 minutes
Cooking Time: 15 minutes
Servings: 6
Ingredients:

- 6 slices of bacon
- 3 eggs
- 1 cup Iceberg lettuce, grated
- 3 cups cooked minced chicken meat
- 2 tomatoes, seeded and minced
- 3/4 cup of blue cheese, crumbled

- 1 avocado - peeled, pitted and diced
- 3 green onions, minced
- 1 bottle (8 oz.) Ranch Vinaigrette

Directions:

1. Put the eggs in a pan and soak them completely with cold water. Boil the water. Cover and remove from heat and let the eggs rest in hot water for 10 to 12 minutes. Remove from hot water, let cool, peel, and chop. Place the bacon in a big, deep-frying pan. Bake over medium heat until smooth. Set aside.
2. Divide the grated lettuce into separate plates. Spread chicken, eggs, tomatoes, blue cheese, bacon, avocado, and green onions in rows on lettuce. Sprinkle with your favorite vinaigrette and enjoy.

Nutrition:

Calories: 525, Fat: 39.9g, Carbohydrates: 10.2g, Protein: 31.7g, Sodium: 54mg, Potassium: 99mg.

570. Broccoli Salad

Preparation Time: 10 minutes
Cooking Time: 15 minutes
Servings: 6
Ingredients:

- 10 slices of bacon
- 1 cup fresh broccoli
- ¼ cup red onion, minced
- ½ cup raisins
- 3 tablespoons white wine vinegar
- 2 tablespoons white sugar
- 1 cup mayonnaise
- 1 cup of sunflower seeds

Directions:

1. Cook the bacon in a deep-frying pan over medium heat. Drain, crumble and set aside. Combine broccoli, onion, and raisins in a medium bowl. Mix vinegar, sugar, and mayonnaise in a small bowl. Pour over the broccoli mixture and mix. Cool for at least two hours.
2. Before serving, mix the salad with crumbled bacon and sunflower seeds.

Nutrition:

Calories: 559, Fat: 48.1g, Carbohydrates: 31g, Protein: 18g, Sodium: 54mg, Potassium: 56mg.

571. Strawberry Spinach Salad

Preparation Time: 10 minutes
Cooking Time: 0 minutes
Servings: 4
Ingredients:

- 2 tablespoons sesame seeds
- 1 tablespoon poppy seeds
- 1/2 cup white sugar
- 1/2 cup olive oil
- 1/4 cup distilled white vinegar
- 1/4 teaspoon paprika
- 1/4 teaspoon Worcestershire sauce
- 1 tablespoon minced onion
- 10 ounces fresh spinach
- 1-quart strawberries - cleaned, hulled and sliced
- 1/4 cup almonds, blanched and slivered

Directions:

1. In a medium bowl, whisk the same seeds, poppy seeds, sugar, olive oil, vinegar, paprika, Worcestershire sauce, and onion. Cover, and chill for one hour.
2. In a large bowl, incorporate spinach, strawberries, and almonds. Drizzle dressing over salad and toss. Refrigerate 10 to 15 minutes before serving.

Nutrition:

Calories: 491, Fat: 35.2g, Carbohydrates: 42.9g, Protein: 6g, Sodium: 67mg, Potassium: 90mg.

572. Pear Salad with Roquefort Cheese

Preparation Time: 20 minutes
Cooking Time: 10 minutes
Servings: 2
Ingredients:

- 1 leaf lettuce, torn into bite-sized pieces
- 3 pears - peeled, cored and diced
- 5 ounces Roquefort, crumbled
- 1 avocado - peeled, seeded and diced
- 1/2 cup chopped green onions
- 1/4 cup white sugar
- 1/2 cup pecan nuts
- 1/3 cup olive oil
- 3 tablespoons red wine vinegar
- 1 1/2 teaspoon of white sugar
- 1 1/2 teaspoon of prepared mustard
- 1/2 teaspoon of salted black pepper
- 1 clove of garlic

Directions:

1. Stir in 1/4 cup of sugar with the pecans in a pan over medium heat. Continue stirring gently until the sugar caramelizes with the nuts. Cautiously transfer the nuts to wax paper. Let it chill and break into pieces.
2. Mix vinaigrette oil, marinade, 1 1/2 teaspoon of sugar, mustard, chopped garlic, salt, and pepper.
3. In a deep bowl, combine lettuce, pears, blue cheese, avocado, and green onions. Put vinaigrette over salad, sprinkle with pecans and serve.

Nutrition:

Calories: 426, Fat: 31.6g, Carbohydrates: 33.1g, Protein: 8g, Sodium: 34mg, Potassium: 23mg.

573. Mexican Bean Salad

Preparation Time: 15 minutes
Cooking Time: 0 minutes
Servings: 6
Ingredients:

- 1 can black beans (15 oz), drained
- 1 can red beans (15 oz), drained
- 1 can white beans (15 oz), drained
- 1 green pepper, minced
- 1 red pepper, minced
- 1 pack of frozen corn kernels
- 1 red onion, minced
- 2 tablespoons fresh lime juice
- 1/2 cup olive oil
- 1/2 cup red wine vinegar
- 1 tablespoon lemon juice
- 1 tablespoon salt
- 2 tablespoons white sugar
- 1 clove of crushed garlic
- 1/4 cup chopped coriander
- 1/2 tablespoon ground cumin
- 1/2 tablespoon ground black pepper
- 1 dash of hot pepper sauce
- 1/2 teaspoon chili powder

Directions:

1. Combine beans, peppers, frozen corn, and red onion in a large bowl. Combine olive oil, lime juice, red wine vinegar, lemon juice, sugar, salt, garlic, coriander, cumin, and black pepper in a small bowl — season with hot sauce and chili powder.
2. Pour the vinaigrette with olive oil over the vegetables; mix well. Cool well and serve cold.

Nutrition:

Calories: 334, Fat: 14.8g, Carbohydrates: 41.7g, Protein: 11.2g, Sodium: 200mg, Potassium: 43mg.

574. Melon-Mozzarella Salad

Preparation Time: 20 minutes
Cooking Time: 0 minutes
Servings: 6
Ingredients:

- ¼ teaspoon sea salt
- ¼ teaspoon black pepper
- 1 tablespoon balsamic vinegar
- 1 cantaloupe, quartered & seeded
- 12 watermelon, small & seedless
- 2 cups mozzarella balls, fresh
- 1/3 cup basil, fresh and torn
- 2 tbsp. olive oil

Directions:

1. Scrape out balls of cantaloupe and place them in a colander over a serving bowl. Use your melon baller to cut the watermelon as well, and then put them in with your cantaloupe.
2. Allow your fruit to drain for ten minutes, and then refrigerate the juice for another recipe. It can even be added to smoothies. Wipe the bowl dry, and then place your fruit in it.
3. Add in your basil, oil, vinegar, mozzarella and tomatoes before seasoning with salt and pepper. Gently mix and serve immediately or chilled.

Nutrition:

Calories: 219, Fat: 13g, Carbohydrates: 9g, Protein: 10g, Sodium: 125mg, Potassium: 876mg.

575. Citrus Celery Salad

Preparation Time: 15 minutes
Cooking Time: 0 minutes
Servings: 6
Ingredients:

- 1 tablespoon lemon juice, fresh
- ¼ teaspoon sea salt, fine
- ¼ teaspoon black pepper
- 1 tablespoon olive brine
- 1 tablespoon olive oil
- ¼ cup red onion, sliced
- ½ cup green olives
- 2 oranges, peeled & sliced

- 3 celery stalks, sliced diagonally in ½ inch slices

Directions:

1. Put your oranges, olives, onion and celery in a shallow bowl. In a different bowl, whisk your oil, olive brine and lemon juice, pour this over your salad. Season with salt and pepper before serving.

Nutrition:

Calories: 65, Fats: 7g, Carbohydrates: 9g, Protein: 2g, Sodium: 231mg, Potassium: 743mg.

576. Oven-Roasted Broccoli Salad

Preparation Time: 20 minutes
Cooking Time: 10 minutes
Servings: 4
Ingredients:

- 1 lb. broccoli, cut into florets & stem sliced
- 3 tablespoons olive oil, divided
- 1-pint cherry tomatoes
- 1 ½ teaspoons honey, raw & divided
- 3 cups cubed bread, whole grain
- 1 tablespoon balsamic vinegar
- ½ teaspoon black pepper
- ¼ teaspoon sea salt, fine
- grated parmesan for serving

Directions:

1. Prepare oven at 450 degrees, and then take out a rimmed baking sheet. Place it in the oven to heat. Drizzle your broccoli with a tablespoon of oil and toss to coat.
2. Remove the baking sheet from the oven and spoon the broccoli on it. Leave oil at the bottom of the bowl and add in your tomatoes, toss to coat, and then toss your tomatoes with a tablespoon of honey. Pour them on the same baking sheet as your broccoli.
3. Roast for fifteen minutes and stir halfway through your cooking time. Add in your bread, and then roast for three more minutes. Whisk two tablespoons of oil, vinegar, and remaining honey. Season with salt and pepper. Pour this over your broccoli mix to serve.

Nutrition:

Calories: 226, Fat: 12g, Carbohydrates: 26g, Protein: 7g,

Sodium: 210mg, Potassium: 324mg.

577. Sun-Dried Tomato Salad

Preparation Time: 20 minutes
Cooking Time: 0 minutes
Servings: 4
Ingredients:
- 1 cucumber, sliced
- ¼ cup sun-dried tomatoes, chopped
- 1 lb. tomatoes, cubed
- ½ cup black olives
- 1 red onion, sliced
- 1 tablespoon balsamic vinegar
- ¼ cup parsley, fresh and chopped
- 2 tablespoons olive oil
- sea salt and black pepper to taste

Directions:
1. Take out a bowl and combine all of your vegetables. To make your dressing, mix all your seasoning, olive oil and vinegar. Toss with your salad and serve fresh.

Nutrition:
Calories: 126, Fat: 9.2g, Carbohydrates: 11.5g, Protein: 2.1g, Sodium: 564mg, Potassium: 231mg.

578. Feta Cheese and Beet Salad

Preparation Time: 15 minutes
Cooking Time: 0 minutes
Servings: 4
Ingredients:
- 6 red beets, cooked & peeled
- 3 ounces feta cheese, cubed
- 2 tablespoons olive oil
- 2 tablespoons balsamic vinegar

Directions:
1. Combine everything, and then serve.

Nutrition:
Calories: 230, Fat: 12g, Carbohydrates: 26.3g, Protein: 7.3g, Sodium: 32mg, Potassium: 54mg.

579. Cauliflower-Tomato Salad

Preparation Time: 15 minutes
Cooking Time: 0 minutes
Servings: 4
Ingredients:

- 1 head cauliflower, chopped
- 2 tablespoons parsley, fresh and chopped
- 2 cups cherry tomatoes, halved
- 2 tablespoons lemon juice, fresh
- 2 tablespoons pine nuts
- sea salt and black pepper to taste

Directions:
1. Mix your lemon juice, cherry tomatoes, cauliflower and parsley together, and then season. Top with pine nuts and mix well before serving.

Nutrition:
Calories: 64, Fat: 3.3g, Carbohydrates: 7.9g, Protein: 2.8g, Sodium: 134mg, Potassium: 87mg.

580. Cheesy and Spiced Pilaf

Preparation Time: 20 minutes
Cooking Time: 10 minutes
Servings: 6
Ingredients:
- 2 cups yellow long grain rice, parboiled
- 1 cup onion
- 4 green onions
- 3 tablespoons butter
- 3 tablespoons vegetable broth
- 2 teaspoons cayenne pepper
- 1 teaspoon paprika
- ½ teaspoon cloves, minced
- 2 tablespoons mint leaves, fresh and chopped
- 1 bunch fresh mint leaves to garnish
- 1 tablespoon olive oil
- sea salt and black pepper to taste

Cheese Cream:
- 3 tablespoons olive oil
- sea salt and black pepper to taste
- 9 ounces cream cheese

Directions:
1. Ready the oven at 360 degrees, and then pull out a pan. Heat your butter and olive oil together and cook your onions and spring onions for two minutes.
2. Add in your salt, pepper, paprika, cloves, vegetable broth, rice and remaining seasoning. Sauté for three minutes. Wrap with foil and bake for another half hour. Allow it to cool.
3. Mix in the cream cheese, cheese, olive oil, salt and pepper. Serve

your pilaf garnished with fresh mint leaves.

Nutrition:
Calories: 364, Fat: 30g, Carbohydrates: 20g, Protein: 5g, Sodium: 156mg, Potassium: 187mg.

581. Oven-Roasted Vegetable Salad

Preparation Time: 10 minutes
Cooking Time: 20 minutes
Servings: 6
Ingredients:
- 1 red onion, sliced
- 2 tablespoons parsley, fresh and chopped
- 1 teaspoon thyme
- 2 cups cherry tomatoes, halved
- sea salt and black pepper to taste
- 1 teaspoon oregano
- 3 tablespoons olive oil
- 1 teaspoon basil
- 3 eggplants, peeled & cubed

Directions:
1. Start by heating your oven to 350F. Season your eggplant with basil, salt, pepper, oregano, thyme and olive oil. Put it on a baking tray and bake for a half hour. Toss with your remaining ingredients before serving.

Nutrition:
Calories: 148, Fat: 7.7g, Carbohydrates: 20.5g, Protein: 3.5g, Sodium: 543mg, Potassium: 98mg.

582. Herb-Roasted Vegetables

Preparation Time: 5 minutes
Cooking Time: 15 minutes
Servings: 12
Ingredients:
- 6 cloves garlic
- 6 tablespoons olive oil
- 1 fennel bulb, diced
- 1 zucchini, diced
- 2 red bell peppers, diced
- 6 potatoes, large and diced
- 2 teaspoons sea salt
- ½ cup balsamic vinegar
- ¼ cup rosemary, chopped and fresh
- 2 teaspoons vegetable bouillon powder

Directions:

1. Start by heating your oven to 400F. Put your potatoes, fennel, zucchini, garlic and fennel on a baking dish, drizzling with olive oil. Sprinkle with salt, bouillon powder, and rosemary. Mix well, and then bake at 450F for thirty to forty minutes. Mix your vinegar into the vegetables before serving.

Nutrition:

Calories: 675, Fat: 21g, Carbohydrates: 112g, Protein: 13g, Sodium: 575mg, Potassium: 98mg.

583. Cheesy Pistachio Salad

Preparation Time: 20 minutes
Cooking Time: 0 minutes
Servings: 6
Ingredients:

- 6 cups kale, chopped
- ¼ cup olive oil
- 2 tablespoons lemon juice, fresh
- ½ teaspoon smoked paprika
- 2 cups arugula
- 1/3 cup pistachios, unsalted and shelled
- 6 tablespoons parmesan cheese, grated

Directions:

1. Take out a salad bowl and combine your oil, lemon, smoked paprika and kale. Gently massage the leaves for half a minute. Your kale should be coated well. Gently mix your arugula and pistachios when ready to serve.

Nutrition:

Calories: 150, Fat: 12g, Carbohydrates: 8g, Protein: 5g, Sodium: 232mg, Potassium: 87mg.

584. Parmesan Barley Risotto

Preparation Time: 10 minutes
Cooking Time: 20 minutes
Servings: 6
Ingredients:

- 1 cup yellow onion, chopped
- 1 tablespoon olive oil
- 4 cups vegetable broth, low sodium
- 2 cups pearl barley, uncooked
- ½ cup dry white wine
- 1 cup parmesan cheese, grated fine & divided

- sea salt and black pepper to taste
- fresh chives, chopped for serving
- lemon wedges for serving

Directions:

1. Add your broth into a saucepan and bring it to a simmer over medium-high heat. Take out a stock pot and put it over medium-high heat as well. Heat your oil before adding in your onion. Cook for eight minutes and stir occasionally. Add in your barley and cook for two minutes more. Stir in your barley, cooking until it's toasted.

2. Pour in the wine, cooking for a minute more. Most of the liquid should have evaporated before adding in a cup of warm broth. Cook and stir for two minutes. Your liquid should be absorbed. Add in the remaining broth by the cup and cook until each cup is absorbed before adding more. It should take about two minutes each time.

3. Pull out from the heat. Add in half a cup of cheese, and top with remaining cheese, chives and lemon wedges.

Nutrition:

Calories: 345, Fat: 7g, Carbohydrates: 56g, Protein: 14g, Sodium: 32mg, Potassium: 98mg.

585. Seafood & Avocado Salad

Preparation Time: 10 minutes
Cooking Time: 0 minutes
Servings: 4
Ingredients:

- 2 lbs. salmon, cooked and chopped
- 2 lbs. shrimp, cooked and chopped
- 1 cup avocado, chopped
- 1 cup mayonnaise
- 4 tablespoons lime juice, fresh
- 2 cloves garlic
- 1 cup sour cream
- sea salt and black pepper to taste
- ½ red onion, minced
- 1 cup cucumber, chopped

Directions:

1. Start by getting out a bowl and combine your garlic, salt, pepper, onion, mayonnaise, sour cream and lime juice,

2. Take out a different bowl and mix your salmon, shrimp, cucumber, and avocado.

3. Add the mayonnaise mixture to your shrimp, and then allow it to sit for twenty minutes in the fridge before serving.

Nutrition:

Calories: 394, Fat: 30g, Carbohydrates: 3g, Protein: 27g, Sodium: 76mg, Potassium: 09mg.

586. Mediterranean Shrimp Salad

Preparation Time: 40 minutes
Cooking Time: 0 minutes
Servings: 6
Ingredients:

- 1 ½ lbs. shrimp, cleaned & cooked
- 2 celery stalks, fresh
- 1 onion
- 2 green onions
- 4 eggs, boiled
- 3 potatoes, cooked
- 3 tablespoons mayonnaise
- sea salt and black pepper to taste

Directions:

1. Start by slicing your potatoes and chopping your celery. Slice your eggs and season. Mix everything. Put your shrimp over the eggs, and then serve with onion and green onions.

Nutrition:

Calories: 207, Fat: 6g, Carbohydrates: 15g, Protein: 17g, Sodium: 43mg, Potassium: 56mg.

587. Chickpea Pasta Salad

Preparation Time: 10 minutes
Cooking Time: 15 minutes
Servings: 6
Ingredients:

- 2 tablespoons olive oil
- 16 ounces rotelle pasta
- ½ cup cured olives, chopped
- 2 tablespoons oregano, fresh and minced
- 2 tablespoons parsley, fresh and chopped
- 1 bunch green onions, chopped
- ¼ cup red wine vinegar
- 15 ounces canned garbanzo beans, drained and rinsed
- ½ cup parmesan cheese, grated
- sea salt and black pepper to taste

Directions:

1. Boil water and put the pasta al dente and follow per package instructions. Drain it and rinse it using cold water.
2. Take out a skillet and heat your olive oil over medium heat. Add in your scallions, chickpeas, parsley, oregano and olives. Lower the heat, and sauté for twenty minutes more. Allow this mixture to cool.
3. Toss your chickpea mixture with your pasta, and then add in your grated cheese, salt, pepper and vinegar. Let it chill for four hours or overnight before serving.

Nutrition:
Calories: 424, Fat: 10g, Carbohydrates: 69g, Protein: 16g, Sodium: 320mg, Potassium: 187mg.

588. Mediterranean Stir Fry

Preparation Time: 10 minutes
Cooking Time: 30 minutes
Servings: 4
Ingredients:

- 2 zucchinis
- 1 onion
- ¼ teaspoon sea salt
- 2 cloves garlic
- 3 teaspoons olive oil, divided
- 1 lb. chicken breasts, boneless
- 1 cup quick cooking barley
- 2 cups water
- ¼ teaspoon black pepper
- 1 teaspoon oregano
- ¼ teaspoon red pepper flakes
- ½ teaspoon basil
- 2 plum tomatoes
- ½ cup Greek olives, pitted
- 1 tablespoon parsley, fresh

Directions:

1. Start by removing the skin from your chicken, and then chop it into smaller pieces. Chop the garlic and parsley, and then chop your olives, zucchini, tomatoes and onions. Take out a saucepan and bring your water to a boil. Mix in your barley, letting it simmer for eight to ten minutes.
2. Turn off the heat. Let it rest for five minutes. Take out a skillet and add in two teaspoons of olive oil. Stir fry your chicken once it's hot, and then remove it from heat. Cook the onion in your remaining oil. Mix in your

remaining ingredients and cook for an additional three to five minutes. Serve warm.

Nutrition:
Calories: 337, Fat: 8.6g, Carbohydrates: 32.3g, Protein: 31.7g, Sodium: 231mg, Potassium: 218mg.

589. Balsamic Cucumber Salad

Preparation Time: 15 minutes
Cooking Time: 0 minutes
Servings: 4
Ingredients:

- 2/3 large English cucumber, halved and sliced
- 2/3 medium red onion, halved and thinly sliced
- 5 1/2 tablespoons balsamic vinaigrette
- 1 1/3 cups grape tomatoes, halved
- 1/2 cup crumbled reduced-fat feta cheese

Directions:

1. In a big bowl, mix cucumber, tomatoes and onion. Add vinaigrette; toss to coating. Refrigerate, covered, till serving. Just before serving, stir in cheese. Serve with a slotted teaspoon.

Nutrition:
Calories: 250, Fats: 12g, Carbohydrates: 15g, Protein: 34g, Sodium: 95mg, Potassium: 65mg.

590. Beef Kefta Patties with Cucumber Salad

Preparation Time: 10 minutes
Cooking Time: 15 minutes
Servings: 2
Ingredients:

- Cooking spray
- 1/2-pound ground sirloin
- 2 tablespoons plus 2 tablespoons chopped fresh flat-leaf parsley, divided
- 1 1/2 teaspoons chopped peeled fresh ginger
- 1 teaspoon ground coriander
- 2 tablespoons chopped fresh cilantro
- 1/4 teaspoon salt

- 1/2 teaspoon ground cumin
- 1/4 teaspoon ground cinnamon
- 1 cup thinly sliced English cucumbers
- 1 tablespoon rice vinegar
- 1/4 cup plain fat-free Greek yogurt
- 1 1/2 teaspoons fresh lemon juice
- 1/4 teaspoon freshly ground black pepper
- 1 (6-inch) pitas, quartered

Directions:

1. Heat a grill skillet over medium-high heat. Coat pan with cooking spray. Combine beef, 1/4 glass parsley, cilantro, and the next 5 elements in a medium bowl.
2. Divide combination into 4 the same portions, shaping each into a 1/2-inch-thick patty. Add patties to pan; cook both sides until the desired degree of doneness.
3. Mix cucumber and vinegar in a medium bowl; toss well. Combine fat-free yogurt, remaining 2 tablespoons parsley, juice, and pepper in a little bowl; stir with a whisk. Set up 1 patty and 1/2 cup cucumber mixture on each of 4 portions.
4. Top each offering with about 2 tablespoons of yogurt spices. Serve each with 2 pita wedges.

Nutrition:
Calories: 116, Fats: 5g, Carbohydrates: 11g, Protein: 28g, Sodium: 36mg, Potassium: 97mg.

591. Chicken and Cucumber Salad with Parsley Pesto

Preparation Time: 15 minutes
Cooking Time: 5 minutes
Servings: 8
Ingredients:

- 2 2/3 cups packed fresh flat-leaf parsley leaves
- 1 1/3 cups fresh baby spinach
- 1 1/2 tablespoons toasted pine nuts
- 1 1/2 tablespoons grated Parmesan cheese
- 2 1/2 tablespoons fresh lemon juice
- 1 1/3 teaspoons kosher salt
- 1/3 teaspoon black pepper

- 1 1/3 medium garlic cloves, smashed
- 2/3 cup extra-virgin olive oil
- 5 1/3 cups shredded rotisserie chicken (from 1 chicken)
- 2 2/3 cups cooked shelled edamame
- 1 1/2 cans 1 (15-oz.) unsalted chickpeas, drained and rinsed
- 1 1/3 cups chopped English cucumbers
- 5 1/3 cups loosely packed arugula

Directions:
1. Combine parsley, spinach, lemon juice, pine nuts, cheese, garlic, salt, and pepper in a food processor; process for about 1 minute. With processor running, add oil; process until smooth, about 1 minute.
2. Stir together chicken, edamame, chickpeas, and cucumber in a large bowl. Add pesto; toss to combine.
3. Place 2/3 cup arugula in each of 6 bowls; top each with 1 cup chicken salad mixture. Serve immediately.

Nutrition:
Calories: 116, Fats: 12g, Carbohydrates: 3g, Protein: 9g, Sodium: 54mg, Potassium: 99mg.

592. Easy Arugula Salad

Preparation Time: 15 minutes
Cooking Time: 0 minutes
Servings: 6
Ingredients:
- 6 cups young arugula leaves, rinsed and dried
- 1 1/2 cups cherry tomatoes, halved
- 6 tablespoons pine nuts
- 3 tablespoons grapeseed oil or olive oil
- 1 1/2 tablespoons rice vinegar
- 3/8 teaspoon freshly ground black pepper to taste
- 6 tablespoons grated Parmesan cheese
- 3/4 teaspoon salt to taste
- 1 1/2 large avocados - peeled, pitted and sliced

Directions:
1. In a sizable plastic dish with a cover, incorporate arugula, cherry tomatoes, pine nut products, oil, vinegar, and Parmesan cheese. Season with

salt and pepper to flavor. Cover, and wring to mix.
2. Separate salad onto portions, and top with slices of avocado.

Nutrition:
Calories: 120, Fats: 12g, Carbohydrates: 14g, Protein: 25g, Sodium: 90mg, Potassium: 43mg.

593. Feta Garbanzo Bean Salad

Preparation Time: 10 minutes
Cooking Time: 0 minutes
Servings: 6
Ingredients:
- 1 1/2 cans (15 ounces) garbanzo beans
- 1 1/2 cans (2-1/4 ounces) sliced ripe olives, drained
- 1 1/2 medium tomatoes
- 6 tablespoons thinly sliced red onions
- 2 1/4 cups 1-1/2 coarsely chopped English cucumbers
- 6 tablespoons chopped fresh parsley
- 4 1/2 tablespoons olive oil
- 3/8 teaspoon salt
- 1 1/2 tablespoons lemon juice
- 3/16 teaspoon pepper
- 7 1/2 cups mixed salad greens
- 3/4 cup crumbled feta cheese

Directions:
1. Transfer all ingredients to a big bowl; toss to combine. Add parmesan cheese.

Nutrition:
Calories: 140, Fats: 16g, Carbohydrates: 10g, Protein: 24g, Sodium: 34mg, Potassium: 67mg.

594. Greek Brown and Wild Rice Bowls

Preparation Time: 15 minutes
Cooking Time: 5 minutes
Servings: 4
Ingredients:
- 2 packages (8-1/2 ounces) ready-to-serve whole grain brown and wild rice medley
- 1 medium ripe avocado, peeled and sliced
- 1 1/2 cups cherry tomatoes, halved
- 1/2 cup Greek vinaigrette, divided

- 1/2 cup crumbled feta cheese
- 1/2 cup pitted Greek olives, sliced
- minced fresh parsley, optional

Directions:
1. Inside a microwave-safe dish, mix the grain mix and 2 tablespoons vinaigrette. Cover and cook on High until warmed through, about 2 minutes. Divide between 2 bowls. Best with avocado, tomato vegetables, cheese, olives, leftover dressing and, if desired, parsley.

Nutrition:
Calories: 116, Fats: 10g, Carbohydrates: 9g, Protein: 26g, Sodium: 76mg, Potassium: 89mg.

595. Greek Dinner Salad

Preparation Time: 10 minutes
Cooking Time: 0 minutes
Servings: 4
Ingredients:
- 2 1/2 tablespoons coarsely chopped fresh parsley
- 2 tablespoons coarsely chopped fresh dill
- 2 teaspoons fresh lemon juice
- 2/3 teaspoon dried oregano
- 2 teaspoons extra virgin olive oil
- 4 cups shredded Romaine lettuce
- 2/3 cup thinly sliced red onions
- 1/2 cup crumbled feta cheese
- 2 cups diced tomatoes
- 2 teaspoons capers
- 2/3 cucumber, peeled, quartered lengthwise, and thinly sliced
- 2/3 (19-ounce) can chickpeas, drained and rinsed
- 4 (6-inch) whole wheat pitas, each cut into 8 wedges

Directions:
1. Combine the first 5 substances in a big dish; stir with a whisk. Add a member of the lettuce family and the next 6 ingredients (lettuce through chickpeas); toss well. Serve with pita wedges.

Nutrition:
Calories: 103, Fats: 12g, Carbohydrates: 8g, Protein: 36g, Sodium: 143mg, Potassium: 98mg.

596. Halibut Salad

Preparation Time: 15 minutes
Cooking Time: 5 minutes
Servings: 2
Ingredients:

- 1/2 teaspoon ground coriander
- 1/4 teaspoon salt
- 1/8 teaspoon freshly ground black pepper
- 2 1/2 teaspoons extra-virgin olive oils, divided
- 1/4 teaspoon ground cumin
- 1 garlic clove, minced
- 2 (6-ounce) halibut fillets
- 1 cup fennel bulb
- 2 tablespoons thinly vertically sliced red onions
- 1 tablespoon fresh lemon juice
- 1 1/2 teaspoons chopped flat-leaf parsley
- 1/2 teaspoon fresh thyme leaves

Directions:

1. Combine the first 4 substances in a little dish. Combine 1/2 teaspoon of spice mixture, 2 teaspoons oil, and garlic in a little bowl; rub garlic clove mixture evenly over fish. Heat 1 teaspoon of oil in a sizable nonstick frying pan over medium-high flame. Add fish to pan; cook 5 minutes on each side or until the desired level of doneness.
2. Combine remaining 3/4 teaspoon of spice mix, remaining 2 teaspoons of oil, fennel light bulb, and remaining substances in a medium bowl, tossing well to coat. Provide salad with seafood.

Nutrition:

Calories: 110, Fats: 9g, Carbohydrates: 11g, Protein: 29g, Sodium: 123mg, Potassium: 76mg.

597. Herbed Greek Chicken Salad

Preparation Time: 10 minutes
Cooking Time: 10 minutes
Servings: 2
Ingredients:

- 1/2 teaspoon dried oregano
- 1/4 teaspoon garlic powder
- 3/8 teaspoon black pepper, divided
- cooking spray
- 1/2-pound skinless, boneless chicken breasts, cut into 1-inch cubes
- 1/4 teaspoon salt, divided
- 1/2 cup plain fat-free yogurt
- 1 teaspoon tahini (sesame-seed paste)
- 2 1/2 tsp. fresh lemon juice
- 1/2 teaspoon bottled minced garlic
- 4 cups chopped Romaine lettuce
- 1/2 cup peeled chopped English cucumbers
- 1/2 cup grape tomatoes, halved
- 3 pitted kalamata olives, halved
- 2 tablespoons (1 ounce) crumbled feta cheese

Directions:

1. Combine oregano, natural garlic powder, 1/2 teaspoon of pepper and 1/4 teaspoon of salt in a bowl. Heat a nonstick skillet over medium-high heat. Coat the pan with cooking spray. Add poultry and spice combination; sauté until poultry is done. Drizzle with 1 teaspoon juice; stir. Remove from skillet.
2. Combine remaining 2 teaspoons of juice, remaining 1/4 teaspoon of sodium, remaining 1/4 teaspoon of pepper, yogurt, tahini and garlic in a small bowl; mix well. Combine lettuce, cucumber, tomatoes and olives. Place 2 1/2 cups of the lettuce mixture on each of 4 plates. Top each serving with 1/2 cup of the chicken combination and 1 teaspoon of the cheese. Drizzle each serving with 3 tablespoons yogurt combination.

Nutrition:

Calories: 116, Fats: 11g, Carbohydrates: 15g, Protein: 28g, Sodium: 98mg, Potassium: 123mg.

598. Greek Couscous Salad

Preparation Time: 10 minutes
Cooking Time: 15 minutes
Servings: 10
Ingredients:

- 1 can (14-1/2 ounces) reduced-sodium chicken broth
- 1 1/2 cups 1-3/4 uncooked whole wheat couscous (about 11 ounces)

Dressing:

- 6 1/2 tablespoons olive oil
- 1 1/4 teaspoons 1-1/2 grated lemon zest
- 3 1/2 tablespoons lemon juice
- 13/16 teaspoon adobo seasonings
- 3/16 teaspoon salt

Salad:

- 1 2/3 cups grape tomatoes, halved
- 5/6 English cucumber, halved lengthwise and sliced
- 3/4 cup coarsely chopped fresh parsley
- 1 can (6-1/2 ounces) sliced ripe olives, drained
- 6 1/2 tablespoons crumbled feta cheese
- 3 1/3 green onions, chopped

Directions:

1. In a big saucepan, bring broth to a boil. Stir in couscous. Remove from heat; let stand, covered, until broth is absorbed, about 5 minutes. Transfer to a big dish; cool completely.
2. Beat together dressing substances. Add cucumber, tomato vegetables, parsley, olives and green onions to couscous; stir in dressing. Gently mix in cheese. Provide immediately or refrigerate and serve frosty.

Nutrition:

Calories: 114, Fats: 13g, Carbohydrates: 18g, Protein: 27g, Sodium: 54mg, Potassium: 88mg.

Chapter 13. Soup

599. Chicken Wild Rice Soup

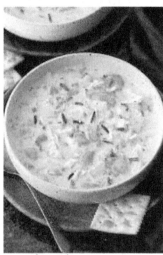

Preparation Time: 10 minutes
Cooking Time: 15 minutes
Servings: 6
Ingredients:
- 2/3 cup wild rice, uncooked
- 1 tablespoon onion, chopped finely
- 1 tablespoon fresh parsley, chopped
- 1 cup carrots, chopped
- 8-ounces chicken breast, cooked
- 2 tablespoon butter
- 1/4 cup all-purpose white flour
- 5 cups low-sodium chicken broth
- 1 tablespoon slivered almonds

Directions:
1. Start by adding rice and 2 cups of broth along with ½ cup of water to a cooking pot. Cook the chicken until the rice is al dente and set it aside. Add butter to a saucepan and melt it.
2. Stir in onion and sauté until soft, then add the flour and the remaining broth.
3. Stir it and then cook for it 1 minute, then add the chicken, cooked rice, and carrots. Cook for 5 minutes on simmer. Garnish with almonds. Serve fresh.

Nutrition:
Calories: 287, Protein: 21g, Fat: 35g, Sodium: 54mg, Potassium: 76mg.

600. Classic Chicken Soup

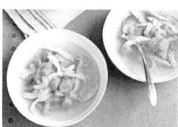

Preparation Time: 10 minutes
Cooking Time: 25 minutes
Servings: 2
Ingredients:
- 1 1/2 cups low-sodium vegetable broth
- 1 cup of water
- 1/4 teaspoon poultry seasoning
- 1/4 teaspoon black pepper
- 1 cup chicken strips
- 1/4 cup carrot
- 2-ounces egg noodles, uncooked

Directions:
1. Gather all the ingredients into a slow cooker and toss it. Cook soup on high heat for 25 minutes.
2. Serve warm.

Nutrition:
Calories: 103, Protein: 8g, Fat: 11g, Sodium: 89mg, Potassium: 44mg.

601. Cucumber Soup

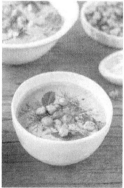

Preparation Time: 10 minutes
Cooking Time: 0 minutes
Servings: 4
Ingredients:
- 2 medium cucumbers

- 1/3 cup sweet white onion
- 1 green onion
- 1/4 cup fresh mint
- 2 tablespoons fresh dill
- 2 tablespoons lemon juice
- 2/3 cup water
- 1/2 cup half and half cream
- 1/3 cup sour cream
- 1/2 teaspoon pepper
- Fresh dill sprigs for garnish

Directions:
1. Situate all the ingredients into a food processor and toss. Puree the mixture and refrigerate for 2 hours. Garnish with dill sprigs. Enjoy fresh.

Nutrition:
Calories: 77, Protein: 2g, Fats: 6g, Sodium: 32mg, Potassium: 80mg.

602. Squash and Turmeric Soup

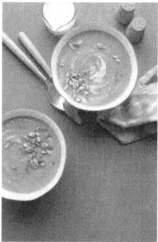

Preparation Time: 10 minutes
Cooking Time: 30 minutes
Servings: 4
Ingredients:
- 4 cups low-sodium vegetable broth
- 2 medium zucchini squash
- 2 medium yellow crookneck squash
- 1 small onion
- 1/2 cup frozen green peas
- 2 tablespoons olive oil
- 1/2 cup plain nonfat Greek yogurt
- 2 teaspoon turmeric

Directions:

1. Warm the broth in a saucepan on medium heat. Toss in onion, squash, and zucchini. Let it simmer for approximately 25 minutes, then add oil and green peas.
2. Cook for another 5 minutes and then allow it to cool. Puree the soup using a handheld blender, then add Greek yogurt and turmeric. Refrigerate it overnight and serve fresh.

Nutrition:
Calories: 100, Protein: 4g, Fat: 10g, Sodium: 45mg, Potassium: 90mg.

603. Leek, Potato, and Carrot Soup

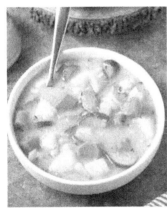

Preparation Time: 15 minutes
Cooking Time: 25 minutes
Servings: 4
Ingredients:
- 1 leek
- ¾ cup diced and boiled potatoes
- ¾ cup diced and boiled carrots
- 1 garlic clove
- 1 tablespoon oil
- Crushed pepper to taste
- 3 cups low sodium chicken stock
- Chopped parsley for garnish
- 1 bay leaf
- ¼ teaspoon ground cumin

Directions:
1. Trim and remove a part of the thick portions of the leek, then delicately reduce and rinse everything in water.
2. Heat the oil in a large pot. Include the leek and garlic, and brown over low heat for two to three minutes, until tender.
3. Add the stock, bay leaf, cumin and pepper. Heat the mixture, stirring constantly. Add the potatoes and carrots and cook

for 10-15 minutes. Modify the taste, remove the bay leaf and serve sprinkled generously with chopped parsley.
4. To make a pureed soup, manner the soup in a blender or nourishment processor till smooth. Come again to the pan. Include milk. Bring to boil and stew for 2-3 minutes.

Nutrition:
Calories: 315, Fat: 8g, Protein: 15g, Sodium: 59mg, Potassium: 56mg.

604. Bell Pepper Soup

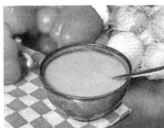

Preparation Time: 30 minutes
Cooking Time: 35 minutes
Servings: 4
Ingredients:
- 4 cups low-sodium chicken broth
- 3 red peppers
- 2 medium onions
- 3 tablespoon lemon juice
- 1 tablespoon finely minced lemon zest
- A pinch cayenne peppers
- ¼ teaspoon cinnamon
- ½ cup finely minced fresh cilantro

Directions:
1. In a medium saucepan, combine all ingredients except cilantro and heat to boiling point over high heat.
2. Reduce the heat and stew, usually under cover, for about 30 minutes, until thickened. Cool slightly. Using a hand blender or food processor, puree the soup. Stir in the cilantro and heat through.

Nutrition:
Calories: 265, Fat: 8g, Protein: 5g, Sodium: 45mg, Potassium: 80mg.

605. Yucatan Soup

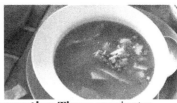

Preparation Time: 10 minutes
Cooking Time: 20 minutes
Servings: 4
Ingredients:
- ½ cup onion, chopped
- 8 cloves garlic, chopped
- 2 Serrano chili peppers, chopped
- 1 medium tomato, chopped
- 1 ½ cups chicken breast, cooked, shredded
- 2 six-inch corn tortillas, sliced
- 1 tablespoon olive oil
- 4 cups chicken broth
- 1 bay leaf
- ¼ cup lime juice
- ¼ cup cilantro, chopped
- 1 teaspoon black pepper

Directions:
1. Spread the corn tortillas on a baking sheet and bake them for 3 minutes at 400°F. Place a suitably-sized saucepan over medium heat and add oil to heat.
2. Toss in chili peppers, garlic, and onion, then sauté until soft. Stir in broth, tomatoes, bay leaf, and chicken.
3. Let this chicken soup cook for 10 minutes on a simmer. Stir in cilantro, lime juice, and black pepper. Garnish with baked corn tortillas. Serve.

Nutrition:
Calories: 215, Protein: 21g, Fat: 32g, Sodium: 56mg, Potassium: 98mg.

606. Zesty Taco Soup

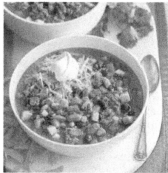

Preparation Time: 10 minutes
Cooking Time: 7 hours
Servings: 2
Ingredients:
- 1 ½ pounds chicken breast
- 15 ½ ounces canned dark red kidney beans
- 15 ½ ounces canned white corn
- 1 cup canned tomatoes
- ½ cup onion
- 15 ½ ounces canned yellow hominy
- ½ cup green bell peppers
- 1 garlic clove
- 1 medium jalapeno
- 1 tablespoon package McCormick
- 2 cups chicken broth

Directions:
1. Add drained beans, hominy, corn, onion, garlic, jalapeno pepper, chicken, and green peppers to a Crockpot.
2. Cover the beans-corn mixture and cook for 1 hour at "high" temperature. Set heat to "low" and continue cooking for 6 hours. Shred the slow-cooked chicken and return to the taco soup. Serve warm.

Nutrition:
Calories: 191, Protein: 21g, Fat: 20g, Sodium: 34mg, Potassium: 54mg.

607. Southwestern Posole

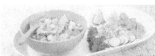

Preparation Time: 10 minutes
Cooking Time: 53 minutes
Servings: 4
Ingredients:
- 1 tablespoon olive oil

- 1-pound pork loin, diced
- ½ cup onion, chopped
- 1 garlic clove, chopped
- 28 ounces canned white hominy
- 4 ounces canned diced green chilis
- 4 cups chicken broth
- ¼ teaspoon black pepper

Directions:
1. Place a suitably-sized cooking pot over medium heat and add oil to heat. Toss in pork pieces and sauté for 4 minutes.
2. Stir in garlic and onion, then stir for 4 minutes, or until onion is soft. Add the remaining ingredients, then cover the pork soup. Cook this for 45 minutes or until the pork is tender. Serve warm.

Nutrition:
Calories: 286, Protein: 25g, Fat: 15g, Sodium: 90mg, Potassium: 76mg.

608. Spring Vegetable Soup

Preparation Time: 10 minutes
Cooking Time: 45 minutes
Servings: 4
Ingredients:
- 1 cup fresh green beans
- ¾ cup celery
- ½ cup onion
- ½ cup carrots
- ½ cup mushrooms
- ½ cup of frozen corn
- 1 medium Roma tomato
- 2 tablespoons olive oil
- ½ cup of frozen corn
- 4 cups vegetable broth
- 1 teaspoon dried oregano leaves
- 1 teaspoon garlic powder

Directions:
1. Place a suitably-sized cooking pot over medium heat and add olive oil to heat. Toss in onion and celery, then sauté until soft. Stir in the corn and rest of the ingredients and cook the soup to boil.
2. Now reduce its heat to a simmer and cook for 45 minutes. Serve warm.

Nutrition:
Calories: 115, Protein: 3g, Fat 13g, Sodium: 43mg, Potassium: 87mg.

609. Seafood Corn Chowder

Preparation Time: 10 minutes
Cooking Time: 12 minutes
Servings: 4
Ingredients:
- 1 tablespoon butter
- 1 cup onion
- 1/3 cup celery
- ½ cup green bell pepper
- ½ cup red bell pepper
- 1 tablespoon white flour
- 14 ounces chicken broth
- 2 cups cream
- 6 ounces evaporated milk
- 10 ounces surimi imitation crab chunks
- 2 cups frozen corn kernels
- ½ teaspoon black pepper
- ½ teaspoon paprika

Directions:
1. Place a suitably-sized saucepan over medium heat and add butter to melt. Toss in onion, green and red peppers, and celery, then sauté for 5 minutes. Stir in flour and whisk well for 2 minutes.
2. Pour in chicken broth and stir until it boils. Add evaporated milk, corn, surimi crab, paprika, black pepper, and creamer. Cook for 5 minutes and serve warm.

Nutrition:
Calories: 175, Protein: 8g, Fat 7g, Sodium: 56mg, Potassium: 89mg.

610. Beef Sage Soup

Preparation Time: 10 minutes
Cooking Time: 20 minutes
Servings: 4
Ingredients:
- ½ pound ground beef
- ½ teaspoon ground sage
- ½ teaspoon black pepper
- ½ teaspoon dried basil
- ½ teaspoon garlic powder
- 4 slices bread, cubed
- 2 tablespoons olive oil
- 1 tablespoon herb seasoning blend
- 2 garlic cloves, minced
- 3 cups chicken broth
- 1 ½ cups water
- 4 tablespoons fresh parsley
- 2 tablespoons parmesan cheese

Directions:
1. Preheat your oven to 375°F. Mix beef with sage, basil, black

pepper, and garlic powder in a bowl, then set it aside. Throw in the bread cubes with olive oil on a baking sheet and bake them for 8 minutes.

2. Meanwhile, sauté the beef mixture in a greased cooking pot until it is browned. Stir in garlic and sauté for 2 minutes, then add parsley, water, and broth. Cover the beef soup and cook for 10 minutes on a simmer. Garnish the soup with parmesan cheese and baked bread. Serve warm.

Nutrition:
Calories: 336, Protein: 26g, Fat: 16g, Sodium: 67mg, Potassium: 98mg.

611. Cabbage Borscht

Preparation Time: 10 minutes
Cooking Time: 90 minutes
Servings: 6
Ingredients:
- 2 pounds beef steaks
- 6 cups cold water
- 2 tablespoons olive oil
- ½ cup tomato sauce
- 1 medium cabbage, chopped
- 1 cup onion, diced
- 1 cup carrots, diced
- 1 cup turnips, peeled and diced
- 1 teaspoon pepper
- 6 tablespoons lemon juice
- 4 tablespoons sugar

Directions:
1. Start by placing steak in a large cooking pot and pour enough water to cover it. Cover the beef pot and cook it on a simmer until it is tender, then shred it using a fork. Add olive oil, onion, tomato sauce, carrots, turnips, and shredded steak to the cooking liquid in the pot.
2. Stir in black pepper, sugar, and lemon juice to season the soup. Cover the cabbage soup and cook on low heat for 1 ½ hour. Serve warm.

Nutrition:
Calories: 212, Protein: 19g, Fat: 10g, Sodium: 43mg, Potassium: 45mg.

612. Ground Beef Soup

Preparation Time: 10 minutes
Cooking Time: 30 minutes
Servings: 4

Ingredients:
- 1-pound lean ground beef
- ½ cup onion, chopped
- 2 teaspoons lemon-pepper seasoning blend
- 1 cup beef broth
- 2 cups of water
- 1/3 cup white rice, uncooked
- 3 cups of frozen mixed vegetables
- 1 tablespoon sour cream

Directions:
1. Spray a saucepan with cooking oil and place it over medium heat. Toss in onion and ground beef, then sauté until brown. Stir in broth and the rest of the ingredients, then boil it.
2. Reduce heat to a simmer, then cover the soup to cook for 30 minutes. Garnish with sour cream. Enjoy.

Nutrition:
Calories: 223, Protein: 20g, Fat: 20g, Sodium: 56mg, Potassium: 88mg.

613. Mexican Tortilla Soup

Preparation Time: 7 minutes
Cooking Time: 40 minutes
Servings: 4
Ingredients:
- 1-pound chicken breasts
- 1 can (15 ounces) whole peeled tomatoes
- 1 can (10 ounces) red enchilada sauce
- 1 and 1/2 teaspoons minced garlic
- 1 yellow onion, diced
- 1 can (4 ounces) fire-roasted diced green chili
- 1 can (15 ounces) black beans
- 1 can (15 ounces) fire-roasted corn
- 1 container (32 ounces) chicken stock
- 1 teaspoon ground cumin
- 2 teaspoons chili powder
- 3/4 teaspoons paprika
- 1 bay leaf
- 1 tablespoon chopped cilantro

Directions:
1. Set your Instant Pot on Sauté mode.
2. Toss olive oil, onion and garlic into the insert of the Instant Pot.
3. Sauté for 4 minutes and then add the chicken and the rest of the ingredients.
4. Mix well and close the lid.

5. Select Manual mode for 7 minutes at high pressure.
6. Once done, release the pressure completely and remove the lid.
7. Adjust seasoning as needed.
8. Garnish with desired toppings.

Nutrition:
Calories: 390, Protein: 29.5g, Fat: 26.5g, Sodium: 23mg, Potassium: 89mg.

614. Chicken Noodle Soup

Preparation Time: 9 minutes
Cooking Time: 35 minutes
Servings: 6
Ingredients:
- 1 tablespoon olive oil
- 1 1/2 cups carrots
- 1 1/2 cup diced celery
- 1 cup chopped yellow onion
- 3 tablespoons minced garlic
- 8 cups low-sodium chicken broth
- 2 teaspoons minced fresh thyme
- 2 teaspoons minced fresh rosemary
- 1 bay leaf
- 2 1/2 lbs. chicken thighs
- 3 cups wide egg noodles
- 1 tablespoon fresh lemon juice
- 1/4 cup chopped fresh parsley

Directions:
1. Preheat olive oil in the Instant Pot on Sauté mode.
2. Add onion, celery, and carrots and sauté them for minutes.
3. Stir in garlic and sauté for 1 minute.
4. Add bay leaf, thyme, broth, rosemary, salt, and pepper.
5. Seal and secure the Instant Pot lid and select Manual mode for 10 minutes at high pressure.
6. Once done, release the pressure completely and remove the lid.
7. Add the noodles to the pan and set the Instant Pot to stir-fry mode.
8. Cook the soup for 6 minutes until the noodles are done.
9. Remove the chicken and shred with a fork.
10. Return the chicken to the soup and add the lemon juice and parsley.

Nutrition:
Calories: 333, Protein: 44.7g, Fat: 13.7g, Sodium: 65mg, Potassium: 78mg.

615. Cheesy Broccoli Soup

Preparation Time: 11 minutes
Cooking Time: 30 minutes
Servings: 4
Ingredients:

- ½ cup heavy whipping cream
- 1 cup broccoli
- 1 cup cheddar cheese
- Salt to taste
- 1½ cups chicken broth

Directions:

1. Cook chicken broth in a large pot and add broccoli.
2. Boil and stir in the rest of the ingredients.
3. Simmer on low heat for 21 minutes.
4. Ladle out into a bowl and serve hot.

Nutrition:

Calories: 188, Fats: 15g, Protein: 9.8g, Sodium: 90mg, Potassium: 76mg.

616. Rich Potato Soup

Preparation Time: 6 minutes
Cooking Time: 30 minutes
Servings: 4
Ingredients:

- 1 tablespoon butter
- 1 medium onion, diced
- 3 cloves garlic, minced
- 3 cups chicken broth
- 1 can/box cream of chicken soup
- 7-8 medium-sized russet potatoes
- 1 1/2 teaspoons salt
- 1 cup milk
- 1 tablespoon flour
- 2 cups shredded cheddar cheese

Garnish:

- 5-6 slices bacon, chopped
- Sliced green onions
- Shredded cheddar cheese

Directions:

1. Heat butter in the Instant Pot on sauté mode.
2. Add onions and sauté for 4 minutes until soft.
3. Stir in garlic and sauté it for 1 minute.
4. Add potatoes, cream of chicken, broth, salt, and pepper to the insert.
5. Mix well, then seal and lock the lid.
6. Cook this mixture for 10 minutes at Manual Mode with high pressure.

7. Meanwhile, mix flour with milk in a bowl and set it aside.
8. Once the Instant Pot beeps, release the pressure completely.
9. Remove the Instant Pot lid and switch the Instant Pot to Sauté mode.
10. Pour in flour slurry and stir cook the mixture for 5 minutes until it thickens.
11. Add 2 cups of cheddar cheese and let it melt.
12. Garnish it as desired.

Nutrition:

Calories784, Protein: 34g, Fat: 46.5g, Sodium: 54mg, Potassium: 43mg.

617. Mediterranean Lentil Soup

Preparation Time: 9 minutes
Cooking Time: 20 minutes
Servings: 4
Ingredients:

- 1 tablespoon olive oil
- 1/2 cup red lentils
- 1 medium yellow or red onion
- 2 garlic cloves
- 1/2 teaspoon ground cumin
- 1/2 teaspoon ground coriander
- 1/2 teaspoon ground sumac
- 1/2 teaspoon red chili flakes
- 1/2 teaspoon dried parsley
- 3/4 teaspoons dried mint flakes
- 2.5 cups water
- juice of 1/2 lime

Directions:

1. Preheat oil in your Instant Pot on Sauté mode.
2. Add onion and sauté until it turns golden brown.
3. Toss in the garlic, parsley sugar, mint flakes, red chili flakes, sumac, coriander, and cumin.
4. Stir cook this mixture for 2 minutes.
5. Add water, lentils, salt, and pepper. Stir gently.
6. Seal and lock the Instant Pot lid and select Manual mode for 8 minutes at high pressure.
7. Once done, release the pressure completely, then remove the lid.
8. Stir well and add lime juice.

Nutrition:

Calories: 525, Protein: 30g, Fat: 19.3g, Sodium: 76mg, Potassium: 75mg.

618. Sausage Kale Soup with Mushrooms

Preparation Time: 8 minutes
Cooking Time: 70 minutes
Servings: 6
Ingredients:

- 2 cups fresh kale
- 6.5 ounces mushrooms, sliced
- 6 cups chicken bone broth
- 1-pound sausage, cooked and sliced

Directions:

1. Heat chicken broth with two cans of water in a large pot and bring to a boil.
2. Stir in the remaining ingredients and allow the soup to simmer on low heat for about 1 hour.
3. Dish out and serve hot.

Nutrition:

Calories: 259, Fats: 20g, Proteins 14g, Sodium: 54mg, Potassium: 88mg.

619. Classic Minestrone

Preparation Time: 12 minutes
Cooking Time: 25 minutes
Servings: 6
Ingredients:

- 2 tablespoons olive oil
- 3 cloves garlic
- 1 onion, diced
- 2 carrots
- 2 stalks celery
- 1 1/2 teaspoons dried basil
- 1 teaspoon dried oregano
- 1/2 teaspoon fennel seed
- 6 cups low sodium chicken broth
- 1 (28-ounce) can tomatoes
- 1 (16-ounce) can kidney beans
- 1 zucchini
- 1 Parmesan rind
- 1 bay leaf
- 1 bunch kale leaves, chopped
- 2 teaspoons red wine vinegar
- 1/3 cup freshly grated Parmesan
- 2 tablespoons chopped fresh parsley leaves

Directions:

1. Preheat olive oil in the Instant Pot on Sauté mode.
2. Add carrots, celery, and onion, sauté for 3 minutes.
3. Stir in fennel seeds, oregano, and basil. Stir cook for 1 minute.
4. Add stock, beans, tomatoes, parmesan, bay leaf, and zucchini.

5. Secure and seal the lid of the Instant Pot and then select the manual mode to cook for minutes at high pressure.
6. Once done, release the pressure completely and remove the lid.
7. Add kale and let it sit for 2 minutes in the hot soup.
8. Stir in red wine, vinegar, pepper, and salt.
9. Garnish with parsley and parmesan.

Nutrition:
Calories: 805, Protein: 124g, Fat: 34g, Sodium: 123mg, Potassium: 213mg.

620. Turkey Meatball and Ditalini Soup

Preparation Time: 15 minutes
Cooking Time: 40 minutes
Servings: 4
Ingredients:
Meatballs:
- 1 pound 93% lean ground turkey
- 1/3 cup seasoned breadcrumbs
- 3 tablespoons grated Pecorino Romano cheese
- 1 large egg, beaten
- 1 clove crushed garlic
- 1 tablespoon fresh minced parsley
- 1/2 teaspoon kosher salt

Soup:
- 1 teaspoon olive oil
- 1/2 cup onion
- 1/2 cup celery
- 1/2 cup carrot
- 3 cloves garlic
- 1 can San Marzano tomatoes
- 4 cups reduced sodium chicken broth
- 4 torn basil leaves
- 2 bay leaves
- 1 cup ditalini pasta
- 1 cup zucchini, diced small
- Parmesan rind, optional
- Grated parmesan cheese, optional for serving

Directions:
1. Thoroughly combine turkey with egg, garlic, parsley, salt, pecorino and breadcrumbs in a bowl.
2. Make 30 equal-sized meatballs out of this mixture.
3. Preheat olive oil in the Instant Pot on Sauté mode.
4. Sear the meatballs in the heated oil in batches until brown.

5. Set the meatballs aside on a plate.
6. Add more oil to the insert of the Instant Pot.
7. Stir in carrots, garlic, celery, and onion. Sauté for 4 minutes.
8. Add basil, bay leaves, tomatoes, and Parmesan rind.
9. Return the seared meatballs to the pot along with the broth.
10. Secure and sear the Instant Pot lid and select Manual mode for 15 minutes at high pressure.
11. Once done, release the pressure completely, then remove the lid.
12. Add zucchini and pasta, cook it for 4 minutes on Sauté mode.
13. Garnish with cheese and basil.

Nutrition:
Calories: 261, Protein: 37g, Fat: 7g, Sodium: 453mg, Potassium: 145mg.

621. Mint Avocado Chilled Soup

Preparation Time: 6 minutes
Cooking Time: 0 minutes
Servings: 2
Ingredients:
- 1 cup coconut milk, chilled
- 1 medium ripe avocado
- 1 tablespoon lime juice
- Salt to taste
- 20 fresh mint leaves

Directions:
1. Put all the ingredients into an immersion blender and blend until a thick mixture is formed.
2. Allow to cool for 10 minutes and serve chilled.

Nutrition:
Calories: 286, Fats: 27g, Proteins 4.2g, Sodium: 154mg, Potassium: 187mg.

622. Split Pea Soup

Preparation Time: 11 minutes
Cooking Time: 30 minutes
Servings: 6
Ingredients:
- 3 tablespoons butter
- 1 onion diced
- 2 ribs celery diced
- 2 carrots diced
- 6 oz. diced ham
- 1 lb. dry split peas sorted and rinsed
- 6 cups chicken stock
- 2 bay leaves

Directions:

1. Set your Instant Pot on Sauté mode and melt butter in it.
2. Stir in celery, onion, carrots, salt, and pepper.
3. Sauté for 5 minutes and then add the split peas, ham bone, chicken broth and bay leaves.
4. Seal and lock the Instant Pot lid, then select Manual mode for 15 minutes at high pressure.
5. Once this is done, release the pressure completely and remove the lid.
6. Remove the ham bone and separate the meat from the bone.
7. Shred the meat and return it to the soup.
8. Rectify seasoning if necessary and serve hot.

Nutrition:
Calories: 190, Protein: 8g, Fat: 3.5g, Sodium: 165mg, Potassium: 198mg.

623. Butternut Squash Soup

Preparation Time: 8 minutes
Cooking Time: 40 minutes
Servings: 4
Ingredients:
- 1 tablespoon olive oil
- 1 medium yellow onion chopped
- 1 large carrot chopped
- 1 celery rib chopped
- 3 cloves of garlic minced
- 2 lbs. butternut squash, peeled chopped
- 2 cups vegetable broth
- 1 green apple peeled, cored, and chopped
- 1/4 teaspoon ground cinnamon
- 1 sprig fresh thyme
- 1 sprig fresh rosemary
- 1 teaspoon kosher salt
- 1/2 teaspoon black pepper
- Pinch of nutmeg optional

Directions:
1. Preheat olive oil in the Instant Pot on Sauté mode.
2. Add celery, carrots, and garlic, sauté for 5 minutes.
3. Stir in squash, broth, cinnamon, apple nutmeg, rosemary, thyme, salt, and pepper.
4. Carefully mix well and then close and secure the lid.
5. Select the manual mode to cook for 10 minutes at high pressure.
6. Once done, release the pressure completely and remove the lid.
7. Puree the soup using an immersion blender.

8. Serve warm.

Nutrition:
Calories: 282, Protein: 13g, Fat: 4.7g, Sodium: 198mg, Potassium: 165mg.

624. Beef Stroganoff Soup

Preparation Time: 9 minutes
Cooking Time: 35 minutes
Servings: 6
Ingredients:
- 1.5 pounds stew meat
- 6 cups beef broth
- 4 tablespoons Worcestershire sauce
- 1/2 teaspoon Italian seasoning blend
- 1 1/2 teaspoons onion powder
- 2 teaspoons garlic powder
- salt and pepper to taste
- 1/2 cup sour cream
- 8 ounces mushrooms, sliced
- 8 ounces short noodles, cooked
- 1/3 cup cold water
- 1/4 cup corn starch

Directions:
1. Add meat, 5 cups broth, Italian seasoning, Worcestershire sauce, garlic powder, salt, pepper, and onion powder to the insert of the Instant Pot.
2. Secure and seal the Instant Pot lid, then select Manual mode for 1 hour at high pressure.
3. Once done, release the pressure completely and remove the lid.
4. Press the instant pot to soup mode and add the sour cream along with 1 cup of broth.
5. Blend well and then add the mushrooms and mix well.
6. Whisk the cornstarch with water and pour this mixture into the pot.
7. Cook this mixture until it thickens and then add the noodles, salt and pepper.
8. Garnish with cheese parsley and black pepper.

Nutrition:
Calories: 320, Protein: 26.9g, Fat: 13.7g, Sodium: 186mg, Potassium: 54mg.

625. Creamy Low Carb Butternut Squash Soup

Preparation Time: 12 minutes
Cooking Time: 70 minutes

Servings: 8
Ingredients:
- 2 tablespoons avocado oil, divided
- 2 pounds butternut squash
- 1 (13.5-oz) can coconut milk
- 4 cups chicken bone broth

Directions:
1. Adjust oven at 400 degrees F and grease a baking sheet.
2. Spread the squash halves open side up on the baking sheet.
3. Pour half of the avocado oil and season with sea salt and black pepper.
4. Flip over and transfer into the oven.
5. Roast the butternut squash.
6. Cook remaining avocado oil over medium heat in a large pot and add the broth and coconut milk.
7. Let it simmer for 22 minutes and scoop the squash out of the shells to transfer into the soup.
8. Puree this mixture in an immersion blender until smooth and serve immediately.

Nutrition:
Calories: 185, Fats: 12.6g, Proteins 4.7g, Sodium: 157mg, Potassium: 176mg.

626. Baked Shrimp Stew

Preparation Time: 13 minutes
Cooking Time: 25 minutes
Servings: 6
Ingredients:
- Greek extra virgin olive oil
- 2 1/2 lb. prawns, peeled
- 1 large red onion
- 5 garlic cloves
- 1 red bell pepper
- 2 15-oz cans diced tomatoes
- 1/2 cup water
- 1 1/2 tsp ground coriander
- 1 tsp sumac
- 1 tsp cumin
- 1 tsp red pepper flakes
- 1/2 tsp ground green cardamom
- Salt and pepper to taste
- 1 cup parsley leaves, stems removed
- 1/3 cup toasted pine nuts
- 1/4 cup toasted sesame seeds
- Lemon or lime wedges to serve

Directions:
1. Preheat the oven to 375 degrees F.
2. Using a frying pan, add 1 tablespoon of olive oil.

3. Sauté the prawns for 2 minutes, until they are barely pink, then remove and set aside.
4. In the same pan over medium-high heat, drizzle a little more olive oil and sauté the chopped onions, garlic and red bell peppers for 5 minutes, stirring regularly.
5. Add in the canned diced tomatoes and water, allow to simmer for 10 minutes, until the liquid reduces, stir occasionally.
6. Turn the heat to medium and return the shrimp to the pan. Add the spices, ground coriander, sumac, cumin, red pepper flakes, green cardamom, salt and pepper, then the toasted pine nuts, sesame seeds and parsley leaves.
7. Transfer the shrimp and sauce to an oven-safe earthenware or stoneware dish, cover tightly with foil. Situate in the oven to bake for minutes, uncover and broil briefly.
8. Allow the dish to cool completely.
9. Distribute among the containers, store for 2-3 days.
10. To Serve: Reheat on the stove for 1-2 minutes or until heated through. Serve with your favorite bread or whole grain. Garnish with a side of lime or lemon wedges.

Nutrition:
Calories: 977, Fat: 20g, Protein: 41g, Sodium: 198mg, Potassium: 186mg.

627. Cinnamon Squash Soup

Preparation Time: 11 minutes
Cooking Time: 1 hour
Servings: 6
Ingredients:
- 1 small butternut squash
- 4 tablespoons extra-virgin olive oil
- 1 small yellow onion
- 2 large garlic cloves
- 1 teaspoon salt, divided
- 1 pinch black pepper
- 1 teaspoon dried oregano
- 2 tablespoons fresh oregano
- 2 cups low sodium chicken stock
- 1 cinnamon stick
- ½ cup canned white kidney beans
- 1 small pear
- 2 tablespoons walnut pieces

- ¼ cup Greek yogurt
- 2 tablespoons parsley

Directions:
1. Preheat oven to 425 degrees F.
2. Place squash in a bowl and season with a ½ teaspoon of salt and tablespoons of olive oil.
3. Arrange squash onto a roasting pan and roast for about 25 minutes until tender.
4. Keep aside squash to let cool.
5. Cook remaining 2 tablespoons of olive oil in a medium-sized pot at medium-high heat.
6. Sauté onions
7. Add dried oregano and garlic and sauté for 1 minute.
8. Mix squash, broth, pear, cinnamon stick, pepper, and remaining salt.
9. Bring mixture to a boil.
10. Once the boiling point is reached, add walnuts and beans.
11. Lower heat and cook for 20 minutes.
12. Remove the cinnamon stick.
13. Use an immersion blender and blend the entire mixture until smooth.
14. Add yogurt gradually while whisking.
15. Season to your taste.
16. Garnish with parsley and fresh oregano.

Nutrition:
Calories: 197, Fat: 11.6g, Protein: 6.1g, Sodium: 165mg, Potassium: 154mg.

628. Bulgarian Lentil Soup

Preparation Time: 8 minutes
Cooking Time: 15 minutes
Servings: 10
Ingredients:
- 2 cups brown lentils
- 2 onions, chopped
- 5-6 cloves garlic, peeled
- 2-3 medium carrots, chopped
- 1-2 small tomatoes, ripe
- 4 tbsp olive oil
- 1 ½ tsp paprika
- 1 tsp summer savory

Directions:
1. Cook oil in a cooking pot; add the onions and carrots. Add the paprika and washed lentils with 4 cups of warm water; continue to simmer.
2. Chop the tomatoes and stir in them to the soup about 15 minutes after the lentils have started to simmer. Add savory

and peeled garlic cloves. Simmer soup. Salt to taste.

Nutrition:
Calories: 201, Fat: 12g, Protein: 5g, Sodium: 132mg, Potassium: 186mg.

629. White Bean Soup

Preparation Time: 13 minutes
Cooking Time: 17 minutes
Servings: 6
Ingredients:
- 1 cup white beans
- 2-3 carrots
- 2 onions, finely chopped
- 1-2 tomatoes, grated
- 1 red bell pepper, chopped
- 4-5 springs of fresh mint and parsley
- 1 tsp paprika
- 3 tbsp sunflower oil

Directions:
1. Submerge beans in cold water for 3-4 hours, drain and discard the water.
2. Cover the beans with cold water. Add the oil, finely chopped carrots, onions and bell pepper. Boil and simmer until tender.
3. Add the grated tomatoes, mint, paprika and salt. Simmer for another 15 minutes. Serve sprinkled with finely chopped parsley.

Nutrition:
Calories: 210, Fat: 11g, Protein: 5g, Sodium: 185mg, Potassium: 164mg.

630. Cauliflower Soup

Preparation Time: 9 minutes
Cooking Time: 40 minutes
Servings: 8
Ingredients:
- 1 large onion finely cut
- 1 medium head cauliflower
- 2-3 garlic cloves, crushed
- 3 cups water
- ½ cup whole cream
- 4 tbsp olive oil

Directions:
1. Cook olive oil in a large pot over medium heat and sauté the onion, cauliflower and garlic. Stir in the water and bring the soup to a boil.
2. Reduce heat, cover, and simmer for 40 minutes. Remove the soup from the heat, add the

cream and blend in a blender. Season with salt and pepper.

Nutrition:
Calories: 221, Fat: 19g, Protein: 8g, Sodium: 154mg, Potassium: 143mg.

631. Moroccan Pumpkin Soup

Preparation Time: 7 minutes
Cooking Time: 54 minutes
Servings: 6
Ingredients:
- 1 leek, white part only
- 3 cloves garlic
- ½ tsp ground ginger
- ½ tsp ground cinnamon
- ½ tsp ground cumin
- 2 carrots
- 2 lb. pumpkin
- 1/3 cup chickpeas
- 5 tbsp olive oil
- juice of ½ lemon

Directions:
1. Put oil in a large saucepan and sauté the leek, garlic and 2 teaspoons of salt, stirring occasionally, until soft. Add the cinnamon, ginger and cumin and stir. Add the carrots, pumpkin and chickpeas. Stir to combine.
2. Add 5 cups of water and bring the soup to a boil, then reduce the heat and simmer for 50 minutes.
3. Remove from the heat. Add the lemon juice and blend the soup. Return to a simmer for 4-5 minutes. Serve with parsley sprigs.

Nutrition:
Calories: 241, Fat: 21g, Protein: 4g, Sodium: 143mg, Potassium: 186mg.

632. Potato Soup

Preparation Time: 16 minutes
Cooking Time: 7 minutes
Servings: 5
Ingredients:
- 4-5 medium potatoes
- 2 carrots
- 1 zucchini
- 1 celery rib
- 3 cups water
- 3 tbsp olive oil
- 1 cup whole milk
- ½ tsp dried rosemary

Directions:

1. Cook olive oil over medium heat and sauté the vegetables for 2-3 minutes. Pour 3 cups of water, add the rosemary and bring the soup to a boil, then lower heat and simmer until tender.
2. Blend the soup in a blender until smooth. Add a cup of warm milk and blend some more. Serve warm, seasoned with black pepper and parsley sprinkled over each serving.

Nutrition:
Calories: 211, Fat: 18g, Protein: 6g, Sodium: 165mg, Potassium: 196mg.

633. Leek, Rice and Potato Soup

Preparation Time: 9 minutes
Cooking Time: 17 minutes
Servings: 6
Ingredients:
- 1/3 cup rice
- 4 cups of water
- 2-3 potatoes, diced
- 1 small onion, cut
- 1 leek, halved lengthwise and sliced
- 3 tbsp olive oil
- lemon juice, to serve

Directions:
1. Heat a soup pot over medium heat. Add olive oil and onion and sauté for 2 minutes. Add leeks and potatoes and stir for a few minutes more. Fill in three cups of water, boil, reduce heat and simmer for 5 minutes.
2. Add the very well washed rice and simmer for 10 minutes. Serve with lemon juice to taste.

Nutrition:
Calories: 180, Fat: 11g, Protein: 5g, Sodium: 130mg, Potassium: 133mg.

634. Carrot and Chickpea Soup

Preparation Time: 9 minutes
Cooking Time: 18 minutes
Servings: 5
Ingredients:
- 3-4 big carrots
- 1 leek, chopped
- 4 cups vegetable broth
- 1 cup canned chickpeas
- ½ cup orange juice
- 2 tbsp olive oil
- ½ tsp cumin

- ½ tsp ginger
- 4-5 tbsp yogurt, to serve

Directions:
1. Cook oil in a huge saucepan over medium heat. Add leek and carrots and sauté until soft. Add orange juice, broth, chickpeas and spices. Bring to a boil.
2. Switch heat to medium-low and simmer for 15 minutes.
3. Blend the soup until smooth; return to pan. Season with salt and pepper. Stir over low heat until heated through. Pour in 4-5 bowls, top with yogurt, and serve.

Nutrition:
Calories: 207, Fat: 13g, Protein: 4g, Sodium: 197mg, Potassium: 143mg.

635. Broccoli, Zucchini and Blue Cheese Soup

Preparation Time: 11 minutes
Cooking Time: 22 minutes
Servings: 6
Ingredients:
- 2 leeks, white part only
- 1 head broccoli
- 2 zucchinis, chopped
- 1 potato, chopped
- 2 cups vegetable broth
- 2 cups water
- 3 tbsp olive oil
- 1 oz blue cheese, crumbled
- 1/3 cup light cream

Directions:
1. Cook oil in a saucepan over medium heat. Sauté the leeks, stirring, for 5 minutes. Stir in bite-sized pieces of broccoli, zucchinis, potato, water and broth and bring to a boil.
2. Reduce heat to low and simmer, stirring occasionally, for 10 minutes, or until vegetables are just tender. Remove from heat and set aside for 5 minutes to cool slightly.
3. Transfer the soup to a blender. Drizzle cheese and blend in batches until smooth. Return to saucepan and place over low heat. Add cream and stir to combine. Season with salt and pepper to taste.

Nutrition:
Calories: 301, Fat: 16g, Protein: 4g, Sodium: 106mg, Potassium: 165mg.

636. Beetroot and Carrot Soup

Preparation Time: 12 minutes
Cooking Time: 32 minutes
Servings: 6
Ingredients:
- 4 beets
- 2 carrots
- 2 potatoes
- 1 medium onion
- 4 cups vegetable broth
- 2 cups water
- 2 tbsp yogurt
- 2 tbsp olive oil

Directions:
1. Peel and chop the beets. Cook olive oil in a saucepan over medium-high heat and sauté the onion and carrot until the onion is tender. Add beets, potatoes, broth and water. Bring to the boil. Switch heat to medium and simmer, partially covered, for 30-40 minutes. Cool slightly.
2. Blend the soup in batches until smooth. Return it to pan over low heat and cook, stirring, for 4 to 5 minutes or until heated through. Season with salt and pepper. Serve soup topped with yogurt and sprinkled with spring onions.

Nutrition:
Calories: 301, Fat: 21g, Protein: 11g, Sodium: 195mg, Potassium: 154mg.

637. Roasted Red Pepper Soup

Preparation Time: 16 minutes
Cooking Time: 23 minutes
Servings: 7
Ingredients:
- 5-6 red peppers
- 1 large brown onion
- 2 garlic cloves
- 4 medium tomatoes
- 3 cups chicken broth
- 3 tbsp olive oil
- 2 bay leaves

Directions:
1. Roast peppers in the oven at 450 F until the skins are a little burnt. Place the roasted peppers in a brown paper bag or a lidded container and leave covered for about 10 minutes. This makes it easier to peel them. Peel the skins and remove the seeds. Cut the peppers into small pieces.

2. Cook oil in a big saucepan over medium-high heat. Add onion and garlic and sauté, stirring, for 3 minutes or until the onion has softened. Add the red peppers, bay leaves, tomato and simmer for 5 minutes.
3. Add in the broth. Season with pepper. Boil, reduce heat and simmer for 23 minutes. Set aside to cool slightly. Blend, in batches, until smooth and serve.

Nutrition:
Calories: 311, Fat: 13g, Protein: 5g, Sodium: 127mg, Potassium: 106mg.

638. Lentil, Barley and Mushroom Soup

Preparation Time: 4 minutes
Cooking Time: 38 minutes
Servings: 6
Ingredients:
- 2 medium leeks
- 10 white mushrooms
- 3 garlic cloves
- 2 bay leaves
- 2 cans tomatoes
- 3/4 cup red lentils
- 1/3 cup barley
- 3 tbsp olive oil
- 1 tsp paprika
- 1 tsp summer savory
- ½ tsp cumin

Directions:
1. Cook oil in a large saucepan over medium-high heat. Sauté leeks and mushrooms for 3 to 4 minutes or until softened. Add cumin, paprika, savory and tomatoes, lentils, barley, and 5 cups cold water. Season with salt and pepper.
2. Cover and bring to boil. Reduce heat to low. Simmer for 37 minutes.

Nutrition:
Calories: 314, Fat: 19g, Protein: 5g, Sodium: 196mg, Potassium: 132mg.

639. Spinach Soup

Preparation Time: 10 minutes
Cooking Time: 21 minutes
Servings: 6
Ingredients:
- 14 oz frozen spinach
- 1 large onion
- 1 carrot

- 4 cups water
- 3-4 tbsp olive oil
- 1/4 cup white rice
- 1-2 cloves garlic, crushed

Directions:
1. Cook oil in a cooking pot, stir in onion and carrot and sauté together for a few minutes until just softened. Add chopped garlic and rice and stir for a minute. Remove from heat.
2. Add in the chopped spinach along with about 2 cups of hot water and season with salt and pepper. Bring back to a boil, then reduce the heat and simmer for around 30 minutes.

Nutrition:
Calories: 291, Fat: 16g, Protein: 7g, Sodium: 120mg, Potassium: 154mg.

640. Spinach and Feta Cheese Soup

Preparation Time: 8 minutes
Cooking Time: 24 minutes
Servings: 4
Ingredients:
- 14 oz frozen spinach
- 10 oz feta cheese
- 1 large onion or 4-5 scallions
- 2-3 tbsp light cream
- 3-4 tbsp olive oil
- 1-2 cloves garlic
- 4 cups water

Directions:
1. Cook oil in a cooking pot, add the onion and spinach and sauté together for a few minutes until softened. Add garlic and stir for a minute. Remove from heat. Fill 2 cups of hot water and season with salt and pepper.
2. Bring back to the boil, then reduce the heat and simmer for around 30 minutes. Blend soup in a blender. Crumble the cheese with a fork. Stir in the crumbled feta cheese and the cream. Serve hot.

Nutrition:
Calories: 251, Fat: 13g, Protein: 5g, Sodium: 165mg, Potassium: 107mg.

641. Nettle Soup

Preparation Time: 4 minutes
Cooking Time: 26 minutes

Servings: 6
Ingredients:
- 1 lb. young top shoots of nettles
- 3-4 tbsp sunflower oil
- 2 potatoes, diced small
- 1 bunch spring onions
- 1 ½ cup freshly boiled water
- 1 tsp salt

Directions:
1. Clean the young nettles, wash and cook them in slightly salted water. Drain, rinse, drain again and then chop or pass through a sieve. Sauté the chopped spring onions and potatoes.
2. Turn off the heat and add the nettles. Then, gradually stir in the water. Simmer until the potatoes are cooked through.

Nutrition:
Calories: 251, Protein: 4g, Sodium: 176mg, Potassium: 214mg.

642. Thick Herb Soup

Preparation Time: 11 minutes
Cooking Time: 23 minutes
Servings: 4
Ingredients:
- 2 oz mint leaves
- 2 oz celery leaves
- 4 tbsp butter or olive oil
- 2 tbsp flour
- 3 cups water
- ½ cup thick yogurt
- juice of a lemon
- 2 egg yolks
- 1 tsp salt

Directions:
1. Rinse the herbs, remove stalks and snip or chop finely. Cook butter or oil in a cooking pot and add the prepared herbs. Cover and simmer gently.
2. When the herbs are tender, add in the flour and stir to combine. Cook for a few moments before slowly adding the water, stirring all the time. Simmer for about 10-15 minutes.
3. Mix separately egg yolks, thick yogurt (or sour cream) and lemon juice. Add to the soup slowly, then stir well.

Nutrition:
Calories: 247, Fat: 13g, Protein: 7g, Sodium: 21mg, Potassium: 65mg.

Chapter 14. Red Meat and Pork

643. Lamb Chops with Rosemary

Preparation Time: 5 minutes
Cooking Time: 15 minutes
Servings: 4
Ingredients:
- 1 lb. lamb chops
- 1/2 tsp. freshly ground black pepper
- 1 tbsp. olive oil
- 5 garlic cloves
- 1 tbsp. chopped fresh rosemary

Directions:
1. Adjust the oven rack to the top third of the oven. Preheat the broiler. Line a baking sheet with foil.
2. Place the garlic, rosemary, pepper, and olive oil into a small bowl and stir well to combine.
3. Place the lamb chops on a baking sheet and brush half of the garlic-rosemary mixture equally between the chops, coating well. Place the sheet beneath the broiler and broil for 4–5 minutes.
4. Remove from oven and carefully flip over the chops. Divide the remaining garlic-rosemary mixture evenly between the chops and spread to coat. Return pan to oven and broil for another 3 minutes.
5. Remove from oven and serve immediately.

Nutrition:
Calories: 185, Fat: 9g, Carbs: 1g, Protein: 23g, Sugars: 0g, Sodium: 72.8mg, Potassium: 216mg.

644. Cane Wrapped Around in Prosciutto

Preparation Time: 3 minutes
Cooking Time: 5 minutes
Servings: 4
Ingredients:
- 80 oz. sliced prosciutto
- 1 lb. thick asparagus

Directions:
1. The first step here is to prepare your Instant Pot by pouring in about 2 cups of water.
2. Take the asparagus and wrap them up in prosciutto spears. Once all the asparagus are wrapped, gently place the processed asparaguses in the cooking basket inside your pot in layers. Turn up the heat to a high temperature and when there is a pressure build up, take down the heat and let it cook for about 2-3 minutes at the high pressure. Once the timer runs out, gently open the cover of the pressure cooker.
3. Take out the steamer basket from the pot instantly and toss the asparaguses on a plate to serve.
4. Eat warm or let them come down to room temperature.

Nutrition:
Calories: 212, Fat: 14g, Carbs: 11g, Protein: 12g, Sugars: 367.6g, Sodium: 0mg, Potassium: 32mg.

645. Beef Veggie Pot Meal

Preparation Time: 45-50 minutes
Cooking Time: 40 minutes
Servings: 2-3
Ingredients:
- 1 tsp. butter
- 1/4 shredded cabbage head
- 2 peeled and sliced carrots
- 1 tbsp. flour
- 4 tbsps. sour cream
- 1 chopped onion
- 10 oz. sliced and boiled beef tenderloin

Directions:
1. In a saucepan, add the butter, cabbage, carrots, and onions.
2. Cook on medium-high heat until the veggies get softened.
3. Add the beef meat and stir the mix.
4. In a mixing bowl, beat the cream with flour until smooth.
5. Add the sauce over the beef.
6. Cover and cook for 40 minutes.
7. Serve warm.

Nutrition:
Calories: 245.5, Fat: 10.2g, Carbs: 18.4g, Protein: 19.0g, Sugars: 5.5g, Sodium: 188.2mg, Potassium: 56mg.

646. Braised Beef Shanks

Preparation Time: 10 minutes
Cooking Time: 4-6 hours
Servings: 2
Ingredients:
- Freshly ground black pepper
- 5 minced garlic cloves
- 11/2 lbs. lean beef shanks
- 2 sprigs fresh rosemary
- 1 c. low-fat, low-sodium beef broth
- 1 tbsp. fresh lime juice

Directions:
1. In a slow cooker, add all ingredients and mix. Set the slow cooker on Low.
2. Cover and cook for 4-6 hours.

Nutrition:
Calories: 50, Fat: 1g, Carbs: 0.8g, Protein: 8g, Sugars: 0g, Sodium: 108mg, Potassium: 234mg.

647. Beef with Mushrooms

Preparation Time: 15 minutes
Cooking Time: 8 hours
Servings: 8
Ingredients:
- 2 c. salt-free tomato paste
- 2 c. sliced fresh mushrooms
- 2 c. low-fat, low-sodium beef broth
- 2 lbs. cubed lean beef stew meat
- 1 c. chopped fresh parsley leaves
- Freshly ground black pepper
- 4 minced garlic cloves

Directions:
1. In a slow cooker, add all ingredients except lemon juice and stir to combine.
2. Set the slow cooker on Low.
3. Cover and cook for about 8 hours.
4. Serve hot with the drizzling of lemon juice

Nutrition:
Calories: 260, Fat: 12g, Carbs: 18g, Protein: 44g, Sugars: 4g, Sodium: 480mg, Potassium: 176mg.

648. Lemony Braised Beef Roast

Preparation Time: 15 minutes
Cooking Time: 6-8 hours
Servings: 6
Ingredients:

- 1 tbsp. minced fresh rosemary
- 1/2 c. low-fat, low-sodium beef broth
- Freshly ground black pepper
- 2 lbs. lean beef pot roast
- 1 sliced onion
- 2 minced garlic cloves
- 1/4 c. fresh lemon juice
- 1 tsp. ground cumin

Directions:

1. In a large slow cooker, add all ingredients and mix well.
2. Set the slow cooker on Low.
3. Cover and cook for about 6-8 hours.

Nutrition:

Calories: 344, Fat: 2.8g, Carbs: 18g, Protein: 32g, Sugars: 2.4g, Sodium: 278mg, Potassium: 187mg.

649. Grilled Fennel-Cumin Lamb Chops

Preparation Time: 10 minutes
Cooking Time: 30 minutes
Servings: 2
Ingredients:

- 1/4 tsp. salt
- 1 minced large garlic clove
- 1/8 tsp. cracked black pepper
- ¾ tsp. crushed fennel seeds
- 1/4 tsp. ground coriander
- 4-6 sliced lamb rib chops
- ¾ tsp. ground cumin

Directions:

1. Trim fat from chops. Place the chops on a plate.
2. In a small bowl, combine the garlic, fennel seeds, cumin, salt, coriander, and black pepper. Sprinkle the mixture evenly over chops; rub in with your fingers. Cover the chops with plastic wrap and marinate in the refrigerator for at least 30 minutes or up to 24 hours.
3. Grill chops on the rack of an uncovered grill directly over medium coals until chops reach desired doneness.

Nutrition:

Calories: 239, Fat: 12g, Carbs: 2g, Protein: 29g, Sugars: 0g,

Sodium: 409mg, Potassium: 123mg.

650. Beef Heart

Preparation Time: 40 minutes
Cooking Time: 30 minutes
Servings: 4
Ingredients:

- 1 chopped large onion
- 1 c. water
- 2 peeled and chopped tomatoes
- 1 boiled beef heart
- 2 tbsps. tomato paste

Directions:

1. Boil the beef heart until half-done.
2. Sauté the onions with tomatoes until soft.
3. Cut the beef heart into cubes and add to tomato and onion mixture. Add water and tomato paste. Stew on low heat for 30 minutes.

Nutrition:

Calories: 138, Fat: 3g, Carbs: 0.1g, Protein: 24.2g, Sugars: 0g, Sodium: 50.2mg, Potassium: 234mg.

651. Jerk Beef and Plantain Kabobs

Preparation Time: 10 minutes
Cooking Time: 15 minutes
Servings: 4
Ingredients:

- 2 peeled and sliced ripe plantains
- 2 tbsps. red wine vinegar
- Lime wedges
- 1 tbsp. cooking oil
- 1 sliced medium red onion
- 12 oz. sliced boneless beef sirloin steak
- 1 tbsp. Jamaican jerk seasoning

Directions:

1. Trim fat from meat. Cut into 1-inch pieces. In a small bowl, stir together red wine vinegar, oil, and jerk seasoning. Toss meat cubes with half of the vinegar mixture. On long skewers, alternately thread meat, plantain chunks, and onion wedges, leaving a 1/4-inch space between pieces.
2. Brush plantains and onion wedges with the remaining vinegar mixture.
3. Place skewers on the rack of an uncovered grill directly over

medium coals. Grill for 12 to 15 minutes or until meat is desired doneness, turning occasionally.

4. Serve with lime wedges.

Nutrition:

Calories: 260, Fat: 7g, Carbs: 21g, Protein: 26g, Sugars: 2.5g, Sodium: 358mg, Potassium: 187mg.

652. Beef Pot

Preparation Time: 10 minutes
Cooking Time: 40 minutes
Servings: 2
Ingredients:

- 4 tbsps. sour cream
- 1/4 shredded cabbage head
- 1 tsp. butter
- 2 peeled and sliced carrots
- 1 chopped onion
- 10 oz. boiled and sliced beef tenderloin
- 1 tbsp. flour

Directions:

1. Sauté the cabbage, carrots and onions in butter.
2. Spray a pot with cooking spray.
3. In layers, place the sautéed vegetables, then beef, then another layer of vegetables.
4. Beat the sour cream with flour until smooth and pour over the beef.
5. Cover and bake at 400F for 40 minutes.

Nutrition:

Calories: 210, Fat: 30g, Carbs: 4g, Protein: 14g, Sugars: 1g, Sodium: 600mg, Potassium: 215mg.

653. Beef with Cucumber Raito

Preparation Time: 10 minutes
Cooking Time: 30 minutes
Servings: 2
Ingredients:

- 1/2 tsp. lemon-pepper seasoning
- 1/4 c. coarsely shredded unpeeled cucumber
- Black pepper and salt
- 1 tbsp. finely chopped red onion
- 1/4 tsp. sugar
- 1 lb. sliced de-boned beef sirloin steak
- 8 oz. plain fat-free yogurt
- 1 tbsp. snipped fresh mint

Directions:

1. Preheat the broiler.
2. In a small bowl, combine yogurt, cucumber, onion, snipped mint, and sugar. Season to taste with salt and pepper; set aside

3. Trim fat from meat. Sprinkle meat with lemon-pepper seasoning.
4. Place meat on the unheated rack of a broiler pan. Broil 3 to 4 inches from heat, turning meat over after half of the broiling time.
5. Allow 15 to 17 minutes for medium-rare (145 degrees F) and 20 to 22 minutes for medium (160 degrees F).
6. Cut steak across the grain into thin slices.
7. Serve and enjoy.

Nutrition:
Calories: 176, Fat: 3g, Carbs: 5g, Protein: 28g, Sugars: 8.9g, Sodium: 88.3mg, Potassium: 87mg.

654. Bistro Beef Tenderloin

Preparation Time: 10 minutes
Cooking Time: 45 minutes
Servings: 12
Ingredients:
- 2 tbsps. extra-virgin olive oil
- 2 tbsps. Dijon mustard
- 1 tsp. kosher salt
- 2/3 c. chopped mixed fresh herbs
- 3 lbs. trimmed beef tenderloin
- 1/2 tsp. freshly ground pepper

Directions:
1. Preheat oven to 400F.
2. Tie kitchen twine around the loin at three points so that it does not get flattened while grilling.
3. Rub the tenderloin with oil; pat on salt and pepper. Place in a large roasting pan.
4. Roast until a thermometer inserted into the thickest part of the tenderloin registers 140F for medium-rare, about 45 minutes, turning two or three times during roasting to ensure even cooking.
5. Transfer to a cutting board; let rest for 10 minutes. Remove the string.
6. Place herbs on a large plate. Coat the tenderloin evenly with mustard; then roll in the herbs, pressing gently to adhere. Slice and serve.

Nutrition:
Calories: 280, Fat: 20.6g, Carbs: 0.9g, Protein: 22.2g, Sugars: 0g, Sodium: 160mg, Potassium: 64mg.

655. The Surprising No "Noodle" Lasagna

Preparation Time: 10 minutes
Cooking Time: 10 minutes
Servings: 8
Ingredients:
- 1/2 c. Parmesan cheese
- 2 minced garlic cloves
- 8 oz. sliced mozzarella
- 1 lb. ground beef
- 25 oz. marinara sauce
- 1 small sized onion
- 1 1/2 c. ricotta cheese
- 1 large-sized egg

Directions:
1. Set your pot to Sauté mode and add garlic, onion and ground beef.
2. Take a small bowl and add ricotta and parmesan with egg and mix.
3. Drain the grease and transfer the beef to a 1 and a 1/2-quart soufflé dish.
4. Add marinara sauce to the browned meat and reserve half.
5. Top the remaining meat sauce with half of your mozzarella cheese.
6. Spread half of the ricotta cheese over the mozzarella layer.
7. Top with the remaining meat sauce.
8. Add a final layer of mozzarella cheese on top.
9. Spread any remaining ricotta cheese mixture over the mozzarella.
10. Carefully add this mixture to your Soufflé Dish.
11. Pour 1 cup of water into your pot.
12. Place it over a trivet.
13. Lock up the lid and cook on HIGH pressure for 10 minutes.
14. Release the pressure naturally over 10 minutes.
15. Serve and enjoy!

Nutrition:
Calories: 607, Fat: 23g, Carbs: 65g, Protein: 33g, Sugars: 0.31g, Sodium: 128mg, Potassium: 187mg.

656. Lamb Chops with Kale

Preparation Time: 10 minutes

Cooking Time: 35 minutes
Servings: 4
Ingredients:
- 1 tbsp. olive oil
- 1 sliced yellow onion
- 1 c. torn kale
- 2 tbsps. low-sodium tomato paste
- 1/4 tsp. black pepper
- 1/2 c. low-sodium veggie stock
- 1 lb. lamb chops

Directions:
1. Grease a roasting pan with the oil, arrange the lamb chops inside, also add the kale and the other ingredients and toss gently.
2. Bake everything at 390F for 35 minutes, divide between plates and serve.

Nutrition:
Calories: 275, Fat: 11.8g, Carbs: 7.3g, Protein: 33.6g, Sugars: 0.1g, Sodium: 280mg, Potassium: 32mg.

657. Beef & Vegetable Stir-Fry

Preparation Time: 20 minutes
Cooking Time: 30 minutes
Servings: 4
Ingredients:
- 1 lb. thinly sliced skirt steak
- 2 tbsps. sesame seeds
- ¾ c. stir-fry sauce
- 1 thinly sliced red bell pepper
- 2 thinly sliced scallions
- 2 tbsps. canola oil
- 1/4 tsp. ground black pepper
- 1 sliced broccoli head
- 1 1/2 c. fluffy brown rice

Directions:
1. Prepare the Stir-Fry Sauce.
2. Heat the canola oil in a large wok or skillet over medium-high heat. Season the steak with black pepper and cook for 4 minutes, until crispy on the outside and pink on the inside. Remove the steak from the skillet and place the broccoli and peppers in the hot oil. Stir-fry for 4 minutes, stirring or tossing occasionally, until crisp and slightly tender.
3. Place the steak back in the skillet with the vegetables. Pour the stir-fry sauce over the steak and vegetables and let simmer for 3 minutes. Remove from the heat.

4. Serve the stir-fry over rice and top with the scallions and sesame seeds.
5. For leftovers, divide the stir-fry evenly into microwaveable airtight containers and store them in the refrigerator for up to 5 days. Reheat in the microwave on high for 2 to 3 minutes, until heated through.

Nutrition:
Calories: 408, Fat: 18g, Carbs: 36g, Protein: 31g, Sugars: 5.5g, Sodium: 197mg, Potassium: 45mg.

658. Simple Veal Chops

Preparation Time: 10 minutes
Cooking Time: 10 minutes
Servings: 4
Ingredients:
- 3 tbsps. essential olive oil
- Zest of 1 grated lemon
- 3 tbsps. whole-wheat flour
- 1 1/2 c. whole-wheat breadcrumbs
- Black pepper
- 1 tbsp. milk
- 4 veal rib chops
- 2 eggs

Directions:
1. Put whole-wheat flour within a bowl.
2. In another bowl, mix eggs with milk and whisk
3. In 1/3 bowl, mix the breadcrumbs with lemon zest.
4. Season veal chops with black pepper, dredge them in flour and dip inside egg mix then in breadcrumbs.
5. Heat a frying pan over medium-high flame, add the veal chops, cook them for 2 minutes on both sides and transfer them to a baking tray. Put them in the oven at 350F, bake them for a quarter of an hour, divide them among the plates and serve them with a side salad.
6. Enjoy!

Nutrition:
Calories: 270, Fat: 6g, Carbs: 10g, Protein: 16g, Sugars: 0g, Sodium: 320mg, Potassium: 36mg.

659. Beef and Barley Farmers Soup

Preparation Time: 10 minutes
Cooking Time: 20 minutes
Servings: 4
Ingredients:
- 1 diced onion
- 15 g sunflower oil
- 15 g balsamic vinegar
- 900 g Campbell's red and white vegetable beef soup bowl
- 2 thinly sliced green onion stalks
- 1 diced carrot
- 340 g cubed lean beef
- 1 Julienned celery stalk
- 1 Minced Garlic Clove
- 85 g pot barley

Directions:
1. Throw a cast iron pan or a deep saucepan on medium heat with the oil and cubed beef to allow the two to cook. Wait till beef is properly browned on all sides, and then add in the diced vegetables. Cover and cook for an additional 3-5 minutes, stirring occasionally.
2. Add in a combination of the broth, vinegar, and barley; reduce the flame and bring to a boil. Continue to cook for about 20 minutes or until thickened to preferred consistency.
3. Top with chopped green onions and serve!

Nutrition:
Calories: 279, Fat: 7.6g, Carbs: 28.91g, Protein: 24.82g, Sugars: 3g, Sodium: 590mg, Potassium: 78mg.

660. Simple Pork and Capers

Preparation Time: 10 minutes
Cooking Time: 10 minutes
Servings: 2
Ingredients:
- 8 oz. cubed pork
- 1 c. low-sodium chicken stock
- Black pepper
- 2 tbsps. organic extra virgin olive oil
- 1 minced garlic oil
- 2 tbsps. capers

Directions:
1. Heat a pan with the oil over medium-high flame. Add the pork season with black pepper and cook for 4 minutes on both sides.

2. Add garlic, capers and stock, stir and cook for 7 minutes more.
3. Divide everything between plates and serve.
4. Enjoy!

Nutrition:
Calories: 224, Fat: 12g, Carbs: 12g, Protein: 10g, Sugars: 5g, Sodium: 5mg, Potassium: 98mg.

661. A "Boney" Pork Chop

Preparation Time: 20 minutes
Cooking Time: 30 minutes
Servings: 4
Ingredients:
- 1 c. baby carrots
- Flavored vinegar
- 3 tbsps. Worcestershire sauce
- Ground pepper
- 1 chopped onion
- 4 ¾ bone-in thick pork chops
- 1/4 c. divided butter
- 1 c. vegetables

Directions:
1. Take a bowl and add pork chops, season with pepper and flavored vinegar.
2. Take a skillet and place it over medium heat. Add 2 teaspoons of butter and melt it.
3. Toss the pork chops and brown them.
4. Each side should take about 3-5 minutes.
5. Set your pot to sauté mode and add 2 tablespoons of butter, add carrots and sauté them.
6. Pour broth and Worcestershire.
7. Add pork chops and lock up the lid.
8. Cook on HIGH pressure for 13 minutes.
9. Release the pressure naturally.
10. Enjoy!

Nutrition:
Calories: 715, Fat: 37.4g, Carbs: 2g, Protein: 20.7g, Sugars: 0g, Sodium: 276mg, Potassium: 88mg.

662. Roast and Mushrooms

Preparation Time: 10 minutes
Cooking Time: 20 minutes
Servings: 4
Ingredients:
- 1 tsp. Italian seasoning
- 12 oz. low-sodium beef stock
- 3 1/2 lbs. pork roast
- 4 oz. sliced mushrooms

Directions:

1. In a roasting pan, combine the roast with mushrooms, stock and Italian seasoning, and toss.
2. Introduce inside the oven and bake at 350F during 20 minutes.
3. Slice the roast, divide it along while using the mushroom mix between plates and serve.
4. Enjoy!

Nutrition:

Calories: 310, Fat: 16g, Carbs: 10g, Protein: 22g, Sugars: 4g, Sodium: 600mg, Potassium: 65mg.

663. Pork and Celery Mix

Preparation Time: 10 minutes
Cooking Time: 30 minutes
Servings: 8
Ingredients:

- 3 tsp. Fenugreek powder
- Black pepper
- 1 tbsp. organic olive oil
- 1 1/2 c. coconut cream
- 26 oz. chopped celery leaves and stalks
- 1 lb. cubed pork meat
- 1 tbsp. chopped onion

Directions:

1. Heat a pan while using oil over medium-high heat. Add the pork as well as the onion, black pepper and Fenugreek. Toss and brown for 5 minutes.
2. Add the celery and coconut cream. Toss, cook over medium heat for twenty minutes, divide everything into bowls and serve.
3. Enjoy!

Nutrition:

Calories: 340, Fat: 5g, Carbs: 8g, Protein: 14g, Sugars: 2.1g, Sodium: 200mg, Potassium: 68mg.

664. Pork and Dates Sauce

Preparation Time: 10 minutes
Cooking Time: 40 minutes
Servings: 6
Ingredients:

- 2 tbsps. water
- 2 tbsps. mustard
- 1/3 c. pitted dates
- Black pepper
- 1/4 tsp. onion powder
- 1/4 c. coconut amino
- 1 1/2 lbs. pork tenderloin
- 1/4 tsp. smoked paprika

Directions:

1. In your blender, mix dates with water, coconut amino, mustard, paprika, pepper and onion powder and blend well.
2. Place the pork loin inside the roasting pan. Add the date sauce, stir to coat perfectly, put everything inside the oven at 400F. Bake for 40 minutes, cut the meat, divide it and the sauce among the plates and serve.
3. Enjoy!

Nutrition:

Calories: 240, Fat: 8g, Carbs: 13g, Protein: 24g, Sugars: 0g, Sodium: 433mg, Potassium: 90mg.

665. Pork Roast and Cranberry Roast

Preparation Time: 10 minutes
Cooking Time: 30 minutes
Servings: 4
Ingredients:

- 2 minced garlic cloves
- 1/2 tsp. grated ginger
- Black pepper
- 1/2 c. low-sodium veggie stock
- 1 1/2 lbs. pork loin roast
- 1 tbsp. coconut flour
- 1/2 c. cranberries
- Juice of 1/2 lemon

Directions:

1. Put the stock in a little pan and heat over medium-high flame. Add black pepper, ginger, garlic, cranberries, fresh freshly squeezed lemon juice and the flour. Whisk well and cook for ten minutes.
2. Put the roast in the pan. Add the cranberry sauce at the very top, introduce inside oven and bake at 375F for an hour and 20 minutes.
3. Slice the roast, divide it along using the sauce between plates and serve.
4. Enjoy!

Nutrition:

Calories: 330, Fat: 13g, Carbs: 13g, Protein: 25g, Sugars: 7g, Sodium: 150mg, Potassium: 45mg.

666. Easy Pork Chops

Preparation Time: 10 minutes
Cooking Time: 10 minutes
Servings: 4

Ingredients:

- 1 c. low-sodium chicken stock
- 1 tsp. sweet paprika
- 4 boneless pork chops
- 1/4 tsp. black pepper
- 1 tbsp. extra-virgin olive oil

Directions:

1. Heat a pan while using the oil over medium-high flame. Add pork chops, brown them for 5 minutes on either side, add paprika, black pepper and stock, toss, cook for fifteen minutes more, divide between plates and serve.
2. Enjoy!

Nutrition:

Calories: 272, Fat: 4g, Carbs: 14g, Protein: 17g, Sugars: 0.2g, Sodium: 68mg, Potassium: 67mg.

667. Pork and Roasted Tomatoes Mix

Preparation Time: 10 minutes
Cooking Time: 15 minutes
Servings: 6
Ingredients:

- 1/2 c. chopped yellow onion
- 2 c. chopped zucchinis
- 1 lb. ground pork meat
- ¾ c. shredded low-fat cheddar cheese
- Black pepper
- 15 oz. no-salt-added, chopped and canned roasted tomatoes

Directions:

1. Heat a pan over medium-high flame. Add pork, onion, black pepper and zucchini, stir and cook for 7 minutes.
2. Add roasted tomatoes, stir, bring to a boil, cook over medium heat for 8 minutes, divide into bowls, sprinkle cheddar on the top and serve.
3. Enjoy!

Nutrition:

Calories: 270, Fat: 5g, Carbs: 10g, Protein: 12g, Sugars: 8g, Sodium: 390mg, Potassium: 90mg.

668. Provence Pork Medallions

Preparation Time: 10 minutes
Cooking Time: 20 minutes
Servings: 4
Ingredients:

- 1 tsp. Herb de Provence

- Pepper.
- 1/2 c. dry white wine
- 16 oz. pork tenderloins
- Salt

Directions:
1. Season pork lightly with salt and pepper.
2. Place the pork between two pieces of parchment paper and pound with a mallet.
3. You need to have 1/4-inch-thick meat.
4. In a large non-stick frying pan, cook the pork over medium-high heat for 2-3 minutes per side.
5. Remove from the heat and sprinkle with herb de Provence. Remove the pork from the skillet and place it aside. Keep warm.
6. Place the skillet over the heat again. Add the wine and cook, stirring to scrape down the bits.
7. Cook until reduced slightly and pour over pork. Serve.

Nutrition:
Calories: 105.7, Fat: 1.7g, Carbs: 0.8g, Protein: 22.6g, Sugars: 0g, Sodium: 67mg, Potassium: 65mg.

669. Garlic Pork Shoulder

Preparation Time: 10 minutes
Cooking Time: 4 hours
Servings: 6
Ingredients:
- 2 tsp. sweet paprika
- 4 lbs. pork shoulder
- 3 tbsps. extra virgin essential olive oil
- Black pepper
- 3 tbsps. minced garlic

Directions:
1. In a bowl, mix extra virgin olive oil with paprika, black pepper and oil and whisk well.
2. Brush pork shoulder with this mix, arrange inside a baking dish and introduce inside the oven at 425F for twenty or so minutes.
3. Reduce heat to 325F and bake for 4 hours.
4. Slice the meat, divide it between plates and serve with a side salad.
5. Enjoy!

Nutrition:
Calories: 321, Fat: 6g, Carbs: 12g, Protein: 18g, Sugars: 0g, Sodium: 470mg, Potassium: 55mg.

670. Grilled Flank Steak with Lime Vinaigrette

Preparation Time: 10 minutes
Cooking Time: 10 minutes
Servings: 6
Ingredients:
- 2 tablespoons lime juice, freshly squeezed
- 2 tablespoons extra virgin olive oil
- ½ teaspoon ground black pepper
- ¼ cup chopped fresh cilantro
- 1 tablespoon ground cumin
- ¼ teaspoon red pepper flakes
- ¾ pound flank steak

Directions:
1. Heat the grill to low-medium heat.
2. In a food processor, place all ingredients except for the cumin, red pepper flakes, and flank steak. Pulse until smooth. This will be the vinaigrette sauce. Set aside.
3. Season the flank steak with ground cumin and red pepper flakes and allow to marinate for at least 10 minutes.
4. Place the steak on the grill rack and cook for 5 minutes on each side. Cut into the center to check the doneness of the meat. You can also insert a meat thermometer to check the internal temperature.
5. Remove from the grill and allow to stand for 5 minutes.
6. Slice the steak to 2 inches long and toss the vinaigrette to flavor the meat.
7. Serve with salad if desired.

Nutrition:
Calories per servings: 103, Protein: 13g, Carbs: 1g, Fat: 5g, Saturated Fat: 1g, Sodium: 73mg, Potassium: 76mg.

671. Asian Pork Tenderloin

Preparation Time: 10 minutes
Cooking Time: 15 minutes
Servings: 4
Ingredients:
- 2 tablespoons sesame seeds
- 1 teaspoon ground coriander
- 1/8 teaspoon cayenne pepper
- 1/8 teaspoon celery seed
- ½ teaspoon minced onion
- ¼ teaspoon ground cumin

- 1/8 teaspoon ground cinnamon
- 1 tablespoon sesame oil
- 1-pound pork tenderloin sliced into 4 equal portions

Directions:
1. Preheat the oven to 400F.
2. In a skillet, toast the sesame seeds over low heat and set them aside. Allow the sesame seeds to cool.
3. In a bowl, combine the rest of the ingredients except for the pork tenderloin. Stir in the toasted sesame seeds.
4. Place the pork tenderloin in a baking dish and rub the spices on both sides.
5. Place the baking dish with the pork in the oven and bake for 15 minutes or until the internal temperature of the meat reaches 170F.
6. Serve warm.

Nutrition:
Calories: 248, Protein: 26g, Carbs: 0g, Fat: 16g, Saturated Fat: 5g, Sodium: 57mg, Potassium: 55mg.

672. Simple Beef Brisket and Tomato Soup

Preparation Time: 10 minutes
Cooking Time: 3 hours
Servings: 8
Ingredients:
- 1 tablespoon olive oil
- 2 ½ pounds beef brisket, trimmed of fat and cut into 8 equal parts
- A dash of ground black pepper
- 1 ½ cups chopped onions
- 4 cloves of garlic, smashed
- 1 teaspoon dried thyme
- 1 cup ripe Roma tomato, chopped
- ¼ cup red wine vinegar
- 1 cup beef stock, low sodium or home made

Directions:
1. In a heavy pot, heat the oil over medium-high heat.
2. Season the brisket with ground black pepper and place in the pot.
3. Cook while stirring constantly until the beef turns brown on all sides.
4. Stir in the onions and cook until fragrant. Add in the garlic and thyme and cook for another minute until fragrant.

5. Pour in the rest of the ingredients and bring to a boil.
6. Cook until the beef is tender. This may take about 3 hours or more.

Nutrition:
Calories: 229, Protein: 31g, Carbs: 6g, Fat: 9g, Saturated Fat: 3g, Sodium: 184mg, Potassium: 44mg.

673. Beef Stew with Fennel and Shallots

Preparation Time: 10 minutes
Cooking Time: 40 minutes
Servings: 6
Ingredients:
- 1 tablespoon olive oil
- 1-pound boneless lean beef stew meat, trimmed from fat and cut into cubes
- ½ fennel bulb, trimmed and sliced thinly
- 3 large shallots, chopped
- ¾ teaspoons ground black pepper
- 2 fresh thyme sprigs
- 1 bay leaf
- 3 cups low sodium beef broth
- ½ cup red wine
- 4 large carrots, peeled and cut into chunks
- 4 large white potatoes, peeled and cut into chunks
- 3 portobello mushrooms, cleaned and cut into chunks
- 1/3 cup Italian parsley, chopped

Directions:
1. Heat oil in a pot over medium heat and stir in the beef cubes for 5 minutes or until all sides turn brown.
2. Stir in the fennel, shallots, black pepper, and thyme for one minute or until the ingredients become fragrant.
3. Stir in the bay leaf, broth, red wine, carrots, white potatoes and mushrooms.
4. Bring to a boil and cook for 30 minutes or until everything is tender.
5. Stir in the parsley last.

Nutrition:
Calories: 244, Protein: 21g, Carbs: 22g, Fat: 8g, Saturated Fat: 2g, Sodium: 184mg, Potassium: 60mg.

674. Rustic Beef and Barley Soup

Preparation Time: 10 minutes
Cooking Time: 40 minutes
Servings: 6
Ingredients:
- 1 teaspoon olive oil
- 1-pound beef round steak, sliced into strips
- 2 cups yellow onion, chopped
- 1 cup diced celery
- 4 cloves of garlic, chopped
- 1 cup diced Roma tomatoes
- ½ cup diced sweet potato
- ½ cup diced mushrooms
- 1 cup diced carrots
- ¼ cup uncooked barley
- 3 cups low sodium vegetable stock
- 1 teaspoon dried sage
- 1 paprika
- A dash of black pepper to taste
- 1 cup chopped kale

Directions:
1. In a large pot, heat the oil over medium flame and stir in the beef. Cook for 5 minutes while stirring constantly until all sides turn brown.
2. Stir in the onion, celery, and garlic until fragrant.
3. Add in the rest of the ingredients except for the kale.
4. Bring to a boil and cook for 30 minutes until everything is tender.
5. Stir in the kale last and cook for another 5 minutes.

Nutrition:
Calories per servings: 246, Protein: 21g, Carbs: 24g, Fat: 4g, Saturated Fat: 1g, Sodium: 13mg, Potassium: 95mg.

675. Beef Stroganoff

Preparation Time: 10 minutes
Cooking Time: 25 minutes
Servings: 4
Ingredients:
- ½ cup chopped onion
- ½ pound boneless beef round steak, cut into ¾ inch thick
- 4 cups pasta noodles
- ½ cup fat-free cream of mushroom soup
- ½ cup water
- ½ teaspoon paprika
- ½ cup fat-free sour cream

Directions:

1. In a non-stick frying pan, sauté the onions over low to medium heat without oil while stirring constantly for about 5 minutes.
2. Stir in the beef and cook for another 5 minutes until the beef is tender and turn brown on all sides. Set aside.
3. In a large pot, fill it with water until ¾ full and bring to a boil. Cook the noodles until done according to package instructions. Drain the noodles and set them aside.
4. In a saucepan, whisk the mushroom soup and water. Bring to a boil over medium heat and stir constantly until the sauce has reduced. Add in paprika and sour cream.
5. Assemble the stroganoff by placing the pasta in a bowl and pouring it over the sauce. Top with the meat.
6. Serve warm.

Nutrition:
Calories: 273, Protein: 20g, Carbs: 37g, Fat: 5g, Saturated Fat: 2g, Sodium: 193mg, Potassium: 43mg.

676. Curried Pork Tenderloin in Apple Cider

Preparation Time: 10 minutes
Cooking Time: 26 minutes
Servings: 6
Ingredients:
- 16 ounces pork tenderloin, cut into 6 pieces
- 1 ½ tablespoons curry powder
- 1 tablespoon extra-virgin olive oil
- 2 medium onions, chopped
- 2 cups apple cider, organic and unsweetened
- 1 tart apple, peeled and chopped into chunks

Directions:
1. In a bowl, season the pork with the curry powder and set it aside.
2. Heat oil in a pot over medium flame.
3. Sauté the onions for one minute until fragrant.
4. Stir in the seasoned pork tenderloin and cook for 5 minutes or until lightly golden.
5. Add in the apple cider and apple chunks.
6. Close the lid and bring to a boil.
7. Allow to simmer for 20 minutes.

Nutrition:
Calories: 244, Protein: 24g, Carbs: 18g, Fat: 8g, Saturated Fat: 2g, Sodium: 70mg, Potassium: 85mg.

677. Pork Medallions with Five Spice Powder

Preparation Time: 10 minutes
Cooking Time: 25 minutes
Servings: 4
Ingredients:

- 1 tablespoon olive oil
- 3 cloves of garlic, minced
- 1-pound pork tenderloin, fat trimmed
- 2 tablespoon low-sodium soy sauce
- 1 tablespoon green onion, minced
- ¾ teaspoon five spice powder
- ½ cup water
- ¼ cup dry white wine
- 1/3 cup chopped onion
- ½ head green cabbage, thinly sliced and wilted
- 1 tablespoon chopped fresh parsley

Directions:

1. In a bowl, combine the olive oil, garlic, pork tenderloin, soy sauce, green onion, and five spice powder. Mix until well combined and allow to marinate in the fridge for at least two hours.
2. Heat the oven to 400F.
3. Remove the pork from the marinade and pat dry.
4. On a skillet, sear the meat on all sides until slightly brown before transferring it into a heat-proof baking dish.
5. Place inside the oven and roast the pork for 20 minutes.
6. Meanwhile, pour the water, dry white wine, and onions in the skillet where you seared the pork and deglaze. Allow to simmer until the sauce has reduced.
7. Serve the pork medallions with wilted cabbages and drizzle the sauce on top.

Nutrition:
Calories: 219, Protein: 25g, Carbs: 5g, Fat: 11g, Saturated Fat: 2g, Sodium: 296mg, Potassium: 97mg.

678. Grilled Pork Fajitas

Preparation Time: 10 minutes
Cooking Time: 15 minutes
Servings: 8
Ingredients:

- ½ teaspoon paprika
- ½ teaspoon oregano
- ¼ teaspoon ground coriander
- ¼ teaspoon garlic powder
- 1 tablespoon chili powder
- 1-pound pork tenderloin, fat trimmed and cut into large strips
- 1 onion, sliced
- 8 whole wheat flour tortillas, warmed
- 4 medium tomatoes, chopped
- 4 cups shredded lettuce

Directions:

1. In a bowl, mix the paprika, oregano, coriander, garlic powder, and chili powder.
2. Sprinkle the spice mixture on the pork tenderloin strips and toss to coat the meat with the spices.
3. Prepare the grill and heat to 400F.
4. Place the meat and onion in a grill basket and broil for 20 minutes or until all sides have browned.
5. Assemble the fajitas by placing in the center of the tortillas the grilled pork and onions. Add in the tomatoes and lettuce before rolling the fajitas.

Nutrition:
Calories: 250, Protein: 20g, Carbs: 29g, Fat: 6g, Saturated Fat: 2g, Sodium: 234mg, Potassium: 46mg.

679. New York Strip Steak with Mushroom Sauce

Preparation Time: 10 minutes
Cooking Time: 20 minutes
Servings: 2
Ingredients:

- 2 New York Strip steaks - 4 ounces each, trimmed from fat
- 3 cloves of garlic, minced
- 2 ounces shiitake mushrooms, sliced
- 2 ounces button mushrooms, sliced
- ¼ teaspoon thyme
- ¼ teaspoon rosemary

- ¼ cup low sodium beef broth

Directions:

1. Heat the grill to 350F.
2. Place the grill rack 6 inches from the heat source.
3. Grill the steaks for 10 minutes on each side or until slightly pink on the inside.
4. Meanwhile, prepare the sauce. In a small nonstick pan, water sauté the garlic, mushrooms, thyme and rosemary for a minute. Pour in the broth and bring to a boil. Allow the sauce to simmer until the liquid is reduced.
5. Top the steaks with the mushroom sauce.
6. Serve warm.

Nutrition:
Calories: 270, Protein: 23g, Carbs: 4g, Fat: 6g, Saturated Fat: 2g, Sodium: 96mg, Potassium: 86mg.

680. Pork Chops with Black Currant Jam

Preparation Time: 10 minutes
Cooking Time: 20 minutes
Servings: 6
Ingredients:

- ¼ cup black currant jam
- 2 tablespoons Dijon mustard
- 1 teaspoon olive oil
- 6 center cut pork loin chops, trimmed from fat
- 1/3 cup wine vinegar
- 1/8 teaspoon ground black pepper
- 6 orange slices

Directions:

1. In a small bowl, mix the jam and mustard. Set aside.
2. In a nonstick pan, heat the oil over medium flames and sear the pork chops for 5 minutes on each side or until all sides turn brown.
3. Brush the pork chops with the mustard mixture and turn the flame to low. Cook for two more minutes on each side. Set aside.
4. Using the same frying pan, pour in the wine vinegar to deglaze the pan. Season with ground black pepper and allow to simmer for at least 5 minutes or until the vinegar has reduced.
5. Pour over the pork chops and garnish with orange slices on top.

Nutrition:

Calories: 198, Protein: 25g, Carbs: 11g, Fat: 6g, Saturated Fat: 2g, Sodium: 188mg, Potassium: 55mg.

681. Pork Medallion with Herbes de Provence

Preparation Time: 10 minutes
Cooking Time: 15 minutes
Servings: 2
Ingredients:
- 8 ounces of pork medallion, trimmed from fat
- Freshly ground black pepper to taste
- ½ teaspoon Herbes de Provence
- ¼ cup dry white wine

Directions:
1. Season the meat with black pepper.
2. Place the meat in between sheets of wax paper and pound on a mallet until about ¼ inch thick.
3. In a nonstick skillet, sear the pork over medium heat for 5 minutes on each side or until the meat is slightly brown.
4. Remove meat from the skillet and sprinkle with Herbes de Provence.
5. Using the same skillet, pour the wine and scrape the sides to deglaze. Allow to simmer until the wine is reduced.
6. Pour the wine sauce over the pork.
7. Serve immediately.

Nutrition:
Calories: 120, Protein: 24g, Carbs: 1g, Fat: 2g, Saturated Fat: 0.5g, Sodium: 62mg, Potassium: 65mg.

682. Pork Tenderloin with Apples and Balsamic Vinegar

Preparation Time: 10 minutes
Cooking Time: 25 minutes
Servings: 4
Ingredients:
- 1 tablespoon olive oil
- 1-pound pork tenderloin, trimmed from fat
- Freshly ground black pepper
- 2 cups chopped onion
- 2 cups chopped apple
- 1 ½ tablespoons fresh rosemary, chopped
- 1 cup low sodium chicken broth
- 1 ½ tablespoons balsamic vinegar

Directions:
1. Heat the oven to 450F.
2. Heat the oil in a large skillet over medium flame.
3. Sear the pork and season with black pepper. Cook the pork for 3 minutes until all sides turn light brown. Remove from the heat and place in a baking pan.
4. Roast the pork for 15 minutes.
5. Meanwhile, place the onion, apples, and rosemary on the skillet where the pork is seared. Continue stirring for 5 minutes. Pour in broth and balsamic vinegar and allow to simmer until the sauce thickens.
6. Serve the roasted pork with the onion and apple sauce.

Nutrition:
Calories: 240, Protein: 26g, Carbs: 17g, Fat: 6g, Saturated Fat: 1g, Sodium: 83mg, Potassium: 69mg.

683. Pork Tenderloin with Apples and Blue Cheese

Preparation Time: 10 minutes
Cooking Time: 25 minutes
Servings: 4
Ingredients:
- 1-pound pork tenderloin, trimmed from fat
- ½ teaspoon white pepper
- 2 teaspoons black pepper
- ¼ teaspoon cayenne pepper
- 1 teaspoon paprika
- 2 apples, sliced
- ½ cup unsweetened apple juice
- ¼ cup crumbled blue cheese

Directions:
1. Heat the oven to 350F.
2. Season the tenderloin with white pepper, black pepper, cayenne pepper, and paprika.
3. Heat a non-stick pan over medium flame and sear the meat for 3 minutes on each side. Transfer to a baking dish and roast in the oven for 20 minutes or until the internal temperature reaches 155F. Remove from the oven to cool.
4. While the pork is roasting, prepare the sauce. Using the same skillet used to sear the meat, sauté the apples for 3 minutes. Add the apple juice and allow the sauce to thicken for at least 10 minutes.
5. Serve the pork with the apple sauce and sprinkle with blue cheese on top.

Nutrition:
Calories: 235, Protein: 26g, Carbs: 17, Fat: 3g, Saturated Fat: 1g, Sodium: 145mg, Potassium: 43mg.

684. Pork Tenderloin with Fennel Sauce

Preparation Time: 10 minutes
Cooking Time: 30 minutes
Servings: 4
Ingredients:
- 4 pork tenderloin fillets, trimmed from fat and cut into 4 portions
- 1 tablespoon olive oil
- 1 teaspoon fennel seeds
- 1 fennel bulb, cored and sliced thinly
- 1 sweet onion, sliced thinly
- ½ cup dry white wine
- 12 ounces low sodium chicken broth
- 1 orange, sliced for garnish

Directions:
1. Place the pork slices in between wax paper and pound with a mallet to about ¼-inch thick.
2. Heat oil in a skillet and fry the fennel seeds for 3 minutes or until fragrant.
3. Stir in the pork and cook on all sides for 3 minutes or until golden brown. Remove the pork from the skillet and set it aside.
4. Using the same skillet, add the fennel bulb slices and onion. Sauté for 5 minutes and set aside.
5. Add the wine and chicken broth to the skillet and bring to a boil until the sauce reduces in half.
6. Return the pork to the skillet and cook for another 5 minutes.
7. Serve the pork with sauce and vegetables.

Nutrition:
Calories: 276, Protein: 29g, Carbs: 13g, Fat: 12g, Saturated Fat: 3g, Sodium: 122mg, Potassium: 78mg.

685. Spicy Beef Kebabs

Preparation Time: 10 minutes
Cooking Time: 10 minutes
Servings: 8
Ingredients:

- 2 yellow onions, minced
- 2 tablespoons fresh lemon juice
- 1 ½ pounds lean ground beef, minced
- ¼ cup bulgur, soaked in water for 30 minutes and then rinsed
- ¼ cup chopped pine nuts
- 2 cloves of garlic, minced
- 1 teaspoon ground cumin
- ½ teaspoon ground cinnamon
- ½ teaspoon ground cardamom
- ½ teaspoon freshly ground black pepper
- 16 wooden skewers, soaked in water for 30 minutes

Directions:

1. In a mixing bowl, combine all ingredients except for the skewers. Mix well.
2. Form a sausage from the meat mixture and thread it into the skewers. If the sausage is crumbly, add a tablespoon of water at a time until it holds well together. Refrigerate the skewered meat sausages until ready to cook.
3. Heat the grill to 350F and place the grill rack 6 inches from the heat source.
4. Place the skewered kebabs on the grill and broil for 5 minutes on each side.
5. Serve with yogurt if desired.

Nutrition:
Calories: 219, Protein: 23g, Carbs: 3g, Fat: 12g, Saturated Fat: 3g, Sodium: 53mg, Potassium: 76mg.

686. Spicy Beef Curry

Preparation Time: 10 minutes
Cooking Time: 40 minutes
Servings: 6
Ingredients:

- 1 medium serrano pepper, cut into thirds
- 4 cloves of garlic, minced
- 1 2-inch piece ginger, peeled and chopped
- 1 yellow onion, chopped
- 2 tablespoon ground coriander
- 2 teaspoons ground cumin
- ½ teaspoon ground turmeric
- 2 teaspoons garam masala

- 1 tablespoon olive oil
- 2 pounds beef, cut into chunks
- 1 cup ripe tomatoes, diced
- 2 cups water
- 1 cup fresh cilantro for garnish

Directions:

1. In a food processor, pulse the serrano peppers, garlic, ginger, onion, coriander, cumin, turmeric, and garam masala until well-combined.
2. Heat oil over medium heat in a skillet and sauté the spice mixture for 2 minutes or until fragrant.
3. Stir in the beef and cook while stirring constantly for three minutes or until the beef turns brown.
4. Stir in the tomatoes and sauté for another three minutes.
5. Add in the water and bring to a boil.
6. Once boiling, turn the heat to low and simmer for thirty minutes or until the meat is tender.
7. Add cilantro last before serving.

Nutrition:
Calories: 181, Protein: 16g, Carbs: 5g, Fat: 8g, Saturated Fat: 2g, Sodium: 74mg, Potassium: 89mg.

687. Pork Tenderloin with Apples and Sweet Potatoes

Preparation Time: 10 minutes
Cooking Time: 30 minutes
Servings: 4
Ingredients:

- ¾ cup apple cider
- ¼ cup apple cider vinegar
- 2 tablespoons maple syrup
- ¼ teaspoon smoked paprika powder
- 1 teaspoon grated ginger
- ¼ teaspoon ground black pepper
- 2 teaspoons olive oil
- 1 12-ounce pork tenderloin
- 1 large sweet potato, cut into cubes
- 1 large apple, cored and into cubes

Directions:

1. Preheat the oven to 375F.
2. In a bowl, combine the apple cider, apple cider vinegar, maple syrup, smoked paprika, ginger, and black pepper. Set aside.

3. Heat the oil in a large skillet and sear the meat for 3 minutes on both sides.
4. Transfer the pork to a baking dish and place the sweet potatoes and apples around the pork. Pour in the apple cider sauce.
5. Place inside the oven and cook for 20 minutes.

Nutrition:
Calories: 267, Protein: 23.5g, Carbs: 31g, Fat: 5g, Saturated Fat: 0.5g, Sodium: 69mg, Potassium: 145mg.

688. Tarragon Pork Steak with Tomatoes

Preparation Time: 10 minutes
Cooking Time: 22 minutes
Servings: 4
Ingredients:

- 4 medium pork steaks
- Black pepper to the taste
- 1 tablespoon olive oil
- 8 cherry tomatoes, halved
- A handful of tarragon, chopped

Directions:

1. Heat a pan with the oil over medium-high flame. Add steaks, season with black pepper, cook them for 6 minutes on each side and divide between plates.
2. Heat the same pan over medium flame. Add the tomatoes and the tarragon, cook for 10 minutes, divide next to the pork and serve.
3. Enjoy!

Nutrition:
Calories: 263, Fat: 4g, Fiber: 6g, Carbs: 12g, Protein: 16g, Sodium: 59mg, Potassium: 198mg.

689. Pork Meatballs

Preparation Time: 10 minutes
Cooking Time: 10 minutes
Servings: 4
Ingredients:

- 1 pound pork, ground
- 1/3 cup cilantro, chopped
- 1 cup red onion, chopped
- 4 garlic cloves, minced
- 1 tablespoon ginger, grated
- 1 Thai chili, chopped
- 2 tablespoons olive oil

Directions:

1. In a bowl, combine the meat with cilantro, onion, garlic, ginger and chili, stir well and shape medium meatballs out of this mix.
2. Heat a pan with the oil over medium-high flame. Add the meatballs, cook them for 5 minutes on each side, divide them between plates and serve with a side salad.
3. Enjoy!

Nutrition:
Calories: 220, Fat: 4g, Fiber: 2g, Carbs: 8g, Protein: 14g, Sodium: 176mg, Potassium: 89mg.

690. Pork with Scallions and Peanuts

Preparation Time: 10 minutes
Cooking Time: 16 minutes
Servings: 4
Ingredients:
- 2 tablespoons lime juice
- 2 tablespoons coconut aminos
- 1 and ½ tablespoons brown sugar
- 5 garlic cloves, minced
- 3 tablespoons olive oil
- Black pepper to the taste
- 1 yellow onion, cut into wedges
- 1 and ½ pound pork tenderloin, cubed
- 3 tablespoons peanuts, chopped
- 2 scallions, chopped

Directions:
1. In a bowl, mix lime juice with aminos and sugar and stir very well.
2. In another bowl, mix garlic with 1 and ½ teaspoon oil and some black pepper and stir.
3. Heat a pan with the rest of the oil over medium-high flame. Add meat, and cook for 3 minutes on each side and transfer to a bowl.
4. Heat the same pan over medium-high flame. Add onion, stir and cook for 3 minutes.

5. Add the garlic mix, return the pork, also add the aminos mix, toss and cook for 6 minutes. Divide between plates, sprinkle scallions and peanuts on top and serve.
6. Enjoy!

Nutrition:
Calories: 273, Fat: 4g, Fiber: 5g, Carbs: 12g, Protein: 18g, Sodium: 35mg, Potassium: 89mg.

691. Mediterranean Lamb Mix

Preparation Time: 10 minutes
Cooking Time: 10 minutes
Servings: 4
Ingredients:
- 1 garlic clove, minced
- 2 red chilies, chopped
- 1 cucumber, sliced
- 2 tablespoons balsamic vinegar
- 1 carrot, sliced
- 1 radish, sliced
- ½ cup mint leaves, chopped
- ½ cup coriander leaves, chopped
- Black pepper to the taste
- 2 tablespoons olive oil
- 3 ounces bean sprouts
- 2 lamb fillets

Directions:
1. Put the chilies in a pan, add garlic and vinegar, bring to a boil, stir well and take off the heat.
2. In a bowl, mix cucumber with radish, carrot, coriander, mint and sprouts.
3. Heat your kitchen grill over medium-high flame. Brush lamb fillets with the oil, season them with pepper and cook for 3 minutes on each side. Slice the meat, add over the veggies, also add the vinegar mix, toss and serve.
4. Enjoy!

Nutrition:
Calories: 231, Fat: 3g, Fiber: 5g, Carbs: 7g, Protein: 17g, Sodium: 90mg, Potassium: 86mg.

692. Pork and Veggies Mix

Preparation Time: 15 minutes
Cooking Time: 1 hour
Servings: 6
Ingredients:
- 4 eggplants, cut into halves lengthwise
- 4 ounces olive oil
- 2 yellow onions, chopped
- 4 ounces pork meat, ground
- 2 green bell peppers, chopped
- 1 pound tomatoes, chopped
- 4 tomato slices
- 2 tablespoons low-sodium tomato paste
- ½ cup parsley, chopped
- 4 garlic cloves, minced
- ½ cup hot water
- Black pepper to the taste

Directions:
1. Heat a pan with the olive oil over medium-high flame. Add eggplant halves, cook for 5 minutes and transfer to a plate.
2. Heat the same pan over medium-high flame. Add onion, stir and cook for 3 minutes.
3. Add bell peppers, pork, tomato paste, pepper, parsley and chopped tomatoes, stir and cook for 7 minutes.
4. Arrange the eggplant halves in a baking tray. Divide garlic in each, spoon meat filling and top with a tomato slice.
5. Pour the water over them. Cover the tray with foil and bake in the oven at 350 degrees F for 40 minutes. Divide between plates and serve.
6. Enjoy!

Nutrition:
Calories: 253, Fat: 3g, Fiber: 2g, Carbs: 12g, Protein: 14g, Sodium: 87mg, Potassium: 156mg.

Chapter 15. Vegetarian

693. Lentil-Stuffed Zucchini Boats

Preparation Time: 15 minutes
Cooking Time: 45 minutes
Servings: 2
Ingredients:
- 2 medium zucchinis, halved lengthwise and seeded
- 2¼ cups water, divided
- 1 cup green or red lentils, dried and rinsed
- 2 teaspoons olive oil
- 1/3 cup diced onion
- 2 tablespoons tomato paste
- ½ teaspoon oregano
- ¼ teaspoon garlic powder
- Pinch salt
- ¼ cup grated part-skim mozzarella cheese

Directions:
1. Preheat the oven to 375°F. Line a baking sheet with parchment paper. Place the zucchini, hollow sides up, on the baking sheet, and set aside.
2. Boil 2 cups of water to a boil over high heat in a medium saucepan and add the lentils. Lower the heat, then simmer within 20 to 25 minutes. Drain and set aside.
3. Heat the olive oil in a medium skillet over medium-low heat. Sauté the onions until they are translucent, about 4 minutes. Lower the heat and add the cooked lentils, tomato paste, oregano, garlic powder, and salt.
4. Add the last quarter cup of water and simmer for 3 minutes, until the liquid reduces and forms a sauce. Remove from heat.
5. Stuff each zucchini half with the lentil mixture, dividing it evenly, and top with cheese. Bake for 25 minutes and serve. The zucchini should be fork-tender, and the cheese should be melted.

Nutrition:
Calories: 479, Fat: 9g, Carbohydrates: 74g, Fiber: 14g, Protein: 31g, Sodium: 206mg, Potassium: 1389mg.

694. Baked Eggplant Parmesan

Preparation Time: 15 minutes
Cooking Time: 35 minutes
Servings: 4
Ingredients:
- 1 small to medium eggplant, cut into ¼-inch slices
- ½ teaspoon salt-free Italian seasoning blend
- 1 tablespoon olive oil
- ¼ cup diced onion
- ½ cup diced yellow or red bell pepper
- 2 garlic cloves, pressed or minced
- 1 (8-ounce) can tomato sauce
- 3 ounces fresh mozzarella, cut into 6 pieces
- 1 tablespoon grated Parmesan cheese, divided
- 5 to 6 fresh basil leaves, chopped

Directions:
1. Preheat an oven-style Air Fryer to 400°F.
2. Working in two batches, place the eggplant slices onto the air-fryer tray and sprinkle them with Italian seasoning. Bake for 7 minutes. Repeat with the remaining slices, then set them aside on a plate.
3. In a medium skillet, heat the oil over medium heat and sauté the onion and peppers until softened, about 5 minutes. Add the garlic and sauté for 1 to 2 more minutes. Add the tomato sauce and stir to combine. Remove the sauce from the heat.
4. Spray a 9-by-6-inch casserole dish with cooking spray. Spread one-third of the sauce into the bottom of the dish. Layer eggplant slices onto the sauce. Sprinkle with half of the Parmesan cheese.
5. Continue layering the sauce and eggplant, ending with the sauce. Place the mozzarella pieces on the top. Sprinkle the remaining Parmesan evenly over the entire dish. Bake in the oven for 20 minutes. Garnish with fresh basil, cut into four servings, and serve.

Nutrition:
Calories: 213, Fat: 12g, Carbohydrates: 20g, Fiber: 7g, Protein: 10g, Sodium: 222mg, Potassium: 763mg.

695. Sweet Potato Rice with Spicy Peanut Sauce

Preparation Time: 15 minutes
Cooking Time: 25 minutes
Servings: 2
Ingredients:
- ½ cup basmati rice
- 2 teaspoons olive oil, divided
- 1 (8-ounce) can chickpeas, drained and rinsed
- 2 medium sweet potatoes, small cubes
- ¼ teaspoon ground cumin
- 1 cup of water
- 1/8 teaspoon salt
- 2 tablespoons chopped cilantro
- 3 tablespoons peanut butter
- 1 tablespoon sriracha
- 2 teaspoons reduced-sodium soy sauce
- ½ teaspoon garlic powder
- ¼ teaspoon ground ginger

Directions:
1. Heat 1 teaspoon of oil in a large nonstick skillet over medium-high heat. Add the chickpeas and heat for 3 minutes. Stir and cook until lightly browned. Transfer the chickpeas to a small bowl.
2. Put the rest of the 1 teaspoon of oil into the skillet. Then add the potatoes and cumin, distributing them evenly. Cook the potatoes until they become lightly browned before turning them.
3. While the potatoes are cooking, boil the water with the salt in a large saucepan over medium-high heat. Put the rice in the boiling water, adjust the heat to low, cover, and simmer for 20 minutes.
4. When the potatoes have fully cooked, about 10 minutes in total, remove the skillet from the heat. Transfer the potatoes and chickpeas to the rice, folding them all gently. Add the chopped cilantro.

5. In a small bowl, whisk the peanut butter, sriracha, soy sauce, garlic powder, and ginger until well blended. Divide the rice mixture between two serving bowls. Drizzle with the sauce and serve.

Nutrition:
   Calories: 667, Fat: 22g, Carbohydrates: 100g, Fiber: 14g, Protein: 20g, Sodium: 563mg, Potassium: 963mg.

696. Vegetable Red Curry

Preparation Time: 15 minutes
Cooking Time: 25 minutes
Servings: 2
Ingredients:
- 2 teaspoons olive oil
- 1 cup sliced carrots
- ½ cup chopped onion
- 1 garlic clove, pressed or minced
- 2 bell peppers, seeded and thinly sliced
- 1 cup chopped cauliflower
- 2/3 cup light coconut milk
- ½ cup low-sodium vegetable broth
- 1 tablespoon tomato paste
- 1 teaspoon curry powder
- ½ teaspoon ground cumin
- ½ teaspoon ground coriander
- ¼ teaspoon turmeric
- 2 cups fresh baby spinach
- 1 cup quick-cooking brown rice

Directions:
1. Heat oil in a large nonstick skillet over medium flame. Add the carrots, onion, and garlic and cook for 2 to 3 minutes. Reduce the heat to medium-low, add the peppers and cauliflower to the skillet, cover, and cook within 5 minutes.
2. Add the coconut milk, broth, tomato paste, curry powder, cumin, coriander, and turmeric, stirring to combine. Simmer, covered (vent the lid slightly), for 10 to 15 minutes until the curry is slightly reduced and thickened.
3. Uncover, add the spinach, and stir for 2 minutes until it is wilted and mixed into the vegetables. Remove from the heat. Cook the rice as stated in the package instructions. Serve the curry over the rice.

Nutrition:
   Calories: 584, Fat: 16g, Carbohydrates: 101g, Fiber: 10g, Protein: 13g, Sodium: 102mg, Potassium: 1430mg.

697. Black Bean Burgers

Preparation Time: 15 minutes
Cooking Time: 20 minutes
Servings: 4
Ingredients:
- ½ cup quick-cooking brown rice
- 2 teaspoons canola oil, divided
- ½ cup finely chopped carrots
- ¼ cup finely chopped onion
- 1 can black beans, drained
- 1 tablespoon salt-free mesquite seasoning blend
- 4 small, hard rolls

Directions:
1. Cook the rice as stated in the package directions and set aside. Heat 1 teaspoon of oil in a large nonstick skillet over medium flame. Add the carrots and onions and cook until the onions are translucent, about 4 minutes. Adjust the heat to low, and cook again for 5 to 6 minutes until the carrots are tender.
2. Add the beans and seasoning to the skillet and continue cooking for 2 to 3 more minutes. Pulse bean mixture in a food processor 3 to 4 times or until the mixture is coarsely blended. Put the batter in a medium bowl and fold in the brown rice until well combined.
3. Divide the mixture evenly and form it into 4 patties with your hands. Heat the remaining oil in the skillet. Cook the patties within 4 to 5 minutes per side, turning once. Serve the burgers on the rolls with your choice of toppings.

Nutrition:
   Calories: 368, Fat: 6g, Carbohydrates: 66g, Fiber: 8g, Protein: 13g, Sodium: 322mg, Potassium: 413mg.

698. Summer Barley Pilaf with Yogurt Dill Sauce

Preparation Time: 15 minutes
Cooking Time: 30 minutes
Servings: 3
Ingredients:

- 2 2/3 cups low-sodium vegetable broth
- 2 teaspoons avocado oil
- 1 small zucchini, diced
- 1/3 cup slivered almonds
- 2 scallions, sliced
- 1 cup barley
- ½ cup plain nonfat Greek yogurt
- 2 teaspoons grated lemon zest
- ¼ teaspoon dried dill

Directions:
1. Boil the broth in a large saucepan. Heat the oil in a skillet. Add the zucchini and sauté for 3 to 4 minutes. Add the almonds and the white parts of the scallions and sauté for 2 minutes. Remove, and transfer it to a small bowl.
2. Add the barley to the skillet and sauté for 2 to 3 minutes to toast. Transfer the barley to the boiling broth and reduce the heat to low, cover, and simmer for 25 minutes or until tender. Remove, and let stand within 10 minutes or until the liquid is absorbed.
3. Simultaneously, mix the yogurt, lemon zest, and dill in a small bowl and set aside. Fluff the barley with a fork. Add the zucchini, almond, and onion mixture and mix gently. To serve, divide the pilaf between two bowls and drizzle the yogurt over each bowl.

Nutrition:
   Calories: 545, Fat: 15g, Carbohydrates: 87g, Fiber: 19g, Protein: 21g, Sodium: 37mg, Potassium: 694mg.

699. Lentil Quinoa Gratin with Butternut Squash

Preparation Time: 15 minutes
Cooking Time: 1 hour and 15 minutes
Servings: 3
Ingredients:
For the Lentils and Squash:
- Nonstick cooking spray
- 2 cups of water
- ½ cup dried green or red lentils, rinsed
- Pinch salt
- 1 teaspoon olive oil, divided
- ½ cup quinoa
- ¼ cup diced shallot

- 2 cups frozen cubed butternut squash
- ¼ cup low-fat milk
- 1 teaspoon chopped fresh rosemary
- Freshly ground black pepper

For the Gratin Topping:
- ¼ cup panko bread crumbs
- 1 teaspoon olive oil
- 1/3 cup shredded Gruyere cheese

Directions:
1. Preheat the oven to 400°F. Grease a 1½-quart casserole dish or an 8-by-8-inch baking dish with cooking spray.
2. In a medium saucepan, stir the water, lentils, and salt and boil over medium-high heat. Lower the heat once the water is boiling. Cover, and simmer for 20 to 25 minutes. Then drain and transfer the lentils to a large bowl and set aside.
3. In the same saucepan, heat ½ teaspoon of oil over medium flame. Add the quinoa and quickly stir for 1 minute to toast it lightly. Cook according to the package directions, about 20 minutes.
4. While the quinoa cooks, heat the remaining olive oil in a medium skillet over medium-low flame. Add the shallots, and sauté them until they are translucent, about 3 minutes. Add the squash, milk, and rosemary and cook for 1 to 2 minutes.
5. Remove, then transfer to the lentil bowl. Add in the quinoa and gently toss all. Season with pepper to taste. Transfer the mixture to the casserole dish.
6. For the gratin topping, mix the panko bread crumbs with the olive oil in a small bowl. Put the bread crumbs over the casserole and top them with the cheese. Bake the casserole for 25 minutes and serve.

Nutrition:
Calories: 576, Fat: 15g, Carbohydrates: 87g, Fiber: 12g, Protein: 28g, Sodium: 329mg, Potassium: 1176mg.

700. Brown Rice Casserole with Cottage Cheese

Preparation Time: 15 minutes
Cooking Time: 45 minutes

Servings: 3
Ingredients:
- Nonstick cooking spray
- 1 cup quick-cooking brown rice
- 1 teaspoon olive oil
- ½ cup diced sweet onion
- 1 (10-ounce) bag of fresh spinach
- 1½ cups low-fat cottage cheese
- 1 tablespoon grated Parmesan cheese
- ¼ cup sunflower seed kernels

Directions:
1. Preheat the oven to 375°F. Grease a small 1½-quart casserole dish with cooking spray. Cook the rice, as stated in the package directions. Set aside.
2. Heat the oil in a large nonstick skillet over medium-low flame. Add the onion and sauté for 3 to 4 minutes. Add the spinach and cover the skillet, cooking for 1 to 2 minutes until the spinach wilts. Remove the skillet from the heat.
3. In a medium bowl, mix the rice, spinach mixture, and cottage cheese. Transfer the mixture to the prepared casserole dish. Top with the Parmesan cheese and sunflower seeds, bake for 25 minutes until lightly browned, and serve.

Nutrition:
Calories: 334, Fat: 9g, Carbohydrates: 47g, Fiber: 5g, Protein: 19g, Sodium: 425mg, Potassium: 553mg.

701. Quinoa-Stuffed Peppers

Preparation Time: 15 minutes
Cooking Time: 35 minutes
Servings: 2
Ingredients:
- 2 large green bell peppers, halved
- 1½ teaspoons olive oil, divided
- ½ cup quinoa
- ½ cup minced onion
- 1 garlic clove, pressed or minced
- 1 cup chopped portobello mushrooms
- 3 tablespoons grated Parmesan cheese, divided
- 4 ounces tomato sauce

Directions:
1. Preheat the oven to 400°F. Put the pepper halves on your prepared baking sheet. Brush the insides of peppers with ½ teaspoon olive oil and bake for 10 minutes.
2. Remove the baking sheet, then set aside. While the peppers bake, cook the quinoa in a large saucepan over medium heat according to the package directions and set aside.
3. Heat the rest of the oil in a medium-size skillet over medium heat. Add the onion and sauté until it's translucent, about 3 minutes. Put the garlic and cook within 1 minute.
4. Put the mushrooms in the skillet, adjust the heat to medium-low, cover, and cook within 5 to 6 minutes. Uncover, and if there's still liquid in the pan, reduce the heat and cook until the liquid evaporates.
5. Add the mushroom mixture, 1 tablespoon of Parmesan, and the tomato sauce to the quinoa and gently stir to combine. Carefully spoon the quinoa mixture into each pepper half and sprinkle with the remaining Parmesan. Return the peppers to the oven, bake for 10 to 15 more minutes until tender, and serve.

Nutrition:
Calories: 292, Fat: 9g, Carbohydrates: 45g, Fiber: 8g, Protein: 12g, Sodium: 154mg, Potassium: 929mg.

702. Greek Flatbread with Spinach, Tomatoes & Feta

Preparation Time: 15 minutes
Cooking Time: 9 minutes
Servings: 2
Ingredients:
- 2 cups fresh baby spinach, coarsely chopped
- 2 teaspoons olive oil
- 2 slices Naan, or another flatbread
- ¼ cup sliced black olives
- 2 plum tomatoes, thinly sliced
- 1 teaspoon salt-free Italian seasoning blend
- ¼ cup crumbled feta

Directions:
1. Preheat the oven to 400°F. Heat 3 tablespoons of water in a small skillet over medium heat. Add the spinach, cover, and steam until wilted, about 2 minutes.

Drain off any excess water, then put it aside.

2. Drizzle the oil evenly onto both flatbreads. Top each evenly with spinach, olives, tomatoes, seasoning, and feta. Bake the flatbreads within 5 to 7 minutes, or until lightly browned. Cut each into four pieces and serve hot.

Nutrition:
Calories: 411, Fat: 15g, Carbohydrates: 53g, Fiber: 7g, Protein: 15g, Sodium: 621mg, Potassium: 522mg.

703. Mushroom Risotto with Peas

Preparation Time: 15 minutes
Cooking Time: 20 minutes
Servings: 2
Ingredients:
- 2 cups low-sodium vegetable or chicken broth
- 1 teaspoon olive oil
- 8 ounces baby portobello mushrooms, thinly sliced
- ½ cup frozen peas
- 1 teaspoon butter
- 1 cup Arborio rice
- 1 tablespoon grated Parmesan cheese

Directions:
1. Pour the broth into a microwave-proof glass measuring cup. Microwave on high for 1½ minutes or until hot. Heat the oil over medium heat in a large saucepan. Add the mushrooms and stir for 1 minute. Cover and cook until soft, about 3 more minutes. Stir in the peas and reduce the heat to low.
2. Put the mushroom batter to the saucepan's sides and add the butter to the middle, heating until melted. Put the rice in the saucepan and stir for 1 to 2 minutes to lightly toast. Add the hot broth, ½ cup at a time, and stir gently.
3. As the broth is cooked into the rice, continue adding more broth, ½ cup at a time, stirring after each addition, until all broth is incorporated. Once all the liquid is absorbed (this should take 15 minutes), remove it from the heat. Serve immediately, topped with Parmesan cheese.

Nutrition:
Calories: 430, Fat: 6g, Carbohydrates: 83g, Fiber: 5g, Protein: 10g, Sodium: 78mg, Potassium: 558mg.

704. Loaded Tofu Burrito with Black Beans

Preparation Time: 15 minutes
Cooking Time: 20 minutes
Servings: 2
Ingredients:
- 4 ounces extra-firm tofu, pressed and cut into 2-inch cubes
- 2 teaspoons mesquite salt-free seasoning, divided
- 2 teaspoons canola oil
- 1 cup thinly sliced bell peppers
- ½ cup diced onions
- 2/3 cup of black beans, drained
- 2 (10-inch) whole-wheat tortillas
- 1 tablespoon sriracha
- Nonfat Greek yogurt, for serving

Directions:
1. Put the tofu and 1 teaspoon of seasoning in a medium zip-top plastic freezer bag and toss until the tofu is well coated.
2. Heat the oil in a medium skillet over medium-high heat. Put the tofu in the skillet. Don't stir; allow the tofu to brown before turning. When lightly browned, about 6 minutes, transfer the tofu from the skillet to a small bowl and set aside.
3. Put the peppers plus onions in the skillet and sauté until tender, about 5 minutes. Lower the heat to medium-low, then put the beans and the remaining seasoning. Cook within 5 minutes.
4. For the burritos, lay each tortilla flat on a work surface. Place half of the tofu in the center of each tortilla, top with half of the pepper-bean mixture, and drizzle with the sriracha.
5. Fold the bottom portion of each tortilla up and over the tofu mixture. Then fold each side into the middle, tuck in, and tightly roll it up toward the open end. Serve with a dollop of yogurt.

Nutrition:
Calories: 327, Fat: 12g, Carbohydrates: 41g, Fiber: 11g, Protein: 16g, Sodium: 282mg, Potassium: 120mg.

705. Southwest Tofu Scramble

Preparation Time: 15 minutes
Cooking Time: 15 minutes
Servings: 1
Ingredients:
- ½ tablespoon olive oil
- ½ red onion, chopped
- 2 cups chopped spinach
- 8 ounces firm tofu, drained well
- 1 teaspoon ground cumin
- ½ teaspoon garlic powder
- Optional for servings: sliced avocado or sliced tomatoes

Directions:
1. Heat the olive oil in a medium skillet over medium flame. Put the onion and cook within 5 minutes. Add the spinach and cover to steam for 2 minutes.
2. Using a spatula, move the veggies to one side of the pan. Crumble the tofu into the open area in the pan, breaking it up with a fork. Add the cumin and garlic to the crumbled tofu and mix well. Sauté for 5 to 7 minutes until the tofu is slightly browned.
3. Serve immediately with whole-grain bread, fruit, or beans. Top with optional sliced avocado and tomato, if using.

Nutrition:
Calories: 267, Fat: 17g, Sodium: 75mg, Carbohydrates: 13g, Protein: 23g, Potassium: 47mg.

706. Black-Bean and Vegetable Burrito

Preparation Time: 15 minutes
Cooking Time: 15 minutes
Servings: 4
Ingredients:
- ½ tablespoon olive oil
- 2 red or green bell peppers, chopped
- 1 zucchini or summer squash, diced
- ½ teaspoon chili powder
- 1 teaspoon cumin
- Freshly ground black pepper
- 2cans black beans drained and rinsed
- 1 cup cherry tomatoes, halved
- 4 (8-inch) whole-wheat tortillas

- Optional for servings: spinach, sliced avocado, chopped scallions, or hot sauce

Directions:

1. Heat the oil in a large sauté pan over medium heat. Add the bell peppers and sauté until crisp-tender, about 4 minutes. Add the zucchini, chili powder, cumin, and black pepper to taste, and continue to sauté until the vegetables are tender, about 5 minutes.
2. Add the black beans and cherry tomatoes and cook within 5 minutes. Divide between 4 burritos and serve topped with optional ingredients as desired. Enjoy immediately.

Nutrition:

Calories: 311, Fat: 6g, Sodium: 499mg, Carbohydrates: 52g, Protein: 19g, Potassium: 79mg.

707. Baked Eggs in Avocado

Preparation Time: 15 minutes
Cooking Time: 15 minutes
Servings: 2
Ingredients:

- 2 avocados
- Juice of 2 limes
- Freshly ground black pepper
- 4 eggs
- 2 (8-inch) whole-wheat or corn tortillas, warmed
- Optional for servings: halved cherry tomatoes and chopped cilantro

Directions:

1. Adjust the oven rack to the middle position and preheat the oven to 450°F. Scrape out the center of halved avocado using a spoon of about 1½ tablespoons.
2. Press lime juice over the avocados and season with black pepper to taste, and then place it on a baking sheet. Crack an egg into the avocado.
3. Bake within 10 to 15 minutes. Remove from oven and garnish with optional cilantro and cherry tomatoes and serve with warm tortillas.

Nutrition:

Calories: 534, Fat: 39g, Sodium: 462mg, Potassium: 1,095mg, Carbohydrates: 30g, Fiber: 20g, Sugars: 3g, Protein: 23g.

708. Red Beans and Rice

Preparation Time: 15 minutes
Cooking Time: 45 minutes
Servings: 2
Ingredients:

- ½ cup dry brown rice
- 1 cup water, plus ¼ cup
- 1 can red beans, drained
- 1 tablespoon ground cumin
- Juice of 1 lime
- 4 handfuls of fresh spinach
- Optional toppings: avocado, chopped tomatoes, Greek yogurt, onions

Directions:

1. Mix rice plus water in a pot and bring to a boil. Cover and reduce heat to a low simmer. Cook within 30 to 40 minutes or according to package directions.
2. Meanwhile, add the beans, ¼ cup of water, cumin, and lime juice to a medium skillet. Simmer within 5 to 7 minutes.
3. Once the liquid is mostly gone, remove it from the heat and add spinach. Cover and let spinach wilt slightly, 2 to 3 minutes. Mix in with the beans. Serve beans with rice. Add toppings if using.

Nutrition:

Calories: 232, Fat: 2g, Sodium: 210mg, Carbohydrates: 41g, Protein: 13g, Potassium: 59mg.

709. Hearty Lentil Soup

Preparation Time: 15 minutes
Cooking Time: 30 minutes
Servings: 4
Ingredients:

- 1 tablespoon olive oil
- 2 carrots, peeled and chopped
- 2 celery stalks, diced
- 1 onion, chopped
- 1 teaspoon dried thyme
- ½ teaspoon garlic powder
- Freshly ground black pepper
- 1 (28-ounce) can no-salt diced tomatoes, drained
- 1 cup dry lentils
- 5 cups of water
- Salt

Directions:

1. Heat the oil in a large Dutch oven or pot over medium heat. Once the oil is simmering, add the carrot, celery, and onion. Cook, often stirring within 5 minutes.

2. Add the thyme, garlic powder, and black pepper. Cook within 30 seconds. Pour in the drained diced tomatoes and cook for a few more minutes, often stirring to enhance their flavor.
3. Put the lentils, water, plus a pinch of salt. Raise the heat and bring to a boil, then partially cover the pot and reduce heat to maintain a gentle simmer.
4. Cook within 30 minutes or until lentils are tender but still hold their shape. Ladle into serving bowls and serve with a fresh green salad and whole-grain bread.

Nutrition:

Calories: 168, Fat: 4g, Sodium: 130mg, Carbohydrates: 35g, Protein: 10g, Potassium: 90mg.

710. Black-Bean Soup

Preparation Time: 15 minutes
Cooking Time: 20 minutes
Servings: 4
Ingredients:

- 1 yellow onion
- 1 tablespoon olive oil
- 2 cans black beans, drained
- 1 cup diced fresh tomatoes
- 5 cups low-sodium vegetable broth
- ¼ teaspoon freshly ground black pepper
- ¼ cup chopped fresh cilantro

Directions:

1. Cook or sauté the onion in the olive oil within 4 to 5 minutes in a large saucepan over medium heat. Put the black beans, tomatoes, vegetable broth, and black pepper. Boil, then adjust heat to simmer within 15 minutes.
2. Remove, then working in batches, ladle the soup into a blender and process until somewhat smooth. Put it back in the pot, add the cilantro, and heat until warmed through. Serve immediately.

Nutrition:

Calories: 234, Fat: 5g, Sodium: 363mg, Carbohydrates: 37g, Protein: 11g, Potassium: 58mg.

711. Loaded Baked Sweet Potatoes

Preparation Time: 15 minutes
Cooking Time: 20 minutes
Servings: 4
Ingredients:

- 4 sweet potatoes
- ½ cup nonfat or low-fat plain Greek yogurt
- Freshly ground black pepper
- 1 teaspoon olive oil
- 1 red bell pepper, cored and diced
- ½ red onion, diced
- 1 teaspoon ground cumin
- 1 (15-ounce) can chickpeas, drained and rinsed

Directions:

1. Prick the potatoes using a fork and cook on your microwave's potato setting until potatoes are soft and cooked through, about 8 to 10 minutes for 4 potatoes. If you don't have a microwave, bake at 400°F for about 45 minutes.
2. Combine the yogurt and black pepper in a small bowl and mix well. Heat the oil in a medium pot over medium heat. Add bell pepper, onion, cumin, and additional black pepper to taste.
3. Add the chickpeas, stir to combine, and heat through about 5 minutes. Slice the potatoes lengthwise down the middle and top each half with a portion of the bean mixture followed by 1 to 2 tablespoons of the yogurt. Serve immediately.

Nutrition:

Calories: 264, Fat: 2g, Sodium: 124mg, Carbohydrates: 51g, Protein: 11g, Potassium: 58mg.

712. White Beans with Spinach and Pan-Roasted Tomatoes

Preparation Time: 15 minutes
Cooking Time: 10 minutes
Servings: 2
Ingredients:

- 1 tablespoon olive oil
- 4 small plum tomatoes, halved lengthwise
- 10 ounces frozen spinach, defrosted and squeezed of excess water

- 2 garlic cloves, thinly sliced
- 2 tablespoons water
- ¼ teaspoon freshly ground black pepper
- 1 can white beans, drained
- Juice of 1 lemon

Directions:

1. Heat the oil in a large skillet over medium-high heat. Put the tomatoes, cut-side down, and cook within 3 to 5 minutes; turn and cook within 1 minute more. Transfer to a plate.
2. Reduce heat to medium and add the spinach, garlic, water, and pepper to the skillet. Cook, tossing until the spinach is heated through, 2 to 3 minutes.
3. Return the tomatoes to the skillet, put the white beans and lemon juice, and toss until heated through 1 to 2 minutes.

Nutrition:

Calories: 293, Fat: 9g, Sodium: 267mg, Carbohydrates: 43g, Protein: 15g, Potassium: 78mg.

713. Black-Eyed Peas and Greens Power Salad

Preparation Time: 15 minutes
Cooking Time: 6 minutes
Servings: 2
Ingredients:

- 1 tablespoon olive oil
- 3 cups purple cabbage, chopped
- 5 cups baby spinach
- 1 cup shredded carrots
- 1 can black-eyed peas, drained
- Juice of ½ lemon
- Salt
- Freshly ground black pepper

Directions:

1. In a medium pan, add the oil and cabbage and sauté for 1 to 2 minutes on medium heat. Add in your spinach, cover for 3 to 4 minutes on medium heat, until greens are wilted. Remove from the heat and add to a large bowl.
2. Add in the carrots, black-eyed peas, and a splash of lemon juice. Season with salt and pepper, if desired. Toss and serve.

Nutrition:

Calories: 320, Fat: 9g, Sodium: 351mg, Potassium: 544mg, Carbohydrates: 49g, Protein: 16g.

714. Butternut-Squash Macaroni and Cheese

Preparation Time: 15 minutes
Cooking Time: 20 minutes
Servings: 2
Ingredients:

- 1 cup whole-wheat ziti macaroni
- 2 cups peeled and cubed butternut squash
- 1 cup nonfat or low-fat milk, divided
- Freshly ground black pepper
- 1 teaspoon Dijon mustard
- 1 tablespoon olive oil
- ¼ cup shredded low-fat cheddar cheese

Directions:

1. Cook the pasta al dente. Put the butternut squash plus ½ cup milk in a medium saucepan and place over medium-high heat. Season with black pepper. Bring it to a simmer. Lower the heat, then cook until fork-tender, 8 to 10 minutes.
2. To a blender, add squash and Dijon mustard. Purée until smooth. Meanwhile, place a large sauté pan over medium heat and add olive oil. Add the squash purée and the remaining ½ cup of milk. Simmer within 5 minutes. Add the cheese and stir to combine.
3. Add the pasta to the sauté pan and stir to combine. Serve immediately.

Nutrition:

Calories: 373, Fat: 10g, Sodium: 193mg, Carbohydrates: 59g, Protein: 14g, Potassium: 56mg.

715. Pasta with Tomatoes and Peas

Preparation Time: 15 minutes
Cooking Time: 15 minutes
Servings: 2
Ingredients:

- ½ cup whole-grain pasta of choice
- 8 cups water, plus ¼ for finishing
- 1 cup frozen peas
- 1 tablespoon olive oil
- 1 cup cherry tomatoes, halved
- ¼ teaspoon freshly ground black pepper
- 1 teaspoon dried basil

- ¼ cup grated Parmesan cheese (low-sodium)

Directions:
1. Cook the pasta al dente. Add the water to the same pot you used to cook the pasta, and when it's boiling, add the peas. Cook within 5 minutes. Drain and set aside.
2. Heat the oil in a large skillet over medium heat. Add the cherry tomatoes, put a lid on the skillet and let the tomatoes soften for about 5 minutes, stirring a few times.
3. Season with black pepper and basil. Toss in the pasta, peas, and ¼ cup of water, stir and remove from the heat. Serve topped with Parmesan.

Nutrition:
Calories: 266, Fat: 12g, Sodium: 320mg, Carbohydrates: 30g, Protein: 13g, Potassium: 67mg.

716. Healthy Vegetable Fried Rice

Preparation Time: 15 minutes
Cooking Time: 10 minutes
Servings: 4
Ingredients:
For the sauce:
- 1/3 cup garlic vinegar
- 1½ tablespoons dark molasses
- 1 teaspoon onion powder

For the fried rice:
- 1 teaspoon olive oil
- 2 lightly beaten whole eggs + 4 egg whites
- 1 cup of frozen mixed vegetables
- 1 cup frozen edamame
- 2 cups cooked brown rice

Directions:
1. Prepare the sauce by combining the garlic vinegar, molasses, and onion powder in a glass jar. Shake well.
2. Heat oil in a large wok or skillet over medium-high heat. Add eggs and egg whites, let cook until the eggs set, for about 1 minute.
3. Break up eggs with a spatula or spoon into small pieces. Add frozen mixed vegetables and frozen edamame. Cook for 4 minutes, stirring frequently.
4. Add the brown rice and sauce to the vegetable-and-egg mixture. Cook for 5 minutes or until

heated through. Serve immediately.

Nutrition:
Calories: 210, Fat: 6g, Sodium: 113mg, Carbohydrates: 28g, Protein: 13g, Potassium: 78mg.

717. Portobello-Mushroom Cheeseburgers

Preparation Time: 15 minutes
Cooking Time: 10 minutes
Servings: 4
Ingredients:
- 4 portobello mushrooms, caps removed and brushed clean
- 1 tablespoon olive oil
- ½ teaspoon freshly ground black pepper
- 1 tablespoon red wine vinegar
- 4 slices reduced-fat Swiss cheese, sliced thin
- 4 whole-wheat 100-calorie sandwich thins
- ½ avocado, sliced thin

Directions:
1. Heat a skillet or grill pan over medium-high flame. Clean the mushrooms and remove the stems. Brush each cap with olive oil and sprinkle with black pepper. Place in skillet cap-side up and cook for about 4 minutes. Flip and cook for another 4 minutes.
2. Sprinkle with the red wine vinegar and flip. Add the cheese and cook for 2 more minutes. For optimal melting, place a lid loosely over the pan. Meanwhile, toast the sandwich thins. Create your burgers by topping each with sliced avocado. Enjoy immediately.

Nutrition:
Calories: 245, Fat: 12g, Sodium: 266mg, Carbohydrates: 28g, Protein: 14g, Potassium: 78mg.

718. And-Rosemary Omelet

Preparation Time: 15 minutes
Cooking Time: 15 minutes
Servings: 2
Ingredients:
- ½ tablespoon olive oil
- 4 eggs
- ¼ cup grated Parmesan cheese
- 1 (15-ounce) can chickpeas, drained and rinsed

- 2 cups packed baby spinach
- 1 cup button mushrooms, chopped
- 2 sprigs rosemary, leaves picked (or 2 teaspoons dried rosemary)
- Salt
- Freshly ground black pepper

Directions:
1. Heat the oven to 400 F and put a baking tray on the middle shelf. Line an 8-inch springform pan with baking paper and grease generously with olive oil. If you don't have a springform pan, grease an oven-safe skillet (or cast-iron skillet) with olive oil.
2. Lightly whisk the eggs and Parmesan. Place chickpeas in the prepared pan. Layer the spinach and mushrooms on top of the beans. Pour the egg mixture on top and scatter the rosemary. Season to taste with salt and pepper.
3. Place the pan on the preheated tray and bake until golden and puffy and the center feels firm and springy, about 15 minutes. Remove from the oven, slice, and serve immediately.

Nutrition:
Calories: 418, Fat: 19g, Sodium: 595mg, Carbohydrates: 33g, Protein: 30g, Potassium: 98mg.

719. Chilled Cucumber-And-Avocado Soup with Dill

Preparation Time: 15 minutes
Cooking Time: 30 minutes
Servings: 4
Ingredients:
- 2 English cucumbers, peeled and diced, plus ¼ cup reserved for garnish
- 1 avocado, peeled, pitted, and chopped, plus ¼ cup reserved for garnish
- 1½ cups nonfat or low-fat plain Greek yogurt
- ½ cup of cold water
- 1/3 cup loosely packed dill, plus sprigs for garnish
- 1 tablespoon freshly squeezed lemon juice
- ¼ teaspoon freshly ground black pepper
- ¼ teaspoon salt
- 1 clove garlic

Directions:

1. Purée ingredients in a blender until smooth. If you prefer a thinner soup, add more water until you reach the desired consistency. Divide soup among 4 bowls. Cover with plastic wrap and refrigerate within 30 minutes. Garnish with cucumber, avocado, and dill sprigs, if desired.

Nutrition:
Calories: 142, Fat: 7g, Sodium: 193mg, Carbohydrates: 12g, Protein: 11g, Potassium: 76mg.

720. Southwestern Bean-And-Pepper Salad

Preparation Time: 6 minutes
Cooking Time: 0 minutes
Servings: 4
Ingredients:
- 1 can pinto beans, drained
- 2 bell peppers, cored and chopped
- 1 cup corn kernels
- Salt
- Freshly ground black pepper
- Juice of 2 limes
- 1 tablespoon olive oil
- 1 avocado, chopped

Directions:
1. Mix beans, peppers, corn, salt, plus pepper in a large bowl. Press fresh lime juice, then mix in olive oil. Let the salad stand in the fridge within 30 minutes. Add avocado just before serving.

Nutrition:
Calories: 245, Fat: 11g, Sodium: 97mg, Carbohydrates: 32g, Protein: 8g, Potassium: 87mg.

721. Cauliflower Mashed Potatoes

Preparation Time: 10 minutes
Cooking Time: 10 minutes
Servings: 4
Ingredients:
- 16 cups water (enough to cover cauliflower)
- 1 head cauliflower (about 3 pounds), trimmed and cut into florets
- 4 garlic cloves
- 1 tablespoon olive oil
- ¼ teaspoon salt
- 1/8 teaspoon freshly ground black pepper

- 2 teaspoons dried parsley

Directions:
1. Boil a large pot of water, then the cauliflower and garlic. Cook within 10 minutes, then strain. Move it back to the hot pan, and let it stand within 2 to 3 minutes with the lid on.
2. Put the cauliflower plus garlic in a food processor or blender. Add the olive oil, salt, pepper, and purée until smooth. Taste and adjust the salt and pepper.
3. Remove, then put the parsley, and mix until combined. Garnish with additional olive oil, if desired. Serve immediately.

Nutrition:
Calories: 87g, Fat: 4g, Sodium: 210mg, Carbohydrates: 12g, Protein: 4g, Potassium: 67mg.

722. Roasted Brussels sprouts

Preparation Time: 5 minutes
Cooking Time: 20 minutes
Servings: 4
Ingredients:
- 1½ pounds Brussels sprouts, trimmed and halved
- 2 tablespoons olive oil
- ¼ teaspoon salt
- ½ teaspoon freshly ground black pepper

Directions:
1. Preheat the oven to 400°F. Combine the Brussels sprouts and olive oil in a large mixing bowl and toss until evenly coated.
2. Turn the Brussels sprouts out onto a large baking sheet and flip them over so that they are cut-side down with the flat part touching the baking sheet. Sprinkle with salt and pepper.
3. Bake within 20 to 30 minutes or until the Brussels sprouts are lightly charred and crisp on the outside and toasted on the bottom. The outer leaves will be extra dark, too. Serve immediately.

Nutrition:
Calories: 134, Fat: 8g, Sodium: 189mg, Carbohydrates: 15g, Protein: 6g, Potassium: 78mg.

723. Broccoli with Garlic and Lemon

Preparation Time: 2 minutes
Cooking Time: 4 minutes
Servings: 4
Ingredients:
- 1 cup of water
- 4 cups broccoli florets
- 1 teaspoon olive oil
- 1 tablespoon minced garlic
- 1 teaspoon lemon zest
- Salt
- Freshly ground black pepper

Directions:
1. Put the broccoli in the boiling water in a small saucepan and cook within 2 to 3 minutes. The broccoli should retain its bright-green color. Drain the water from the broccoli.
2. Put the olive oil in a small sauté pan over medium-high heat. Add the garlic and sauté for 30 seconds. Put the broccoli, lemon zest, salt, plus pepper. Combine well and serve.

Nutrition:
Calories: 38g, Fat: 1g, Sodium: 24mg, Carbohydrates: 5g, Protein: 3g, Potassium: 78mg.

724. Brown Rice Pilaf

Preparation Time: 5 minutes
Cooking Time: 10 minutes
Servings: 4
Ingredients:
- 1 cup low-sodium vegetable broth
- ½ tablespoon olive oil
- 1 clove garlic, minced
- 1 scallion, thinly sliced
- 1 tablespoon minced onion flakes
- 1 cup instant brown rice
- 1/8 teaspoon freshly ground black pepper

Directions:
1. Mix the vegetable broth, olive oil, garlic, scallion, and minced onion flakes in a saucepan and boil. Put rice, then boil it again, adjust the heat and simmer within 10 minutes. Remove and let stand within 5 minutes. Fluff with a fork and season with black pepper.

Nutrition:
Calories: 100g, Fat: 2g, Sodium: 35mg, Carbohydrates: 19g, Protein: 2g, Potassium: 89mg.

725. Chunky Black-Bean Dip

Preparation Time: 5 minutes
Cooking Time: 1 minute
Servings: 2
Ingredients:
- 1 (15-ounce) can black beans, drained, with liquid reserved
- ½-can of chipotle peppers in adobo sauce
- ¼ cup plain Greek yogurt
- Freshly ground black pepper

Directions:
1. Combine beans, peppers, and yogurt in a food processor or blender and process until smooth. Add some of the bean liquid, 1 tablespoon at a time, for a thinner consistency. Season to taste with black pepper. Serve.

Nutrition:
Calories: 70g, Fat: 1g, Sodium: 159mg, Carbohydrates: 11g, Protein: 5g, Potassium: 25mg.

726. Classic Hummus

Preparation Time: 5 minutes
Cooking Time: 0 minutes
Servings: 6–8
Ingredients:
- 1 (15-ounce) can chickpeas, drained and rinsed
- 3 tablespoons sesame tahini
- 2 tablespoons olive oil
- 3 garlic cloves, chopped
- Juice of 1 lemon
- Salt
- Freshly ground black pepper

Directions:
1. Mix all the ingredients until smooth but thick in a food processor or blender. Add water if necessary to produce smoother hummus. Store covered for up to 5 days.

Nutrition:
Calories: 147g, Fat: 10g, Sodium: 64mg, Carbohydrates: 11g, Protein: 6g. Potassium: 89mg.

727. Crispy Potato Skins

Preparation Time: 2 minutes
Cooking Time: 19 minutes
Servings: 2
Ingredients:
- 2 russet potatoes
- Cooking spray
- 1 teaspoon dried rosemary
- 1/8 teaspoon freshly ground black pepper

Directions:
1. Preheat the oven to 375°F. Prick or pierce the potatoes all over using a fork. Put on a plate. Cook on full power in the microwave within 5 minutes. Flip over, and cook again within 3 to 4 minutes more, or until soft.
2. Carefully—the potatoes will be very hot—scoop out the pulp of the potatoes, leaving a 1/8 inch of potato pulp attached to the skin. Set aside.
3. Spray the inside of each potato with cooking spray. Press in the rosemary and pepper. Place the skins on a baking sheet and bake in a preheated oven for 5 to 10 minutes until slightly browned and crispy. Serve immediately.

Nutrition:
Calories 114, Fat: 0g, Sodium: 0mg, Carbohydrates: 27g, Protein: 3g, Potassium: 89mg.

728. Roasted Chickpeas

Preparation Time: 5 minutes
Cooking Time: 30 minutes
Servings: 2
Ingredients:
- 1 (15-ounce can) chickpeas, drained and rinsed
- ½ teaspoon olive oil
- 2 teaspoons of your favorite herbs or spice blend
- ¼ teaspoon salt

Directions:
1. Preheat the oven to 400°F.
2. Wrap a rimmed baking sheet with paper towels, place the chickpeas on it in an even layer, and blot with more paper towels until most of the liquid is absorbed.
3. In a medium bowl, gently toss the chickpeas and olive oil until combined. Sprinkle the mixture with the herbs and salt and toss again.
4. Place the chickpeas back on the baking sheet and spread in an even layer. Bake for 30 to 40 minutes, until crunchy and golden brown. Stir halfway through. Serve.

Nutrition:
Calories: 175g, Fat: 3g, Sodium: 474mg, Carbohydrates: 29g, Protein: 11g, Potassium: 90mg.

729. Carrot-Cake Smoothie

Preparation Time: 5 minutes
Cooking Time: 0 minutes
Servings: 2
Ingredients:
- 1 frozen banana, peeled and diced
- 1 cup carrots, diced (peeled if preferred)
- 1 cup nonfat or low-fat milk
- ½ cup nonfat or low-fat vanilla Greek yogurt
- ½ cup ice
- ¼ cup diced pineapple, frozen
- ½ teaspoon ground cinnamon
- Pinch nutmeg
- Optional toppings: chopped walnuts, grated carrots

Directions:
1. Process all the fixings to a blender. Serve immediately with optional toppings as desired.

Nutrition:
Calories: 180g, Fat: 1g, Sodium: 114mg, Carbohydrates: 36g, Protein: 10g, Potassium: 67mg.

730. Vegetable Cheese Calzone

Preparation Time: 15 minutes
Cooking Time: 20 minutes
Servings: 4
Ingredients:
- 3 asparagus stalks, cut into pieces
- 1/2 cup spinach, chopped
- 1/2 cup broccoli, chopped
- 1/2 cup sliced
- 2 tablespoons garlic, minced
- 2 teaspoons olive oil, divided
- 1/2 lb. frozen whole-wheat bread dough, thawed
- 1 medium tomato, sliced
- 1/2 cup mozzarella, shredded
- 2/3 cup pizza sauce

Directions:
1. Prepare the oven to 400 degrees F to preheat. Grease a baking sheet with cooking oil and set it aside. Toss asparagus with mushrooms, garlic, broccoli, and spinach in a bowl. Stir in 1 teaspoon olive oil and mix well. Heat a greased skillet on medium heat.

2. Stir in vegetable mixture and sauté for 5 minutes. Set these vegetables aside. Cut the bread dough into quarters.
3. Spread each bread quarter on a floured surface into an oval. Add sautéed vegetables, 2 tablespoons of cheese, and tomato slice to half of each oval.
4. Wet the edges of each oval and fold the dough over the vegetable filling. Pinch and press the two edges.
5. Place these calzones on the baking sheet. Brush each calzone with foil and bake for 10 minutes. Heat pizza sauce in a saucepan for a minute. Serve the calzone with pizza sauce.

Nutrition:
  Calories: 198, Fat: 8g, Sodium: 124mg, Carbs: 36g, Protein: 12g, Potassium: 89mg.

731. Mixed Vegetarian Chili

Preparation Time: 10 minutes
Cooking Time: 36 minutes
Servings: 4
Ingredients:
- 1 tablespoon olive oil
- 14 oz. canned black beans, rinsed and drained
- ½ cup yellow onion, chopped
- 12 oz. extra-firm tofu, cut into pieces
- 14 oz. canned kidney beans, rinsed and drained
- 2 cans (14 oz.) diced tomatoes
- 3 tablespoons chili powder
- 1 tablespoon oregano
- 1 tablespoon chopped cilantro (fresh coriander)

Directions:
1. Take a soup pot and heat olive oil in it over medium heat. Add onions and sauté for 6 minutes until soft. Add tomatoes, beans, chili powder, oregano, and beans. Boil it first, then reduce the heat to a simmer. Cook for 30 minutes, then add cilantro. Serve warm.

Nutrition:
  Calories: 314, Fat: 6g, Sodium: 119mg, Carbs: 46g, Protein: 19g, Potassium: 68mg.

732. Zucchini Pepper Kebabs

Preparation Time: 15 minutes
Cooking Time: 40 minutes

Servings: 2
Ingredients:
- 1 small zucchini, sliced into 8 pieces
- 1 red onion, cut into 4 wedges
- 1 green bell pepper, cut into 4 chunks
- 8 cherry tomatoes
- 8 button mushrooms
- 1 red bell pepper, cut into 4 chunks
- 1/2 cup Italian dressing, fat-free
- 1/2 cup brown rice
- 1 cup of water
- 4 wooden skewers, soaked and drained

Directions:
1. Toss tomatoes with zucchini, onion, peppers, and mushrooms in a bowl. Stir in Italian dressing and mix well to coat the vegetables. Marinate them for 10 minutes. Boil water with rice in a saucepan, then reduce the heat to a simmer.
2. Cover the rice and cook for 30 minutes until rice is done. Meanwhile, prepare the grill and preheat it on medium heat. Grease the grilling rack with cooking spray and place it 4 inches above the heat.
3. Thread 2 mushrooms, 2 tomatoes, and 2 zucchini slices along with 1 onions wedge, 1 green and red pepper slice on each skewer. Grill these kebabs for 5 minutes per side. Serve warm with boiled rice.

Nutrition:
  Calories: 335, Fat: 8.2g, Sodium: 516mg, Carbs: 67g, Protein: 8.8g, Potassium: 76mg.

733. Asparagus Cheese Vermicelli

Preparation Time: 10 minutes
Cooking Time: 15 minutes
Servings: 4
Ingredients:
- 2 teaspoons olive oil, divided
- 6 asparagus spears, cut into pieces
- 4 oz. dried whole-grain vermicelli
- 1 medium tomato, chopped
- 1 tablespoon garlic, minced
- 2 tablespoons fresh basil, chopped
- 4 tablespoons Parmesan, freshly grated, divided

- 1/8 teaspoon black pepper, ground

Directions:
1. Add 1 teaspoon of oil to a skillet and heat it. Stir in asparagus and sauté until golden brown.
2. Cut the sautéed asparagus into 1-inch pieces. Fill a sauce pot with water up to ¾ full. After boiling the water, add pasta and cook for 10 minutes until it is all done.
3. Drain and rinse the pasta under tap water. Add pasta to a large bowl, then toss in olive oil, tomato, garlic, asparagus, basil, garlic, and parmesan. Serve with black pepper on top.

Nutrition:
  Calories: 325, Fat: 8g, Sodium: 350mg, Carbs: 48g, Protein: 7.3g, Potassium: 98mg.

734. Corn Stuffed Peppers

Preparation Time: 10 minutes
Cooking Time: 35 minutes
Servings: 4
Ingredients:
- 4 red or green bell peppers
- 1 tablespoon olive oil
- ¼ cup onion, chopped
- 1 green bell pepper, chopped
- 2 1/2 cups fresh corn kernels
- 1/8 teaspoon chili powder
- 2 tablespoons chopped fresh parsley
- 3 egg whites
- 1/2 cup skim milk
- 1/2 cup water

Directions:
1. Prepare the oven to 350F to preheat. Layer a baking dish with cooking spray. Cut the bell peppers from the top and remove their seeds from the inside. Put the peppers in your prepared baking dish with their cut side up.
2. Add oil to a skillet, then heat it on medium flame. Stir in onion, corn, and green pepper. Sauté for 5 minutes. Add cilantro and chili powder. Switch the heat to low. Mix milk plus egg whites in a bowl. Pour this mixture into the skillet and cook for 5 minutes while stirring.
3. Divide this mixture into each pepper. Add some water to the baking dish. Cover the stuffed peppers with an aluminum sheet. Bake for 15 minutes and serve hot.

Nutrition:
Calories: 197, Fat: 5g, Sodium: 749mg, Carbs: 29g, Protein: 9g, Potassium: 65mg.

735. Stuffed Eggplant Shells

Preparation Time: 10 minutes
Cooking Time: 25 minutes
Servings: 2
Ingredients:
- 1 medium eggplant
- 1 cup of water
- 1 tablespoon olive oil
- 4 oz. cooked white beans
- 1/4 cup onion, chopped
- 1/2 cup red, green, or yellow bell peppers, chopped
- 1 cup canned unsalted tomatoes
- 1/4 cup tomatoes liquid
- 1/4 cup celery, chopped
- 1 cup fresh mushrooms, sliced
- 3/4 cup whole-wheat breadcrumbs
- Freshly ground black pepper to taste

Directions:
1. Prepare the oven to 350 degrees F to preheat. Grease a baking dish with cooking spray and set it aside. Trim and cut the eggplant in half, lengthwise. Scoop out the pulp using a spoon and leave the shell about ¼ inch thick.
2. Place the shells in the baking dish with their cut side up. Add water to the bottom of the dish. Dice the eggplant pulp into cubes and set them aside. Add oil to an iron skillet and heat it over medium heat. Stir in onions, peppers, chopped eggplant, tomatoes, celery, mushrooms, and tomato juice.
3. Cook for 10 minutes on simmering heat, then stir in beans, black pepper, and breadcrumbs. Divide this mixture into the eggplant shells. Cover the shells with a foil sheet and bake for 15 minutes. Serve warm.

Nutrition:
Calories: 334, Fat: 10g, Sodium: 142mg, Carbs: 35g, Protein: 26g, Potassium: 45mg.

736. Southwestern Vegetables Tacos

Preparation Time: 10 minutes
Cooking Time: 20 minutes
Servings: 4
Ingredients:
- 1 tablespoon olive oil
- 1 cup red onion, chopped
- 1 cup yellow summer squash, diced
- 1 cup green zucchini, diced
- 3 large garlic cloves, minced
- 4 medium tomatoes, seeded and chopped
- 1 jalapeno chili, seeded and chopped
- 1 cup fresh corn kernels
- 1 cup canned pinto, rinsed and drained
- 1/2 cup fresh cilantro, chopped
- 8 corn tortillas
- 1/2 cup smoke-flavored salsa

Directions:
1. Add olive oil to a saucepan, then heat it over medium flame. Stir in onion and sauté until soft. Add zucchini and summer squash. Cook for 5 minutes.
2. Stir in corn kernels, jalapeno, garlic, beans, and tomatoes. Cook for another 5 minutes. Stir in cilantro, then remove the pan from the heat.
3. Warm each tortilla in a dry nonstick skillet for 20 seconds per side. Place the tortilla on the serving plate. Spoon the vegetable mixture in each tortilla. Top the mixture with salsa. Serve.

Nutrition:
Calories: 310, Fat: 6g, Sodium: 97mg, Carbs: 54g, Protein: 10g, Potassium: 64mg.

737. Lentil Quiche

Preparation Time: 15 minutes
Cooking Time: 35 minutes
Servings: 2
Ingredients:
- 1 cup green lentils, boiled
- ½ cup carrot, grated
- 1 onion, diced
- 1 tablespoon olive oil
- ¼ cup flax seeds meal
- 1 teaspoon ground black pepper
- ¼ cup of soy milk

Directions:
1. Cook the onion with olive oil in the skillet until light brown.
2. Then mix cooked onion, lentils, and carrot.
3. Add flax seeds meal, ground black pepper, and soy milk. Stir the mixture until homogenous.
4. After this, transfer it to the baking pan and flatten it.
5. Bake the quiche for 35 minutes at 375F.

Nutrition:
Calories: 351, Protein: 17.1g, Carbohydrates: 41.6g, Fat: 13.1g, Fiber: 23.3g, Cholesterol: 0mg, Sodium: 29mg, Potassium: 88mg.

738. Corn Patties

Preparation Time: 15 minutes
Cooking Time: 10 minutes
Servings: 1
Ingredients:
- ½ cup chickpeas, cooked
- 1 cup corn kernels, cooked
- 1 tablespoon fresh parsley, chopped
- 1 teaspoon chili powder
- ½ teaspoon ground coriander
- 1 tablespoon tomato paste
- 1 tablespoon almond meal
- 1 tablespoon olive oil

Directions:
1. Mash the cooked chickpeas and combine them with corn kernels, parsley, chili powder, ground coriander, tomato paste, and almond meal.
2. Stir the mixture until homogenous.
3. Make the small patties.
4. After this, heat olive oil in the skillet.
5. Put the prepared patties in the hot oil and cook them for 3 minutes per side or until they are golden brown.
6. Dry the cooked patties with the help of a paper towel if needed.

Nutrition:
Calories: 168, Protein: 6.7g, Carbohydrates: 23.9g, Fat: 6.3g, Fiber: 6g, Cholesterol: 0mg, Sodium: 23mg, Potassium: 67mg.

739. Tofu Stir Fry

Preparation Time: 15 minutes
Cooking Time: 10 minutes
Servings: 2
Ingredients:
- 9 oz. firm tofu, cubed
- 3 tablespoons low-sodium soy sauce

- 1 teaspoon sesame seeds
- 1 tablespoon sesame oil
- 1 cup spinach, chopped
- ¼ cup of water

Directions:
1. In the mixing bowl, mix soy sauce and sesame oil.
2. Dip the tofu cubes in the soy sauce mixture and leave for 10 minutes to marinate.
3. Heat a skillet and put the tofu cubes inside. Roast them for 1.5 minutes from each side.
4. Then add water, remaining soy sauce mixture, and chopped spinach.
5. Close the lid and cook the meal for 5 minutes more.

Nutrition:
Calories: 118, Protein: 8.5g, Carbohydrates: 3.1g, Fat: 8.6g, Fiber: 1.1g, Cholesterol: 0mg, sodium 406mg, Potassium: 78mg.

740. Mac Stuffed Sweet Potatoes

Preparation Time: 20 minutes
Cooking Time: 25 minutes
Servings: 2
Ingredients:
- 1 sweet potato
- ¼ cup whole-grain penne pasta
- 1 teaspoon tomato paste
- 1 teaspoon olive oil
- ¼ teaspoon minced garlic
- 1 tablespoon soy milk

Directions:
1. Cut the sweet potato in half and pierce it 3-4 times with the help of the fork.
2. Sprinkle the sweet potato halves with olive oil and bake in the preheated to 375F oven for 25-30 minutes or until the vegetables are tender.
3. Meanwhile, mix penne pasta, tomato paste, minced garlic, and soy milk.
4. When the sweet potatoes are cooked, scoop out the vegetable meat and mix it with a penne pasta mixture.
5. Fill the sweet potatoes with the pasta mixture.

Nutrition:
Calories: 105, Protein: 2.7g, Carbohydrates: 17.8g, Fat: 2.8g, Fiber: 3g, Cholesterol: 0mg, Sodium: 28mg, Potassium: 98mg.

741. Tofu Tikka Masala

Preparation Time: 10 minutes
Cooking Time: 25 minutes
Servings: 2
Ingredients:
- 8 oz. tofu, chopped
- ½ cup of soy milk
- 1 teaspoon garam masala
- 1 teaspoon olive oil
- 1 teaspoon ground paprika
- ½ cup tomatoes, chopped
- ½ onion, diced

Directions:
1. Heat olive oil in the saucepan.
2. Add diced onion and cook it until light brown.
3. Then add tomatoes, ground paprika, and garam masala. Bring the mixture to a boil.
4. Add soy milk and stir well. Simmer it for 5 minutes.
5. Then add chopped tofu and cook the meal for 3 minutes.
6. Leave the cooked meal for 10 minutes to rest.

Nutrition:
Calories: 155, Protein: 12.2g, Carbohydrates: 20.7g, Fat: 8.4g, Fiber: 2.9g, Cholesterol: 0mg, Sodium: 51mg, Potassium: 345mg.

742. Tofu Parmigiana

Preparation Time: 15 minutes
Cooking Time: 8 minutes
Servings: 2
Ingredients:
- 6 oz. firm tofu, roughly sliced
- 1 teaspoon coconut oil
- 1 teaspoon tomato sauce
- ½ teaspoon Italian seasonings

Directions:
1. In the mixing bowl, mix tomato sauce and Italian seasonings.
2. Then brush the sliced tofu with the tomato mixture well and leave for 10 minutes to marinate.
3. Heat coconut oil.
4. Then put the sliced tofu in the hot oil and roast it for 3 minutes per side or until tofu is golden brown.

Nutrition:
Calories: 83, Protein: 7g, Carbohydrates: 1.7g, Fat: 6.2g, Fiber: 0.8, Cholesterol: 1mg, Sodium: 24mg, Potassium: 65mg.

743. Mushroom Stroganoff

Preparation Time: 10 minutes
Cooking Time: 20 minutes
Servings: 2
Ingredients:
- 2 cups mushrooms, sliced
- 1 teaspoon whole-grain wheat flour
- 1 tablespoon coconut oil
- 1 onion, chopped
- 1 teaspoon dried thyme
- 1 garlic clove, diced
- 1 teaspoon ground black pepper
- ½ cup of soy milk

Directions:
1. Heat coconut oil in the saucepan.
2. Add mushrooms and onion and cook them for 10 minutes. Stir the vegetables from time to time.
3. After this, sprinkle them with ground black pepper, thyme, and garlic.
4. Add soy milk and bring the mixture to a boil.
5. Then add flour and stir it well until homogenous.
6. Cook the mushroom stroganoff until it thickens.

Nutrition:
Calories: 70, Protein: 2.6g, Carbohydrates: 6.9g, Fat: 4.1g, Fiber: 1.5g, Cholesterol: 0mg, Sodium: 19mg, Potassium: 54mg.

744. Eggplant Croquettes

Preparation Time: 15 minutes
Cooking Time: 5 minutes
Servings: 2
Ingredients:
- 1 eggplant, peeled, boiled
- 2 potatoes, mashed
- 2 tablespoons almond meal
- 1 teaspoon chili pepper
- 1 tablespoon coconut oil
- 1 tablespoon olive oil
- ¼ teaspoon ground nutmeg

Directions:
1. Blend the eggplant until smooth.
2. Then mix it up with mashed potato, chili pepper, coconut oil, and ground nutmeg.
3. Make the croquettes from the eggplant mixture.
4. Heat olive oil in the skillet.

5. Put the croquettes in the hot oil and cook them for 2 minutes per side or until light brown.

Nutrition:
Calories: 180, Protein: 3.6g, Carbohydrates: 24.3g, Fat: 8.8g, Fiber: 7.1g, Cholesterol: 0mg, Sodium: 9mg, Potassium: 49mg.

745. Stuffed Portobello Mushrooms 2

Preparation Time: 10 minutes
Cooking Time: 20 minutes
Servings: 2
Ingredients:
- 4 Portobello mushroom caps
- ½ zucchini, grated
- 1 tomato, diced
- 1 teaspoon olive oil
- ½ teaspoon dried parsley
- ¼ teaspoon minced garlic

Directions:
1. In the mixing bowl, mix diced tomato, grated zucchini, dried parsley, and minced garlic.
2. Then fill the mushroom caps with zucchini mixture and transfer them to the lined baking paper tray.
3. Bake the vegetables for 20 minutes or until they are soft.

Nutrition:
Calories: 24, Protein: 1.2g, Carbohydrates: 2.9g, Fat: 1.3g, Fiber: 0.9g, Cholesterol: 0mg, Sodium: 5mg, Potassium: 78mg.

746. Chile Relents

Preparation Time: 10 minutes
Cooking Time: 30 minutes
Servings: 2
Ingredients:
- 2 chili peppers
- 2 oz. vegan Mozzarella cheese, shredded
- 2 oz. tomato puree
- 1 tablespoon coconut oil
- 2 tablespoons whole-grain wheat flour
- 1 tablespoon potato starch
- ¼ cup of water
- ½ teaspoon chili flakes

Directions:
1. Bake the chili peppers for 15 minutes in the preheated to 375F oven.
2. Meanwhile, pour tomato puree into the saucepan.

3. Add chili flakes and bring the mixture to a boil. Remove it from the heat.
4. After this, mix potato starch, flour, and water.
5. When the chili peppers are cooked, make the cuts in them and remove the seeds.
6. Then fill the peppers with shredded cheese and secure the cuts with toothpicks.
7. Heat coconut oil in the skillet.
8. Dip the chili peppers in the flour mixture and roast in the coconut oil until golden brown.
9. Sprinkle the cooked chilies with tomato puree mixture.

Nutrition:
Calories: 187, Protein: 4.2g, Carbohydrates: 16g, Fat: 12g, Fiber: 3.7g, Cholesterol: 0mg, Sodium: 122mg, Potassium: 68mg.

747. Carrot Cakes

Preparation Time: 10 minutes
Cooking Time: 10 minutes
Servings: 4
Ingredients:
- 1 cup carrot, grated
- 1 tablespoon semolina
- 1 egg, beaten
- 1 teaspoon Italian seasonings
- 1 tablespoon sesame oil

Directions:
1. In the mixing bowl, mix grated carrot, semolina, egg, and Italian seasonings.
2. Heat sesame oil in the skillet.
3. Make the carrot cakes with the help of 2 spoons and put them in the skillet.
4. Roast the cakes for 4 minutes per side.

Nutrition:
Calories: 70, Protein: 1.9g, Carbohydrates: 4.8g, Fat: 4.9g, Fiber: 0.8g, Cholesterol: 42mg, Sodium: 35mg, Potassium: 108mg.

748. Vegan Chili

Preparation Time: 10 minutes
Cooking Time: 25 minutes
Servings: 4
Ingredients:
- ½ cup bulgur
- 1 cup tomatoes, chopped
- 1 chili pepper, chopped
- 1 cup red kidney beans, cooked
- 2 cups low-sodium chicken broth

- 1 teaspoon tomato paste
- ½ cup celery stalk, chopped

Directions:
1. Put all ingredients in the big saucepan and stir well.
2. Close the lid and simmer the chili for 25 minutes over medium-low heat.

Nutrition:
Calories: 234, Protein: 14.1g, Carbohydrates: 44.4g, Fat: 0.9g, Fiber: 1g, Cholesterol: 0mg, Sodium: 57mg, Potassium: 52mg.

749. Spinach Casserole

Preparation Time: 5 minutes
Cooking Time: 30 minutes
Servings: 3
Ingredients:
- 2 cups spinach, chopped
- 4 oz. artichoke hearts, chopped
- ¼ cup low-fat yogurt
- 1 teaspoon Italian seasonings
- 2 oz. vegan mozzarella, shredded

Directions:
1. Mix all ingredients in the casserole mold and cover it with foil.
2. Then transfer it in the preheated to 365F oven and bake it for 30 minutes.

Nutrition:
Calories: 102, Protein: 3.7g, Carbohydrates: 11g, Fat: 4.9g, Fiber: 2.5g, Cholesterol: 2mg, Sodium: 206mg, Potassium: 300mg.

750. Tofu Turkey

Preparation Time: 15 minutes
Cooking Time: 75 minutes
Servings: 6
Ingredients:
- 1 onion, diced
- 1 cup mushrooms, chopped
- 1 bell pepper, chopped
- 12 oz. firm tofu, crumbled
- 1 teaspoon dried rosemary
- 1 tablespoon avocado oil
- ½ cup marinara sauce
- 1 teaspoon miso paste

Directions:
1. Sauté onion, mushrooms, bell pepper, rosemary, miso paste, and avocado oil in the saucepan until the ingredients are cooked (appx. 10-15 minutes).
2. Then put ½ part of tofu in the round baking pan. Press well

and make the medium whole in the center.

3. Put the mushroom mixture in the tofu whole and top it with marinara sauce.
4. Add remaining tofu and press it well. Cover the meal with foil.
5. Bake the tofu turkey for 60 minutes at 395F.

Nutrition:
Calories: 80, Protein: 5.9g, Carbohydrates: 7.9g, Fat: 3.4, Fiber: 2.1g, Cholesterol: 0mg, Sodium: 130mg, Potassium: 262mg.

751. Cauliflower Tots

Preparation Time: 15 minutes
Cooking Time: 20 minutes
Servings: 4
Ingredients:
- 1 cup cauliflower, shredded
- 3 oz. vegan Parmesan, grated
- 1/3 cup flax seeds meal
- 1 egg, beaten
- 1 teaspoon Italian seasonings
- 1 teaspoon olive oil

Directions:
1. In the bowl, mix shredded cauliflower, vegan Parmesan, flax seeds meal, egg, and Italian seasonings.
2. Knead the cauliflower mixture. Add water if needed.
3. After this, make the cauliflower tots from the mixture.
4. Line the baking tray with baking paper and place the cauliflower tots inside.
5. Drizzle with the olive oil and place in a preheated oven at 375F.
6. Bake the meal for 15-20 minutes or until golden brown.

Nutrition:
Calories: 109, Protein: 6.1g, Carbohydrates: 6.3g, Fat: 6.6g, Fiber: 3.7g, Cholesterol: 42mg, Sodium: 72mg, Potassium: 158mg.

752. Aromatic Whole Grain Spaghetti

Preparation Time: 5 minutes
Cooking Time: 10 minutes
Servings: 2
Ingredients:
- 1 teaspoon dried basil
- ¼ cup of soy milk
- 6 oz. whole-grain spaghetti
- 2 cups of water
- 1 teaspoon ground nutmeg

Directions:
1. Bring the water to boil, add spaghetti and cook them for 8-10 minutes.
2. Meanwhile, bring the soy milk to boil.
3. Drain the cooked spaghetti and mix them up with soy milk, ground nutmeg, and dried basil.
4. Stir the meal well.

Nutrition:
Calories: 128, Protein: 5.6g, Carbohydrates: 25g, Fat: 1.4g, Fiber: 4.3g, Cholesterol: 0mg, Sodium: 25mg, Potassium: 81mg.

753. Chunky Tomatoes

Preparation Time: 5 minutes
Cooking Time: 15 minutes
Servings: 3
Ingredients:
- 2 cups plum tomatoes, roughly chopped
- ½ cup onion, diced
- ½ teaspoon garlic, diced
- 1 teaspoon Italian seasonings
- 1 teaspoon canola oil
- 1 chili pepper, chopped

Directions:
1. Heat canola oil in the saucepan.
2. Add chili pepper and onion. Cook the vegetables for 5 minutes. Stir them from time to time.
3. After this, add tomatoes, garlic, and Italian seasonings.
4. Close the lid and sauté the meal for 10 minutes.

Nutrition:
Calories: 550, Protein: 1.7g, Carbohydrates: 8.4g, Fat: 2.3g, Fiber: 1.8g, Cholesterol: 1mg, Sodium: 17mg, Potassium: 279mg.

754. Baked Falafel

Preparation Time: 10 minutes
Cooking Time: 25 minutes
Servings: 6
Ingredients:
- 2 cups chickpeas, cooked
- 1 yellow onion, diced
- 3 tablespoons olive oil
- 1 cup fresh parsley, chopped
- 1 teaspoon ground cumin
- ½ teaspoon coriander
- 2 garlic cloves, diced

Directions:
1. Put all ingredients in the food processor and blend until smooth.
2. Preheat the oven to 375F.
3. Then line the baking tray with the baking paper.
4. Make the balls from the chickpeas mixture and press them gently in the shape of the falafel.
5. Put the falafel in the tray and bake in the oven for 25 minutes.

Nutrition:
Calories: 316, Protein: 13.5g, Carbohydrates: 43.3g, Fat: 11.2g, Fiber: 12.4g, Cholesterol: 0mg, Sodium: 23mg, Potassium: 676mg.

755. Paella

Preparation Time: 10 minutes
Cooking Time: 25 minutes
Servings: 6
Ingredients:
- 1 teaspoon dried saffron
- 1 cup short-grain rice
- 1 tablespoon olive oil
- 2 cups of water
- 1 teaspoon chili flakes
- 6 oz. artichoke hearts, chopped
- ½ cup green peas
- 1 onion, sliced
- 1 cup bell pepper, sliced

Directions:
1. Pour water into the saucepan. Add rice and cook it for 15 minutes.
2. Meanwhile, heat olive oil in the skillet.
3. Add dried saffron, chili flakes, onion, and bell pepper.
4. Roast the vegetables for 5 minutes.
5. Add them to the cooked rice.
6. Then add artichoke hearts and green peas. Stir the paella well and cook it for 10 minutes over low heat.

Nutrition:
Calories: 170, Protein: 4.2g, Carbohydrates: 32.7g, Fat: 2.7g, Fiber: 3.2g, Cholesterol: 0mg, Sodium: 33mg, Potassium: 237mg.

756. Mushroom Cakes

Preparation Time: 15 minutes
Cooking Time: 10 minutes
Servings: 4
Ingredients:

- 2 cups mushrooms, chopped
- 3 garlic cloves, chopped
- 1 tablespoon dried dill
- 1 egg, beaten
- ¼ cup of rice, cooked
- 1 tablespoon sesame oil
- 1 teaspoon chili powder

Directions:
1. Grind the mushrooms in the food processor.
2. Add garlic, dill, egg, rice, and chili powder.
3. Blend the mixture for 10 seconds.
4. After this, heat sesame oil for 1 minute.
5. Make the medium size mushroom cakes and put them in the hot sesame oil.
6. Cook the mushroom cakes for 5 minutes per side on medium heat.

Nutrition:
Calories: 103, Protein: 3.7g, Carbohydrates: 12g, Fat: 4.8g, Fiber: 0.9g, Cholesterol: 41mg, Sodium: 27mg, Potassium: 187mg.

757. Glazed Eggplant Rings

Preparation Time: 10 minutes
Cooking Time: 10 minutes
Servings: 4
Ingredients:
- 3 eggplants, sliced
- 1 tablespoon liquid honey
- 1 teaspoon minced ginger
- 2 tablespoons lemon juice
- 3 tablespoons avocado oil
- ½ teaspoon ground coriander
- 3 tablespoons water

Directions:
1. Rub the eggplants with ground coriander.
2. Then heat the avocado oil in the skillet for 1 minute.
3. When the oil is hot, add the sliced eggplant and arrange it in one layer.
4. Cook the vegetables for 1 minute per side.
5. Transfer the eggplant to the bowl.
6. Then add minced ginger, liquid honey, lemon juice, and water in the skillet.
7. Bring it to a boil and add cooked eggplants.
8. Coat the vegetables in the sweet liquid well and cook for 2 minutes more.

Nutrition:

Calories: 136, Protein: 4.3g, Carbohydrates: 29.6g, Fat: 2.2g, Fiber: 15.1g, Cholesterol: 0mg, Sodium: 11mg, Potassium: 93mg.

758. Sweet Potato Balls

Preparation Time: 15 minutes
Cooking Time: 10 minutes
Servings: 4
Ingredients:
- 1 cup sweet potato, mashed, cooked
- 1 tablespoon fresh cilantro, chopped
- 1 egg, beaten
- 3 tablespoons ground oatmeal
- 1 teaspoon ground paprika
- ½ teaspoon ground turmeric
- 2 tablespoons coconut oil

Directions:
1. In the bowl, mix mashed sweet potato, fresh cilantro, egg, ground oatmeal, paprika, and turmeric.
2. Stir the mixture until smooth and make the small balls.
3. Heat the coconut oil in the saucepan.
4. When the coconut oil is hot, add the sweet potato balls.
5. Cook them until golden brown.

Nutrition:
Calories: 133, Protein: 2.8g, Carbohydrates: 13.1g, Fat: 8.2g, Fiber: 2.2g, Cholesterol: 41mg, Sodium: 44mg, Potassium: 283mg.

759. Chickpea Curry

Preparation Time: 10 minutes
Cooking Time: 10 minutes
Servings: 4
Ingredients:
- 1 ½ cup chickpeas, boiled
- 1 teaspoon curry powder
- ½ teaspoon garam masala
- 1 cup spinach, chopped
- 1 teaspoon coconut oil
- ¼ cup of soy milk
- 1 tablespoon tomato paste
- ½ cup of water

Directions:
1. Heat coconut oil in the saucepan.
2. Add curry powder, garam masala, tomato paste, and soy milk.

3. Whisk the mixture until smooth and bring it to a boil.
4. Add water, spinach, and chickpeas.
5. Stir the meal and close the lid.
6. Cook it for 5 minutes over medium heat.

Nutrition:
Calories: 298, Protein: 15.4g, Carbohydrates: 47.8g, Fat: 6.1g, Fiber: 13.6g, Cholesterol: 0mg, Sodium: 37mg, Potassium: 765mg.

760. Quinoa Bowl

Preparation Time: 15 minutes
Cooking Time: 15 minutes
Servings: 4
Ingredients:
- 1 cup quinoa
- 2 cups of water
- 1 cup tomatoes, diced
- 1 cup sweet pepper, diced
- ½ cup of rice, cooked
- 1 tablespoon lemon juice
- ½ teaspoon lemon zest, grated
- 1 tablespoon olive oil

Directions:
1. Mix water and quinoa and cook it for 15 minutes. Then remove it from the heat and leave it to rest for 10 minutes.
2. Transfer the cooked quinoa to the big bowl.
3. Add tomatoes, sweet pepper, rice, lemon juice, lemon zest, and olive oil.
4. Stir the mixture well and transfer it to the serving bowls.

Nutrition:
Calories: 290, Protein: 8.4g, Carbohydrates: 49.9g, Fat: 6.4g, Fiber: 4.3g, Cholesterol: 0mg, Sodium: 11mg, Potassium: 435mg.

761. Vegan Meatloaf

Preparation Time: 10 minutes
Cooking Time: 30 minutes
Servings: 6
Ingredients:
- 1 cup chickpeas, cooked
- 1 onion, diced
- 1 tablespoon ground flax seeds
- ½ teaspoon chili flakes
- 1 tablespoon coconut oil
- ½ cup carrot, diced
- ½ cup celery stalk, chopped
- 1 tablespoon tomato paste

Directions:

1. Heat coconut oil in the saucepan.
2. Add carrot, onion, and celery stalk. Cook the vegetables for 8 minutes or until they are soft.
3. Then add chickpeas, chili flakes, and ground flax seeds.
4. Blend the mixture until smooth with the help of the immersion blender.
5. Then line the loaf mold with baking paper and transfer the blended mixture inside.
6. Flatten it well and spread with tomato paste.
7. Bake the meatloaf in the preheated to 365F oven for 20 minutes.

Nutrition:

Calories: 162, Protein: 7.1g, Carbohydrates: 23.9g, Fat: 4.7g, Fiber: 7g, Cholesterol: 0mg, Sodium: 25mg, Potassium: 407mg.

Chapter 16. Poultry

762. Salsa Chicken

Preparation Time: 50 minutes
Cooking Time: 5 minutes
Servings: 4
Ingredients:
- 1 pound chicken breast, boneless and skinless
- 16 ounce scanned Salsa Verde
- Black pepper to the taste
- A pinch of sea salt
- 1 tablespoon olive oil
- 1 and ½ cups fat-free Monterey jack cheese, shredded
- ¼ cup cilantro, chopped
- Wild rice, cooked for serving
- Juice from 1 lime

Directions:
1. Mix chicken with salt, pepper, and oil and toss to coat.
2. Spread salsa in a baking dish. Add chicken on top, introduce in the oven at 400 degrees F and bake for 40 minutes.
3. Take chicken out of the oven. Add cheese, introduce everything in preheated broiler and broil for 3 minutes.
4. Add lime juice, divide between plates, sprinkle cilantro and serve with white rice.

Nutrition:
Calories: 150, Fat: 1g, Fiber: 4g, Carbs: 20g, Sodium: 36mg, Potassium: 176mg.

763. Pear Chicken Casserole

Preparation Time: 10 minutes
Cooking Time: 5 minutes
Servings: 8
Ingredients:
- 2 tablespoons olive oil
- 2 pounds chicken breasts, skinless and boneless
- 2 carrots, chopped
- Black pepper to the taste
- 1 yellow onion, chopped
- 1 teaspoon Cajun seasoning
- ¼ cup flour
- ½ cup orange juice
- 1 can low sodium chicken stock
- 1 cup peas
- ½ cup parsley, chopped
- 2 tablespoons dill, chopped
- ½ cup fat-free yogurt

- 2 and ½ cups cornflakes

Directions:
1. Put water in a pot, add chicken, bring to a boil over medium heat, simmer for 10 minutes, drain and leave aside for now.
2. Heat a pan with the oil over medium-high flame. Add onion, carrots and pepper. Stir and cook for 10 minutes.
3. Add Cajun seasoning and flour, stir and cook for 1 minute.
4. Add stock and orange juice stirring all the time and bring to a boil.
5. Add chicken, dill, peas and half of the parsley, stir and take off the heat.
6. Add yogurt, stir and transfer everything to a baking dish. Introduce in the oven at 375 degrees F and bake for 15 minutes.
7. Meanwhile, in a bowl, mix cornflakes with the rest of the parsley and stir.
8. Take chicken out of the oven, sprinkle cornflakes all over, introduce in the oven again and bake for 6 more minutes.
9. Take the dish out of the oven, leave aside for 10 minutes, divide between plates and serve.

Nutrition:
Calories: 130, Fat: 3g, Fiber: 3g, Carbs: 9g, Protein: 5g, Sodium: 129mg, Potassium: 178mg.

764. Poached Chicken with Rice

Preparation Time: 10 minutes
Cooking Time: 40 minutes
Servings: 4
Ingredients:
- ½ tablespoon ginger, finely grated
- 3 garlic cloves, minced
- 1 tablespoon low sodium soy sauce
- 1 teaspoon black peppercorns
- 8 chicken legs
- 4 bok choy, halved
- Black pepper to the taste
- 2 bunches spring onions, chopped
- 3 tablespoons sesame oil

- Brown rice, already cooked for serving

Directions:
1. In a saucepan, mix ginger with half of the soy sauce, garlic, peppercorns and chicken.
2. Add water to cover, season with black pepper to taste, place on heat, bring to a boil over medium-high heat, reduce heat to low and simmer for 30 minutes.
3. Heat a skillet with the oil over medium-high flame. Add the onions, stir and cook for 1 minute.
4. Remove the pan from the heat. Add the soy sauce, stir well to make a sauce and set aside for now.
5. Remove the chicken from the pan and let it cool on a plate as well.
6. Add the bok choy to the chicken liquid, return it to the heat and cook for 4 minutes.
7. Strain bok choy, discard solids and reserve cooking liquid.
8. Discard skin and bones from chicken legs, shred meat and divide in bowls.
9. Add rice on the side, bok choy, the relish you've made and some of the reserved cooking liquid.

Nutrition:
Calories: 200, Fat: 2g, Fiber: 4g, Carbs: 7g, Protein: 10g, Sodium: 67mg, Potassium: 59mg.

765. Hawaiian Chicken

Preparation Time: 4 hours and 10 minutes
Cooking Time: 12 minutes
Servings: 4
Ingredients:
- 2 tablespoons tomato paste
- ¼ cup canned pineapple juice
- 2 tablespoons low sodium soy sauce
- 2 garlic cloves, minced
- 1 and ½ teaspoons ginger, grated
- 4 chicken breast halves, skinless and boneless
- Cooking spray
- Black pepper to the taste
- ¼ cup cilantro, chopped

- 2 cups brown rice, already cooked

Directions:

1. In a bowl, mix pineapple juice with tomato paste, soy sauce, garlic and ginger and stir well.
2. Reserve ¼ cup of mix and transfer the rest to a zip-top bag. Add chicken, seal bag, shake and keep in the fridge for 4 hours.
3. Heat a pan after you've sprayed some cooking oil in it over medium-high flame. Add marinated chicken and season with black pepper to the taste.
4. Add the reserved marinade, stir and cook chicken for 6 minutes on each side.
5. Add rice and cilantro, stir gently, take off the heat and divide between plates.

Nutrition:

Calories: 140, Fat: 1g, Fiber: 4g, Carbs: 9g, Protein: 12g, Sodium: 69mg, Potassium: 189mg.

766. Fruity Chicken Bites

Preparation Time: 10 minutes
Cooking Time: 10 minutes
Servings: 4
Ingredients:

- 20 ounces canned pineapple slices
- A drizzle of olive oil
- 3 cups chicken thighs, boneless, skinless and cut into medium pieces
- 1 tablespoon smoked tea rub

Directions:

1. Heat a pan over medium-high flame. Add pineapple slices, grill them for a few minutes on each side, transfer to a cutting board, cool them down and cut into medium cubes.
2. Heat a pan with a drizzle of oil over medium-high heat. Rub chicken pieces with smoked tea rub, place them in the pan and cook them for 10 minutes, flipping from time to time.
3. Arrange chicken cubes on a platter. Add a pineapple piece on top and stick a toothpick in each.
4. Serve right away!

Nutrition:

Calories: 120, Fat: 3g, Fiber: 1g, Carbs: 5g, Protein: 2g, Sodium: 68mg, Potassium: 98mg.

767. Fruity Chicken Salad

Preparation Time: 10 minutes
Cooking Time: 30 minutes
Servings: 4
Ingredients:

- 1 whole chicken, chopped
- 8 black tea bags
- 4 scallions, chopped
- 2 celery ribs, chopped
- 1 cup mandarin orange, chopped
- ½ cup fat-free yogurt
- 1 cup cashews, toasted and chopped
- Black pepper to the taste

Directions:

1. Put chicken pieces in a pot. Add water to cover, also add tea bags, bring to a boil over medium heat and cook for 25 minutes until chicken is tender.
2. Discard liquid and tea bags but reserve about 4 ounces.
3. Transfer chicken to a cutting board. Leave aside to cool down, discard bones, shred meat and put it in a bowl.
4. Add celery, orange pieces, cashews, scallion and reserved liquid and toss everything.
5. Add salt, pepper, mayo and yogurt, toss to coat well and keep in the fridge until you serve it.

Nutrition:

Calories: 150, Fat: 3g, Fiber: 3g, Carbs: 7g, Protein: 6g, Sodium: 64mg, Potassium: 188mg.

768. Chicken Corn Chili

Preparation Time: 10 minutes
Cooking Time: 1 hour and 10 minutes
Servings: 6
Ingredients:

- 1 cup white flour
- 1 tablespoon lemon juice
- Salt and black pepper to the taste
- 4 pounds chicken breast, skinless, boneless and cubed
- 4 ounces olive oil
- 4 ounces celery, chopped
- 1 tablespoon garlic, minced
- 8 ounces onion, chopped
- 5 ounces red bell pepper, chopped
- 7 ounces poblano pepper, chopped
- ¼ teaspoon cumin, ground
- 2 cups corn

- A pinch of cayenne pepper
- 1-quart chicken stock
- 1 teaspoon chili powder
- 16 ounces canned beans, drained
- ¼ cup cilantro, chopped

Directions:

1. Put flour in a bowl, add chicken pieces and toss well.
2. Heat a pan with the oil over medium-high flame. Add chicken, cook for 5 minutes on each side, transfer to a bowl and leave aside.
3. Heat the pan again over medium-high flame. Add onion, celery, garlic, bell pepper, poblano pepper and corn, stir and cook for 2 minutes more.
4. Add stock, cumin, chili powder, beans, cayenne, cumin, salt, pepper, chicken pieces and lemon juice, stir, bring to a simmer, reduce heat to medium low, cover and cook for 1 hour.
5. Add cilantro, stir, divide into bowls and serve right away!

Nutrition:

Calories: 345, Fat: 2g, Fiber: 3g, Carbs: 9g, Protein: 4g, Sodium: 134mg, Potassium: 156mg.

769. Sweet Chicken and Peaches

Preparation Time: 10 minutes
Cooking Time: 1 hour and 10 minutes
Servings: 4
Ingredients:

- 6 green tea and peach tea bags
- 1 whole chicken, cut into medium pieces
- ¾ cup water
- 1/3 cup honey
- Salt and black pepper to the taste
- ¼ cup olive oil
- 4 peaches, halved

Directions:

1. Put the water in a pot and bring to a simmer over medium heat. Add tea bags, reduce heat to low and simmer for 10 minutes.
2. Discard tea bags, add pepper and honey, whisk really well and leave aside.
3. Rub chicken pieces with the oil. Season with salt and pepper, place on preheated grill over medium-high heat, brush with tea marinade, cover grill and cook for 15 minutes,

4. Brush chicken with some more marinade, cook for 15 minutes more and then flip again.
5. Brush again with the tea marinade, cover and cook for 20 minutes more.
6. Divide chicken pieces on plates and keep warm.
7. Brush peaches with what's left of the tea and honey marinade. Place them on your grill and cook for 4 minutes.
8. Flip again and cook for 3 minutes more.
9. Divide between plates next to chicken pieces and serve.

Nutrition:
Calories: 500, Fat: 1g, Fiber: 3g, Carbs: 15g, Protein: 10g, Sodium: 43mg, Potassium: 523mg.

770. Pineapple Glazed Chicken

Preparation Time: 10 minutes
Cooking Time: 1 hour and 10 minutes
Servings: 4
Ingredients:
- ½ cup apricot preserves
- ½ cup pineapple preserves
- 1 tablespoon low sodium soy sauce
- 1 onion, chopped
- ¼ teaspoon red pepper flakes
- 1 tablespoon vegetable oil
- Black pepper to the taste
- 6 chicken legs

Directions:
1. In a bowl, mix soy sauce, pepper flakes, apricot and pineapple preserves and whisk really well.
2. Heat a pan with the oil over medium-high flame. Add chicken pieces, cook them for 5 minutes on each side and transfer to a bowl.
3. Spread onion on the bottom of a baking dish and add chicken pieces on top.
4. Season with black pepper. Drizzle the tea glaze on top, cover dish, introduce in the oven at 350 degrees F and bake for 30 minutes.
5. Uncover the dish and bake for 20 minutes more.
6. Divide chicken on plates and keep warm.
7. Pour cooking juices into a pan. Heat over medium-high flame, cook until sauce is reduced and drizzle it over chicken pieces.

Nutrition:

Calories: 198, Fat: 1g, Fiber: 1g, Carbs: 4g, Protein: 19g, Sodium: 145mg, Potassium: 167mg.

771. Teriyaki Chicken Wings

Preparation Time: 15 minutes
Cooking Time: 30 minutes
Servings: 6
Ingredients:
- 3 pounds of chicken wings (15 – 20)
- 1/3 cup lemon juice
- ¼ cup of soy sauce
- ¼ cup of vegetable oil
- 3 tablespoons chili sauce
- 1 garlic clove, finely chopped
- ¼ teaspoon fresh ground pepper
- ¼ teaspoon celery seed
- Dash liquid mustard

Directions:
1. Prepare the marinade. Combine lemon juice, soy sauce, chili sauce, oil, celery seed, garlic, pepper, and mustard. Stir well, set aside. Rinse and dry the chicken wings.
2. Pour marinade over the chicken wings. Coat thoroughly. Refrigerate for 2 hours. After 2 hours. Preheat the broiler in the oven. Drain off the excess sauce.
3. Place the wings on a cookie sheet with parchment paper. Broil on each side for 10 minutes. Serve immediately.

Nutrition:
Calories: 96, Protein: 15g, Carbohydrates: 63g, Fat: 15g, Sodium: 145mg, Potassium: 78mg

772. Hot Chicken Wings

Preparation Time: 15 minutes
Cooking Time: 25 minutes
Servings: 4
Ingredients:
- 10 - 20 chicken wings
- ½ stick margarine
- 1 bottle Durkee hot sauce
- 2 Tablespoons honey
- 10 shakes Tabasco sauce
- 2 Tablespoons cayenne pepper

Directions:
1. Warm canola oil in a deep pot. Deep-fry the wings until cooked, approximately 20 minutes. Mix the hot sauce, honey, Tabasco, and cayenne pepper in a medium bowl. Mix well.

2. Place the cooked wings on paper towels. Drain the excess oil. Mix the chicken wings in the sauce until coated evenly.

Nutrition:
Calories: 102, Protein: 23g, Carbohydrates: 55g, Sugars: 0.1g, Fat: 14g, Sodium: 140mg, Potassium: 157mg.

773. Crispy Cashew Chicken

Preparation Time: 15 minutes
Cooking Time: 30 minutes
Servings: 5
Ingredients:
- 2 chicken breasts, skinless, boneless
- 2 egg whites
- 1 cup cashew nuts
- ¼ cup bread crumbs
- 2 cups of peanut oil or vegetable oil
- ¼ cup of corn starch
- 1 teaspoon brown sugar
- 2 teaspoons salt
- 1 teaspoon dry sherry

Directions:
1. Heat the oven to 400 F. Put the cashews in a blender. Pulse until they are finely chopped. Place in a shallow bowl and stir in the bread crumbs.
2. Wash the chicken breasts. Pat them dry. Cut into small cubes. In a separate shallow bowl, mix the salt, corn starch, brown sugar, and sherry. In a separate bowl, beat the egg white.
3. Put the oil into a large, deep pot. Heat to high temp. Place the chicken pieces on a plate. Arrange the bowls in a row; flour, eggs, cashews & bread crumbs. Prepare a baking tray with parchment paper.
4. Dunk the chicken pieces in the flour, then the egg, and then the cashew mixture. Shake off the excess mixture. Gently place the chicken in the oil. Fry on each side for 2 minutes. Place on the baking tray.
5. Once done, slide the baking tray into the oven. Cook for an additional 4 minutes, flip, cook for an additional 4 minutes, until golden brown. Serve immediately, or cold, with your favorite low-fat dip.

Nutrition:

Calories: 86, Protein: 21g, Carbohydrates: 50g, Sugars: 0.1g, Fat: 16g, Sodium: 139mg, Potassium: 78mg.

774. Chicken Tortellini Soup

Preparation Time: 15 minutes
Cooking Time: 30 minutes
Servings: 5
Ingredients:

- 2 chicken breasts, boneless, skinless; diced into cubes
- 1 Tablespoon flavorless oil (olive oil, canola, sunflower)
- 1 teaspoon butter
- 2 cups cheese tortellini
- 2 cups frozen broccoli
- 2 cans cream of chicken soup
- 4 cups of water
- 1 large onion, diced
- 2 garlic cloves, minced
- 2 large carrots, sliced
- 1 celery stick, sliced
- 1 teaspoon Oregano
- ½ teaspoon Basil

Directions:

1. Pull the broccoli out of the freezer. Set in a bowl. Rinse and pat dry the chicken breasts. Dice into cubes. In a large pot, heat the oil. Fry the cubes of chicken breast. Pull from the pot, place on paper to drain off the oil.
2. Add the teaspoon of butter to the hot pot. Sauté the onion, garlic, carrots, celery, and broccoli. Once the vegetables are al dente, add the chicken soup and water. Stir the ingredients until they are combined. Bring it to a simmer.
3. Add the chicken and tortellini back to the pot. Cook on low within 10 minutes, or until the tortellini is cooked. Serve immediately.

Nutrition:
Calories: 79, Protein: 15g, Carbohydrates: 55g, Sugars: 0g, Fat: 13g, Sodium: 179mg, Potassium: 156mg.

775. Chicken Divan

Preparation Time: 15 minutes
Cooking Time: 30 minutes
Servings: 4
Ingredients:

- 1/2-pound cooked chicken, boneless, skinless, diced in bite-size pieces
- 1 cup broccoli, cooked, diced into bite-size pieces
- 1 cup extra sharp cheddar cheese, grated
- 1 can mushroom soup
- ½ cup of water
- 1 cup croutons

Directions:

1. Heat the oven to 350F. In a large pot, heat the soup and water. Add the chicken, broccoli, and cheese. Combine thoroughly. Pour into a greased baking dish. Place the croutons over the mixture. Bake within 30 minutes or until the casserole is bubbling and the croutons are golden brown.

Nutrition:
Calories: 380, Protein: 25g, Carbohydrates: 10g, Sugars: 1g, Fat: 22g, Sodium: 397mg, Potassium: 58mg.

776. Creamy Chicken Fried Rice

Preparation Time: 15 minutes
Cooking Time: 45 minutes
Servings: 4
Ingredients:

- 2 pounds of chicken; white and dark meat (diced into cubes)
- 2 Tablespoons butter or margarine
- 1 ½ cups instant rice
- 1 cup mixed frozen vegetables
- 1 can condensed cream of chicken soup
- 1 cup of water
- 1 cube instant chicken bouillon
- Salt and pepper to taste

Directions:

1. Take the vegetables out of the freezer. Set aside. Warm large, deep skillet over medium heat. Add the butter or margarine. Place the chicken in the skillet, season with salt and pepper. Fry until both sides are brown.
2. Remove the chicken, then adjust the heat and add the rice. Add the water and bouillon. Cook the rice, then add the chicken and the vegetables. Mix in the soup, then simmer until the vegetables are tender. Serve immediately.

Nutrition:
Calories: 119, Protein: 22g, Carbohydrates: 63g, Fat: 18g, Sodium: 180mg, Potassium: 98mg.

777. Chicken Tikka

Preparation Time: 15 minutes
Cooking Time: 20 minutes
Servings: 6
Ingredients:

- 4 chicken breasts, skinless, boneless; cubed
- 2 large onions, cubed
- 10 cherry tomatoes
- 1/3 cup plain non-fat yogurt
- 4 garlic cloves, crushed
- 1 ½ inch fresh ginger, peeled and chopped
- 1 small onion, grated
- 1 ½ teaspoon chili powder
- 1 Tablespoon ground coriander
- 1 teaspoon salt
- 2 tablespoons of coriander leaves

Directions:

1. In a large bowl, combine the non-fat yogurt, crushed garlic, ginger, chili powder, coriander, salt, and pepper. Add the cubed chicken, stir until the chicken is coated. Cover with plastic film, place in the fridge. Marinate 2 – 4 hours. Heat the broiler or barbecue.
2. After marinating the chicken, get some skewers ready. Alternate pieces of chicken cubes, cherry tomatoes, and cubed onions onto the skewers.
3. Grill within 6 – 8 minutes on each side. Once the chicken is cooked through, pull the meat and vegetables off the skewers onto plates. Garnish with coriander. Serve immediately.

Nutrition:
Calories: 117, Protein: 19g, Carbohydrates: 59g, Fat: 19g, Sodium: 203mg, Potassium: 156mg.

778. Honey Spiced Cajun Chicken

Preparation Time: 15 minutes
Cooking Time: 20 minutes
Servings: 4
Ingredients:

- 2 chicken breasts, skinless, boneless
- 1 tablespoon butter or margarine
- 1 pound of linguini

- 3 large mushrooms, sliced
- 1 large tomato, diced
- 2 tablespoons regular mustard
- 4 tablespoons honey
- 3 ounces low-fat table cream
- Parsley, roughly chopped

Directions:
1. Wash and dry the chicken breasts. Warm 1 tablespoon of butter or margarine in a large pan. Add the chicken breasts. Season with salt and pepper. Heat on each side 6 – 10 minutes, until cooked thoroughly. Pull the chicken breasts from the pan. Set aside.
2. Cook the linguine in a large pot following instructions on the package. Save 1 cup of the pasta water. Drain the linguine. Add the mushrooms, tomatoes to the pan from cooking the chicken. Heat until they are tender.
3. Add the honey, mustard, and cream. Combine thoroughly. Add the chicken and linguine to the pan. Stir until coated. Garnish with parsley. Serve immediately.

Nutrition:
Calories: 112, Protein: 12g, Carbohydrates: 56g, Fat: 20g, Sodium: 158mg, Potassium: 145mg.

779. Italian Chicken

Preparation Time: 15 minutes
Cooking Time: 35 minutes
Servings: 4
Ingredients:
- 4 chicken breasts, skinless boneless
- 1 large jar of pasta sauce, low sodium
- 1 Tablespoon flavorless oil (olive, canola, or sunflower)
- 1 large onion, diced
- 1 large green pepper, diced
- ½ teaspoon garlic salt
- Salt and pepper to taste
- 1 cup low-fat mozzarella cheese, grated
- Spinach leaves, washed, dried, rough chop

Directions:
1. Wash the chicken breasts, pat dry. In a large pot, heat the oil. Add the onion, cook until it sweats and becomes translucent. Add the chicken. Season with salt, pepper, and

garlic salt. Cook the chicken. 6 – 10 minutes on each side.
2. Add the peppers. Cook for 2 minutes. Pour the pasta sauce over the chicken. Mix well. Simmer on low for 20 minutes. Serve on plates, sprinkle the cheese over each piece. Garnish with spinach.

Nutrition:
Calories: 142, Protein: 17g, Carbohydrates: 51g, Fat: 15g, Sodium: 225mg, Potassium: 134mg.

780. Lemon-Parsley Chicken Breast

Preparation Time: 15 minutes
Cooking Time: 15 minutes
Servings: 2
Ingredients:
- 2 chicken breasts, skinless, boneless
- 1/3 cup white wine
- 1/3 cup lemon juice
- 2 garlic cloves, minced
- 3 tablespoons bread crumbs
- 2 tablespoons flavorless oil (olive, canola, or sunflower)
- ¼ cup fresh parsley

Directions:
1. Mix the wine, lemon juice, plus garlic in a measuring cup. Pound each chicken breast until they are ¼ inch thick. Coat the chicken with bread crumbs and heat the oil in a large skillet.
2. Fry the chicken within 6 minutes on each side until they turn brown. Stir in the wine mixture over the chicken. Simmer for 5 minutes. Pour any extra juices over the chicken. Garnish with parsley.

Nutrition:
Calories: 117, Protein: 14g, Carbohydrates: 74g, Fat: 12g, Sodium: 189mg, Potassium: 134mg.

781. Parmesan and Chicken Spaghetti Squash

Preparation Time: 15 minutes
Cooking Time: 20 minutes
Servings: 6
Ingredients:
- 16 oz. mozzarella

- 1 spaghetti squash piece
- 1 lb. cooked cube chicken
- 1 c. Marinara sauce

Directions:
1. Split up the squash in halves and remove the seeds. Arrange or put one cup of water in your pot, then put a trivet on top.
2. Add the squash halves to the trivet. Cook within 20 minutes at HIGH pressure. Remove the squashes and shred them using a fork into spaghetti portions.
3. Pour sauce over the squash and give it a nice mix. Top them up with the cubed-up chicken and top with mozzarella. Broil for 1-2 minutes and broil until the cheese has melted

Nutrition:
Calories: 237, Fat: 10g, Carbs: 32g, Protein: 11g, Sodium: 500mg, Potassium: 76mg.

782. Apricot Chicken

Preparation Time: 15 minutes
Cooking Time: 6 minutes
Servings: 4
Ingredients:
- 1 bottle creamy French dressing
- ¼ c. flavorless oil
- White cooked rice
- 1 large jar Apricot preserve
- 4 lbs. boneless and skinless chicken
- 1 package onion soup mix

Directions:
1. Rinse and pat dry the chicken. Dice into bite-size pieces. In a large bowl, mix the apricot preserve, creamy dressing, and onion soup mix. Stir until thoroughly combined. Place the chicken in the bowl. Mix until coated.
2. In a large skillet, heat the oil. Place the chicken in the oil gently. Cook 4 – 6 minutes on each side until golden brown. Serve over rice.

Nutrition:
Calories: 202, Fat: 12g, Carbs: 75g, Protein: 20g, Sugars: 10g, Sodium: 630mg, Potassium: 123mg.

783. Oven-Fried Chicken Breasts

Preparation Time: 15 minutes

Cooking Time: 30 minutes
Servings: 8
Ingredients:
- ½ pack Ritz crackers
- 1 c. plain non-fat yogurt
- 8 boneless, skinless, and halved chicken breasts

Directions:
1. Preheat the oven to 350F. Rinse and pat dry the chicken breasts. Pour the yogurt into a shallow bowl. Dip the chicken pieces in the yogurt, then roll in the cracker crumbs. Place the chicken in a single layer in a baking dish. Bake within 15 minutes per side. Serve.

Nutrition:
Calories: 200, Fat: 13g, Carbs: 98g, Protein: 19g, Sodium: 217mg, Potassium: 43mg.

784. Rosemary Roasted Chicken

Preparation Time: 15 minutes
Cooking Time: 20 minutes
Servings: 8
Ingredients:
- 8 rosemary springs
- 1 minced garlic clove
- Black pepper
- 1 tbsp. chopped rosemary
- 1 chicken
- 1 tbsp. organic olive oil

Directions:
1. In a bowl, mix garlic with rosemary, rub the chicken with black pepper, the oil and rosemary mix, place it inside roasting pan, introduce inside the oven at 350F, and roast for 20 minutes. Carve chicken, divide between plates and serve using a side dish. Enjoy!

Nutrition:
Calories: 325, Fat: 5g, Carbs: 15g, Protein: 14g, Sodium: 950mg, Potassium: 46mg.

785. Artichoke and Spinach Chicken

Preparation Time: 15 minutes
Cooking Time: 5 minutes
Servings: 4
Ingredients:
- 10 oz. baby spinach
- ½ tsp. crushed red pepper flakes
- 14 oz. chopped artichoke hearts

- 28 oz. no-salt-added tomato sauce
- 2 tbsps. Essential olive oil
- 4 boneless and skinless chicken breasts

Directions:
1. Heat a pan with the oil over medium-high flame. Add chicken and red pepper flakes and cook for 5 minutes. Add spinach, artichokes, and tomato sauce. Toss, cook for ten minutes more, divide between plates and serve. Enjoy!

Nutrition:
Calories: 212, Fat: 3g, Carbs: 16g, Protein: 20g, Sugars: 5g, Sodium: 418mg, Potassium: 45mg.

786. Pumpkin and Black Beans Chicken

Preparation Time: 15 minutes
Cooking Time: 25 minutes
Servings: 4
Ingredients:
- 1 tbsp. essential olive oil
- 1 tbsp. chopped cilantro
- 1 c. coconut milk
- 15 oz. canned black beans, drained
- 1 lb. skinless and boneless chicken breasts
- 2 c. water
- ½ c. pumpkin flesh

Directions:
1. Heat a pan when using oil over medium-high flame. Add the chicken and cook for 5 minutes. Add the water, milk, pumpkin, and black beans. Toss, cover the pan, reduce heat to medium and cook for 20 minutes. Add cilantro, toss, divide between plates and serve. Enjoy!

Nutrition:
Calories: 254, Fat: 6g, Carbs: 16g, Protein: 22g, Sodium: 92mg, Potassium: 126mg.

787. Chicken Thighs and Apples Mix

Preparation Time: 15 minutes
Cooking Time: 60 minutes
Servings: 4
Ingredients:
- 3 cored and sliced apples
- 1 tbsp. apple cider vinegar treatment

- ¾ c. natural apple juice
- ¼ tsp. pepper and salt
- 1 tbsp. grated ginger
- 8 chicken thighs
- 3 tbsps. Chopped onion

Directions:
1. In a bowl, mix chicken with salt, pepper, vinegar, onion, ginger, and apple juice, toss well, cover, keep within the fridge for ten minutes, transfer with a baking dish, and include apples. Introduce inside the oven at 400F for just 1 hour. Divide between plates and serve. Enjoy!

Nutrition:
Calories: 214, Fat: 3g, Carbs: 14g, Protein: 15g, Sodium: 405mg, Potassium: 145mg.

788. Thai Chicken Thighs

Preparation Time: 15 minutes
Cooking Time: 1 hour & 5minutes
Servings: 6
Ingredients:
- ½ c. Thai chili sauce
- 1 chopped green onions bunch
- 4 lbs. chicken thighs

Directions:
1. Heat a pan over medium-high heat. Add chicken thighs, brown them for 5 minutes on both sides. Transfer to some baking dish, then add chili sauce and green onions and toss.
2. Introduce in the oven and bake at 400F for 60 minutes. Divide everything between plates and serve. Enjoy!

Nutrition:
Calories: 220, Fat: 4g, Carbs: 12g, Protein: 10g, Sodium: 870mg, Potassium: 136mg.

789. Falling "Off" The Bone Chicken

Preparation Time: 15 minutes
Cooking Time: 40 minutes
Servings: 4
Ingredients:
- 6 peeled garlic cloves
- 1 tbsp. organic extra virgin coconut oil
- 2 tbsps. Lemon juice
- 1 ½ c. pacific organic bone chicken broth
- ¼ tsp. freshly ground black pepper
- ½ tsp. sea flavored vinegar

- 1 whole organic chicken piece
- 1 tsp. paprika
- 1 tsp. dried thyme

Directions:
1. Take a small bowl and toss in the thyme, paprika, pepper, and flavored vinegar and mix them. Use the mixture to season the chicken properly. Pour down the oil in your Instant Pot and heat it to shimmering, toss in the chicken with breast downward and let it cook for about 6-7 minutes.
2. After 7 minutes, flip over the chicken and pour down the broth, garlic cloves, and lemon juice. Cook within 25 minutes on a high setting. Remove the dish from the cooker and let it stand for about 5 minutes before serving.

Nutrition:
Calories: 664, Fat: 44g, Carbs: 44g, Protein: 27g, Sugars: 0.1g, Sodium: 800mg, Potassium: 135mg.

790. Feisty Chicken Porridge

Preparation Time: 15 minutes
Cooking Time: 30 minutes
Servings: 4
Ingredients:
- 1 ½ c. fresh ginger
- 1 lb. cooked chicken legs
- Green onions
- Toasted cashew nuts
- 5 c. chicken broth
- 1 cup jasmine rice
- 4 c. water

Directions:
1. Place the rice in your fridge and allow it to chill 1 hour before cooking. Take the rice out and add them to your Instant Pot. Pour broth and water. Lock up the lid and cook on Porridge mode.
2. Separate the meat from the chicken legs and add the meat to your soup. Stir well over sauté mode. Season with a bit of flavored vinegar and enjoy with a garnish of nuts and onion.

Nutrition:
Calories: 206, Fat: 8g, Carbs: 8g, Protein: 23g, Sugars: 0g, Sodium: 950mg, Potassium: 214mg.

791. The Ultimate Faux-Tisserie Chicken

Preparation Time: 15 minutes
Cooking Time: 35 minutes
Servings: 5
Ingredients:
- 1 c. low sodium broth
- 2 tbsps. olive oil
- ½ quartered medium onion
- 2 tbsps. favorite seasoning
- 2 ½ lbs. whole chicken
- Black pepper
- 5 large fresh garlic cloves

Directions:
1. Massage the chicken with 1 tablespoon of olive oil and sprinkle pepper on top. Place onion wedges and garlic cloves inside the chicken. Take a butcher's twin and secure the legs
2. Set your pot to Sauté mode. Put olive oil in your pan on medium heat, allow the oil to heat. Add chicken and sear both sides for 4 minutes per side. Sprinkle your seasoning over the chicken, remove the chicken and place a trivet at the bottom of your pot
3. Sprinkle seasoning over the chicken, making sure to rub it. Transfer the chicken to the trivet with the breast side facing up, lock up the lid. Cook on HIGH pressure for 25 minutes. Allow it to rest and serve!

Nutrition:
Calories: 1010, Fat: 64g, Carbs: 47g, Protein: 60g, Sodium: 209mg, Potassium: 125mg.

792. Oregano Chicken Thighs

Preparation Time: 15 minutes
Cooking Time: 20 minutes
Servings: 6
Ingredients:
- 12 chicken thighs
- 1 tsp. dried parsley
- ¼ tsp. pepper and salt
- ½ c. extra virgin essential olive oil
- 4 minced garlic cloves
- 1 c. chopped oregano
- ¼ c. low-sodium veggie stock

Directions:
1. In your food processor, mix parsley with oregano, garlic, salt, pepper, and stock and pulse. Put chicken thighs within the bowl. Add oregano paste,

toss, cover, and then leave aside within the fridge for 10 minutes.
2. Heat the kitchen grill over medium flame. Add chicken pieces, close the lid and cook for twenty or so minutes with them. Divide between plates and serve!

Nutrition:
Calories: 254, Fat: 3g, Carbs: 7g, Protein: 17g, Sugars: 0.9g, Sodium: 730mg, Potassium: 130mg.

793. Pesto Chicken Breasts with Summer Squash

Preparation Time: 15 minutes
Cooking Time: 10 minutes
Servings: 4
Ingredients:
- 4 medium boneless, skinless chicken breast halves
- 1 tbsp. olive oil
- 2 tbsps. Homemade pesto
- 2 c. finely chopped zucchini
- 2 tbsps. Finely shredded Asiago

Directions:
1. Cook your chicken in hot oil on medium heat within 4 minutes in a large nonstick skillet. Flip the chicken and then put the zucchini.
2. Cook within 4 to 6 minutes more or until the chicken is tender and no longer pink (170 F), and squash is crisp-tender, stirring squash gently once or twice. Transfer chicken and squash to 4 dinner plates. Spread pesto over chicken; sprinkle with Asiago.

Nutrition:
Calories: 230, Fat: 9g, Carbs: 8g, Protein: 30g, Sodium: 578mg, Potassium: 129mg.

794. Chicken, Tomato and Green Beans

Preparation Time: 15 minutes
Cooking Time: 25 minutes
Servings: 4
Ingredients:
- 6 oz. low-sodium canned tomato paste
- 2 tbsps. olive oil
- ¼ tsp. black pepper

- 2 lbs. trimmed green beans
- 2 tbsps. chopped parsley
- 1 ½ lbs. boneless, skinless, and cubed chicken breasts
- 25 oz. no-salt-added canned tomato sauce

Directions:
1. Heat a pan with 50 % of the oil over medium flame. Add chicken, stir, cover, and cook within 5 minutes on both sides and transfer to a bowl. Heat inside the same pan while using rest through the oil over medium heat. Add green beans, stir and cook for 10 minutes.
2. Return chicken for that pan, add black pepper, tomato sauce, tomato paste, and parsley. Stir, cover, cook for 10 minutes more, divide between plates and serve. Enjoy!

Nutrition:
Calories: 190, Fat: 4g, Carbs: 12g, Protein: 9g, Sodium: 168mg, Potassium: 100mg.

795. Chicken Tortillas

Preparation Time: 15 minutes
Cooking Time: 5 minutes
Servings: 4
Ingredients:
- 6 oz. boneless, skinless, and cooked chicken breasts
- Black pepper
- 1/3 c. fat-free yogurt
- 4 heated up whole-wheat tortillas
- 2 chopped tomatoes

Directions:
1. Heat a pan over medium flame. Add one tortilla, heat, and hang them on the working surface. Spread yogurt on each tortilla, add chicken and tomatoes, roll, divide between plates and serve. Enjoy!

Nutrition:
Calories: 190, Fat: 2g, Carbs: 12g, Protein: 6g, Sodium: 300mg, Potassium: 100mg.

796. Chicken with Potatoes, Olives & Sprouts

Preparation Time: 15 minutes
Cooking Time: 35 minutes
Servings: 4
Ingredients:

- 1 lb. chicken breasts, skinless, boneless, and cut into pieces
- ¼ cup olives, quartered
- 1 tsp. oregano
- 1 ½ tsp. Dijon mustard
- 1 lemon juice
- 1/3 cup vinaigrette dressing
- 1 medium onion, diced
- 3 cups potatoes cut into pieces
- 4 cups Brussels sprouts, trimmed and quartered
- ¼ tsp. pepper
- ¼ tsp. salt

Directions:
1. Heat oven to 400 F. Place chicken in the center of the baking tray, then place potatoes, sprouts, and onions around the chicken.
2. In a small bowl, mix vinaigrette, oregano, mustard, lemon juice, and salt and pour over chicken and veggies. Sprinkle olives and season with pepper.
3. Bake in preheated oven for 20 minutes. Transfer chicken to a plate. Stir the vegetables and roast for 15 minutes more. Serve and enjoy.

Nutrition:
Calories: 397, Fat: 13g, Protein: 38.3g, Carbs: 31.4g, Sodium: 175mg, Potassium: 120mg.

797. Garlic Mushroom Chicken

Preparation Time: 15 minutes
Cooking Time: 15 minutes
Servings: 4
Ingredients:
- 4 chicken breasts, boneless and skinless
- 3 garlic cloves, minced
- 1 onion, chopped
- 2 cups mushrooms, sliced
- 1 tbsp. olive oil
- ½ cup chicken stock
- ¼ tsp. pepper
- ½ tsp. salt

Directions:
1. Season chicken with pepper and salt. Warm oil in a pan on medium heat, then put season chicken in the pan and cook for 5-6 minutes on each side. Remove and place on a plate.
2. Add onion and mushrooms to the pan and sauté until tender, about 2-3 minutes. Add garlic and sauté for a minute. Add stock and bring to boil. Stir well

and cook for 1-2 minutes. Pour over chicken and serve.

Nutrition:
Calories: 331, Fat: 14.5g, Protein: 43.9g, Carbs: 4.6, Sodium: 420mg, Potassium: 89mg.

798. Grilled Chicken

Preparation Time: 15 minutes
Cooking Time: 15 minutes
Servings: 4
Ingredients:
- 4 chicken breasts, skinless and boneless
- 1 ½ tsp. dried oregano
- 1 tsp. paprika
- 5 garlic cloves, minced
- ½ cup fresh parsley, minced
- ½ cup olive oil
- ½ cup fresh lemon juice
- Pepper
- Salt

Directions:
1. Add lemon juice, oregano, paprika, garlic, parsley, and olive oil to a large zip-lock bag. Season chicken with pepper and salt and add to bag. Seal bag and shake well to coat chicken with marinade. Let sit chicken in the marinade for 20 minutes.
2. Remove chicken from marinade and grill over medium-high heat for 5-6 minutes on each side. Serve and enjoy.

Nutrition:
Calories: 512, Fat: 36.5g, Protein: 43.1g, Carbs: 3g, Sodium: 110mg, Potassium: 90mg.

799. Delicious Lemon Chicken Salad

Preparation Time: 15 minutes
Cooking Time: 5 minutes
Servings: 4
Ingredients:
- 1 lb. chicken breast, cooked and diced
- 1 tbsp. fresh dill, chopped
- 2 tsp. olive oil
- 1/4 cup low-fat yogurt
- 1 tsp. lemon zest, grated
- 2 tbsp. onion, minced
- ¼ tsp. pepper
- ¼ tsp. salt

Directions:

1. Put all your fixing into the large mixing bowl and toss well. Season with pepper and salt. Cover and place in the refrigerator. Serve chilled and enjoy.

Nutrition:
Calories: 165, Fat: 5.4g, Protein: 25.2g, Carbs: 2.2g, Sodium: 153mg, Potassium: 120mg.

800. Healthy Chicken Orzo

Preparation Time: 15 minutes
Cooking Time: 15 minutes
Servings: 4
Ingredients:
- 1 cup whole wheat orzo
- 1 lb. chicken breasts, sliced
- ½ tsp. red pepper flakes
- ½ cup feta cheese, crumbled
- ½ tsp. oregano
- 1 tbsp. fresh parsley, chopped
- 1 tbsp. fresh basil, chopped
- ¼ cup pine nuts
- 1 cup spinach, chopped
- ¼ cup white wine
- ½ cup olives, sliced
- 1 cup grape tomatoes, cut in half
- ½ tbsp. garlic, minced
- 2 tbsp. olive oil
- ½ tsp. pepper
- ½ tsp. salt

Directions:
1. Add water in a small saucepan and bring to boil. Heat 1 tablespoon of olive oil in a pan over medium heat. Season chicken with pepper and salt and cook in the pan for 5-7 minutes on each side. Remove from pan and set aside.
2. Add orzo to boiling water and cook according to the packet directions. Heat remaining olive oil in a pan on medium heat, then put garlic in the pan and sauté for a minute. Stir in white wine and cherry tomatoes and cook on High for 3 minutes.
3. Add cooked orzo, spices, spinach, pine nuts, and olives and stir until well combined. Add chicken on top of orzo and sprinkle with feta cheese. Serve and enjoy.

Nutrition:
Calories: 518, Fat: 27.7g, Protein: 40.6g, Carbs: 26.2g, Sodium: 121mg, Potassium: 100mg.

801. Lemon Garlic Chicken

Preparation Time: 15 minutes
Cooking Time: 12 minutes
Servings: 3
Ingredients:
- 3 chicken breasts, cut into thin slices
- 2 lemon zest, grated
- ¼ cup olive oil
- 4 garlic cloves, minced
- Pepper
- Salt

Directions:
1. Heat olive oil in a pan over medium heat. Add garlic to the pan and sauté for 30 seconds. Put the chicken in the pan and sauté within 10 minutes. Add lemon zest and lemon juice and bring to boil. Remove from heat and season with pepper and salt. Serve and enjoy.

Nutrition:
Calories: 439, Fat: 27.8g, Protein: 42.9g, Carbs: 4.9g, Sodium: 306mg, Potassium: 200mg.

802. Simple Mediterranean Chicken

Preparation Time: 15 minutes
Cooking Time: 15 minutes
Servings: 12
Ingredients:
- 2 chicken breasts, skinless and boneless
- 1 ½ cup grape tomatoes, cut in half
- ½ cup olives
- 2 tbsp. olive oil
- 1 tsp. Italian seasoning
- ¼ tsp. pepper
- ¼ tsp. salt

Directions:
1. Season chicken with Italian seasoning, pepper, and salt. Heat olive oil in a pan over medium heat. Add season chicken to the pan and cook for 4-6 minutes on each side. Transfer chicken on a plate.
2. Put tomatoes plus olives in the pan and cook for 2-4 minutes. Pour olive and tomato mixture on top of the chicken and serve.

Nutrition:
Calories: 468, Fat: 29.4g, Protein: 43.8g, Carbs: 7.8g, Sodium: 410mg, Potassium: 130mg.

803. Roasted Chicken Thighs

Preparation Time: 15 minutes
Cooking Time: 55 minutes
Servings: 4
Ingredients:
- 8 chicken thighs
- 3 tbsp. fresh parsley, chopped
- 1 tsp. dried oregano
- 6 garlic cloves, crushed
- ¼ cup capers, drained
- 10 oz. roasted red peppers, sliced
- 2 cups grape tomatoes
- 1 ½ lbs. potatoes, cut into small chunks
- 4 tbsp. olive oil
- Pepper
- Salt

Directions:
1. Heat the oven to 400 F. Season chicken with pepper and salt. Heat 2 tablespoons of olive oil in a pan over medium heat. Add chicken to the pan and sear until lightly golden brown from all the sides.
2. Transfer chicken onto a baking tray. Add tomato, potatoes, capers, oregano, garlic, and red peppers around the chicken. Season with pepper and salt and drizzle with remaining olive oil. Bake in preheated oven for 45-55 minutes. Garnish with parsley and serve.

Nutrition:
Calories: 848, Fat: 29.1g, Protein: 91.3g, Carbs: 45.2g, Sodium: 110mg, Potassium: 140mg.

804. Mediterranean Turkey Breast

Preparation Time: 15 minutes
Cooking Time: 4 minutes & 30 minutes
Servings: 6
Ingredients:
- 4 lbs. turkey breast
- 3 tbsp. flour
- ¾ cup chicken stock
- 4 garlic cloves, chopped
- 1 tsp. dried oregano
- ½ fresh lemon juice
- ½ cup sun-dried tomatoes, chopped
- ½ cup olives, chopped
- 1 onion, chopped
- ¼ tsp. pepper

- ½ tsp. salt

Directions:
1. Add turkey breast, garlic, oregano, lemon juice, sun-dried tomatoes, olives, onion, pepper, and salt to the slow cooker. Add half stock. Cook on high within 4 hours.
2. Whisk remaining stock and flour in a small bowl and add to slow cooker. Cover and cook for 30 minutes more. Serve and enjoy.

Nutrition:
Calories: 537, Fat: 9.7g, Protein: 79.1g, Carbs: 29.6g, Sodium: 330mg, Potassium: 140mg.

805. Olive Capers Chicken

Preparation Time: 15 minutes
Cooking Time: 16 minutes
Servings: 4
Ingredients:
- 2 lbs. chicken
- 1/3 cup chicken stock
- 1 oz. Capers
- 6 oz. olives
- 1/4 cup fresh basil
- 1 tbsp. olive oil
- 1 tsp. oregano
- 2 garlic cloves, minced
- 2 tbsp. red wine vinegar
- 1/8 tsp. pepper
- 1/4 tsp. salt

Directions:
1. Put olive oil in your Instant Pot and set the pot on sauté mode. Add chicken to the pot and sauté for 3-4 minutes. Add remaining ingredients and stir well. Seal pot with the lid and select manual and set timer for 12 minutes. Serve and enjoy.

Nutrition:
Calories: 433, Fat: 15.2g, Protein: 66.9g, Carbs: 4.8g, Sodium: 244mg, Potassium: 100mg.

806. Chicken with Mushrooms

Preparation Time: 15 minutes
Cooking Time: 6 hours & 10 minutes
Servings: 2
Ingredients:
- 2 chicken breasts, skinless and boneless
- 1 cup mushrooms, sliced
- 1 onion, sliced
- 1 cup chicken stock

- 1/2 tsp. thyme, dried
- Pepper
- Salt

Directions:
1. Add all ingredients to the slow cooker. Cook on low within 6 hours. Serve and enjoy.

Nutrition:
Calories: 313, Fat: 11.3g, Protein: 44.3g, Carbs: 6.9g, Sodium: 541mg, Potassium: 100mg.

807. Baked Chicken

Preparation Time: 15 minutes
Cooking Time: 35 minutes
Servings: 4
Ingredients:
- 2 lbs. chicken tenders
- 1 large zucchini
- 1 cup grape tomatoes
- 2 tbsp. olive oil
- 3 dill sprigs

For topping:
- 2 tbsp. feta cheese, crumbled
- 1 tbsp. olive oil
- 1 tbsp. fresh lemon juice
- 1 tbsp. fresh dill, chopped

Directions:
1. Heat the oven to 200 C/ 400 F. Drizzle the olive oil on a baking tray, then place chicken, zucchini, dill, and tomatoes on the tray. Season with salt. Bake chicken within 30 minutes.
2. Meanwhile, in a small bowl, stir all topping ingredients. Place chicken on the serving tray, then top with veggies and discard dill sprigs. Sprinkle topping mixture on top of chicken and vegetables. Serve and enjoy.

Nutrition:
Calories: 557, Fat: 28.6g, Protein: 67.9g, Carbs: 5.2g, Sodium: 760mg, Potassium: 190mg.

808. Garlic Pepper Chicken

Preparation Time: 15 minutes
Cooking Time: 21 minutes
Servings: 2
Ingredients:
- 2 chicken breasts, cut into strips
- 2 bell peppers, cut into strips
- 5 garlic cloves, chopped
- 3 tbsp. water
- 2 tbsp. olive oil
- 1 tbsp. paprika

- 2 tsp. black pepper
- 1/2 tsp. salt

Directions:
1. Heat olive oil in a large saucepan over medium heat. Add garlic and sauté for 2-3 minutes. Add peppers and cook for 3 minutes. Add chicken and spices and stir to coat. Add water and stir well. Bring to boil. Cover and simmer for 10-15 minutes. Serve and enjoy.

Nutrition:
Calories: 462, Fat: 25.7g, Protein: 44.7g, Carbs: 14.8g, Sodium: 720mg, Potassium: 120mg.

809. Mustard Chicken Tenders

Preparation Time: 15 minutes
Cooking Time: 20 minutes
Servings: 4
Ingredients:
- 1 lb. chicken tenders
- 2 tbsp. fresh tarragon, chopped
- 1/2 cup whole grain mustard
- 1/2 tsp. paprika
- 1 garlic clove, minced
- 1/2 oz. fresh lemon juice
- 1/2 tsp. pepper
- 1/4 tsp. kosher salt

Directions:
1. Heat the oven to 425 F. Add all ingredients except chicken to the large bowl and mix well. Put the chicken in the bowl, then stir until well coated. Place chicken on a baking dish and cover. Bake within 15-20 minutes. Serve and enjoy.

Nutrition:
Calories: 242, Fat: 9.5g, Protein: 33.2g, Carbs: 3.1g, Sodium: 240mg, Potassium: 100mg.

810. Salsa Chicken Chili

Preparation Time: 15 minutes
Cooking Time: 20 minutes
Servings: 8
Ingredients:
- 2 1/2 lbs. chicken breasts, skinless and boneless
- 1/2 tsp. cumin powder
- 3 garlic cloves, minced
- 1 onion, diced
- 16 oz. salsa
- 1 tsp. oregano
- 1 tbsp. olive oil

Directions:

1. Add oil into the Instant Pot and set the pot on sauté mode. Add onion to the pot and sauté until softened, about 3 minutes. Add garlic and sauté for a minute. Add oregano and cumin and sauté for a minute. Add half salsa and stir well. Place chicken and pour remaining salsa over chicken.
2. Seal pot with the lid and select manual and set timer for 10 minutes. Remove chicken and shred. Move it back to the pot, then stir well to combine. Serve and enjoy.

Nutrition:
Calories: 308, Fat: 12.4g, Protein: 42.1g, Carbs: 5.4g, Sodium: 656mg, Potassium: 139mg.

811. Honey Crusted Chicken

Preparation Time: 10 minutes
Cooking Time: 25 minutes
Servings: 2
Ingredients:

- 1 teaspoon paprika
- 8 saltine crackers, 2 inches square
- 2 chicken breasts, each 4 ounces
- 4 tsp. honey

Directions:

1. Set the oven to heat at 375 degrees F. Grease a baking dish with cooking oil. Smash the crackers in a Ziplock bag and toss them with paprika in a bowl. Brush chicken with honey and add it to the crackers.
2. Mix well and transfer the chicken to the baking dish. Bake the chicken for 25 minutes until golden brown. Serve.

Nutrition:
Calories: 219, Fat: 17g, Sodium: 456mg, Carbs 12.1g, Protein: 31g, Potassium: 120mg.

812. Paella with Chicken, Leeks, and Tarragon

Preparation Time: 10 minutes
Cooking Time: 20 minutes
Servings: 2
Ingredients:

- 1 teaspoon extra-virgin olive oil
- 1 small onion, sliced

- 2 leeks (whites only), thinly sliced
- 3 garlic cloves, minced
- 1-pound boneless, skinless chicken breast, cut into strips 1/2-inch-wide and 2 inches long
- 2 large tomatoes, chopped
- 1 red pepper, sliced
- 2/3 cup long-grain brown rice
- 1 teaspoon tarragon, or to taste
- 2 cups fat-free, unsalted chicken broth
- 1 cup frozen peas
- 1/4 cup chopped fresh parsley
- 1 lemon, cut into 4 wedges

Directions:

1. Preheat a nonstick pan with olive oil over medium heat. Toss in leeks, onions, chicken strips, and garlic. Sauté for 5 minutes. Stir in red pepper slices and tomatoes. Stir and cook for 5 minutes.
2. Add tarragon, broth, and rice. Let it boil, then reduce the heat to a simmer. Continue cooking for 10 minutes, then add peas and continue cooking until the liquid is thoroughly cooked. Garnish with parsley and lemon. Serve.

Nutrition:
Calories: 388, Fat: 15.2g, Sodium: 572mg, Carbs 5.4g, Protein: 27g, Potassium: 146mg.

813. Southwestern Chicken and Pasta

Preparation Time: 10 minutes
Cooking Time: 10 minutes
Servings: 2
Ingredients:

- 1 cup uncooked whole-wheat rigatoni
- 2 chicken breasts, cut into cubes
- 1/4 cup of salsa
- 1 1/2 cups of canned unsalted tomato sauce
- 1/8 tsp. garlic powder
- 1 tsp. cumin
- 1/2 tsp. chili powder
- 1/2 cup canned black beans, drained
- 1/2 cup fresh corn
- 1/4 cup Monterey Jack and Colby cheese, shredded

Directions:

1. Fill a pot with water up to ¾ full and boil it. Add pasta to cook until it is al dente, then drain the pasta while rinsing under

cold water. Preheat a skillet with cooking oil, then cook the chicken for 10 minutes until golden from both sides.
2. Add tomato sauce, salsa, cumin, garlic powder, black beans, corn, and chili powder. Cook the mixture while stirring, then toss in the pasta. Serve with 2 tablespoons of cheese on top. Enjoy.

Nutrition:
Calories: 245, Fat: 16.3g, Sodium: 515mg, Carbs 19.3g, Protein: 33.3g, Potassium: 170mg.

814. Stuffed Chicken Breasts

Preparation Time: 15 minutes
Cooking Time: 30 minutes
Servings: 4
Ingredients:

- 3 tbsp. seedless raisins
- 1/2 cup of chopped onion
- 1/2 cup of chopped celery
- 1/4 tsp. garlic, minced
- 1 bay leaf
- 1 cup apple with peel, chopped
- 2 tbsp. chopped water chestnuts
- 4 large chicken breast halves, 5 ounces each
- 1 tablespoon olive oil
- 1 cup fat-free milk
- 1 teaspoon curry powder
- 2 tablespoons all-purpose (plain) flour
- 1 lemon, cut into 4 wedges

Directions:

1. Set the oven to heat at 425 degrees F. Grease a baking dish with cooking oil. Soak raisins in warm water until they swell. Grease a heated skillet with cooking spray.
2. Add celery, garlic, onions, and bay leaf. Sauté for 5 minutes. Discard the bay leaf, then toss in apples. Stir cook for 2 minutes. Drain the soaked raisin and pat them dry to remove excess water.
3. Add raisins and water chestnuts to the apple mixture. Pull apart the chicken's skin and stuff the apple raisin mixture between the skin and the chicken. Preheat olive oil in another skillet and sear the breasts for 5 minutes per side.
4. Place the chicken breasts in the baking dish and cover the dish. Bake for 15 minutes until

temperature reaches 165 degrees F. Prepare sauce by mixing milk, flour, and curry powder in a saucepan.

5. Stir cook until the mixture thickens, about 5 minutes. Pour this sauce over the baked chicken. Bake again in the covered dish for 10 minutes. Serve.

Nutrition:
Calories: 357, Fat: 32.7g, Sodium: 277mg, Carbs 17.7g, Protein: 31.2g, Potassium: 100mg.

815. Buffalo Chicken Salad Wrap

Preparation Time: 10 minutes
Cooking Time: 10 minutes
Servings: 4
Ingredients:
- 3-4 ounces chicken breasts
- 2 whole chipotle peppers
- 1/4 cup white wine vinegar
- 1/4 cup low-calorie mayonnaise
- 2 stalks celery, diced
- 2 carrots, cut into matchsticks
- 1 small yellow onion, diced
- 1/2 cup thinly sliced rutabaga or another root vegetable
- 4 ounces spinach, cut into strips
- 2 whole-grain tortillas (12-inch diameter)

Directions:
1. Set the oven or a grill to heat at 375 degrees F. Bake the chicken first for 10 minutes per side. Blend chipotle peppers with mayonnaise and wine vinegar in the blender. Dice the baked chicken into cubes or small chunks.
2. Mix the chipotle mixture with all the ingredients except tortillas and spinach. Spread 2 ounces of spinach over the tortilla and scoop the stuffing on top. Wrap the tortilla and cut it in half. Serve.

Nutrition:
Calories: 300, Fat: 16.4g, Sodium: 471mg, Carbs 8.7g, Protein: 38.5g, Potassium: 100mg.

816. Chicken Sliders

Preparation Time: 10 minutes
Cooking Time: 10 minutes
Servings: 4

Ingredients:
- 10 ounces ground chicken breast
- 1 tablespoon black pepper
- 1 tablespoon minced garlic
- 1 tablespoon balsamic vinegar
- 1/2 cup minced onion
- 1 fresh chili pepper, minced
- 1 tablespoon fennel seed, crushed
- 4 whole-wheat mini buns
- 4 lettuce leaves
- 4 tomato slices

Directions:
1. Combine all the ingredients except the wheat buns, tomato, and lettuce. Mix well and refrigerate the mixture for 1 hour. Divide the mixture into 4 patties.
2. Broil these patties in a greased baking tray until golden brown. Place the chicken patties in the wheat buns along with lettuce and tomato. Serve.

Nutrition:
Calories: 224, Fat: 4.5g, Sodium: 212mg, Carbs 10.2g, Protein: 67.4g, Potassium: 140mg.

817. White Chicken Chili

Preparation Time: 20 minutes
Cooking Time: 15 minutes
Servings: 4
Ingredients:
- 1 can white chunk chicken
- 2 cans low-sodium white beans, drained
- 1 can low-sodium diced tomatoes
- 4 cups of low-sodium chicken broth
- 1 medium onion, chopped
- 1/2 medium green pepper, chopped
- 1 medium red pepper, chopped
- 2 garlic cloves, minced
- 2 teaspoons chili powder
- 1 teaspoon ground cumin
- 1 teaspoon dried oregano
- Cayenne pepper to taste
- 8 tablespoons shredded reduced-fat Monterey Jack cheese
- 3 tablespoons chopped fresh cilantro

Directions:
1. In a soup pot, add beans, tomatoes, chicken, and chicken broth. Cover this soup pot and let it simmer over medium heat. Meanwhile, grease a nonstick

pan with cooking spray. Add peppers, garlic, and onions. Sauté for 5 minutes until soft.
2. Transfer the mixture to the soup pot. Add cumin, chili powder, cayenne pepper, and oregano. Cook for 10 minutes, then garnish the chili with cilantro and 1 tablespoon cheese. Serve.

Nutrition:
Calories: 225, Fat: 12.9g, Sodium: 480mg, Carbs 24.7g, Protein: 25.3g, Potassium: 178mg.

818. Sweet Potato-Turkey Meatloaf

Preparation Time: 15 minutes
Cooking Time: 25 minutes
Servings: 4
Ingredients:
- 1 large sweet potato, peeled and cubed
- 1-pound ground turkey (breast)
- 1 large egg
- 1 small sweet onion, finely chopped
- 2 cloves garlic, minced
- 2 slices whole-wheat bread, crumbs
- ¼ cup honey barbecue sauce
- ¼ cup ketchup
- 2 tablespoons Dijon Mustard
- 1 tablespoon fresh ground pepper
- ½ tablespoon salt

Directions:
1. Heat the oven to 350F. Grease a baking dish. In a large pot, boil a cup of lightly salted water, add the sweet potato. Cook until tender. Drain the water. Mash the potato.
2. Mix the honey barbecue sauce, ketchup, and Dijon mustard in a small bowl. Mix thoroughly. In a large bowl, mix the turkey and the egg. Add the sweet onion, garlic. Pour in the combined sauces. Add the bread crumbs. Season the mixture with salt and pepper.
3. Add the sweet potato. Combine thoroughly with your hands. If the mixture feels wet, add more bread crumbs. Shape the mixture into a loaf. Place in the loaf pan. Bake for 25 – 35 minutes until the meat is cooked through. Broil for 5 minutes. Slice and serve.

Nutrition:

Calories: 133, Protein: 85g, Carbohydrates: 50g, Fat: 34g, Sodium: 202mg, Potassium: 189mg.

819. Oaxacan Chicken

Preparation Time: 15 minutes
Cooking Time: 28 minutes
Servings: 2
Ingredients:
- 1 4-ounce chicken breast, skinned and halved
- ½ cup uncooked long-grain rice
- 1 teaspoon of extra-virgin olive oil
- ½ cup low-sodium salsa
- ½ cup chicken stock, mixed with 2 tablespoons water
- ¾ cup baby carrots
- 2 tablespoons green olives, pitted and chopped
- 2 tablespoons dark raisins
- ½ teaspoon ground cinnamon
- 2 tablespoons fresh cilantro or parsley, coarsely chopped

Directions:
1. Heat the oven to 350F. In a large saucepan that can fit in the oven, heat the olive oil. Add the rice. Sauté the rice until it begins to pop, approximately 2 minutes.
2. Add the salsa, baby carrots, green olives, dark raisins, halved chicken breast, chicken stock, and ground cinnamon. Bring the mix to a simmer, stir once.
3. Cover the mixture tightly. Bake in the oven until the chicken stock has been completely absorbed, approximately 25 minutes. Sprinkle fresh cilantro or parsley, mix. Serve immediately.

Nutrition:
Calories: 143, Protein: 102g, Carbohydrates: 66g. Fat: 18g.

Sodium: 97mg, Potassium: 189mg.

820. Spicy Chicken with Minty Couscous

Preparation Time: 15 minutes
Cooking Time: 25 minutes
Servings: 2
Ingredients:
- 2 small chicken breasts, sliced
- 1 red chili pepper, finely chopped
- 1 garlic clove, crushed
- ginger root, 2 cm long peeled and grated
- 1 teaspoon ground cumin
- ½ teaspoon turmeric
- 2 tablespoons extra-virgin olive oil
- 1 pinch sea salt
- ¾ cup couscous
- Small bunch mint leaves, finely chopped
- 2 lemons, grate the rind and juice them

Directions:
1. In a large bowl, place the chicken breast slices and chopped chili pepper. Sprinkle with crushed garlic, ginger, cumin, turmeric, and a pinch of salt. Add the grated rind of both lemons and the juice from 1 lemon. Pour 1 tablespoon of the olive oil over the chicken, coat evenly.
2. Cover the dish with plastic and refrigerate within 1 hour. After 1 hour, coat a skillet with olive oil and fry the chicken. As the chicken is cooking, pour the couscous into a bowl and pour hot water over it, let it absorb the water (approximately 5 minutes).
3. Fluff the couscous. Add some chopped mint, the other tablespoon of olive oil, and juice from the second lemon. Top the

couscous with the chicken. Garnish with chopped mint. Serve immediately.
Nutrition:
Calories: 166, Protein: 106g, Carbohydrates: 52g, Sugars: 0.1g, Fat: 17g, Sodium: 108mg, Potassium: 267mg.

821. Chicken, Pasta and Snow Peas

Preparation Time: 15 minutes
Cooking Time: 20 minutes
Servings: 2
Ingredients:
- 1-pound chicken breasts
- 2 ½ cups penne pasta
- 1 cup snow peas, trimmed and halved
- 1 teaspoon olive oil
- 1 standard jar tomato and basil pasta sauce
- Fresh ground pepper

Directions:
1. In a medium frying pan, heat the olive oil. Flavor the chicken breasts with salt and pepper. Heat the chicken breasts until cooked through (approximately 5 – 7 minutes on each side).
2. Cook the pasta, as stated in the instructions of the package. Cook the snow peas with the pasta. Scoop 1 cup of the pasta water. Drain the pasta and peas, set them aside.
3. Once the chicken is cooked, slice diagonally. Return the chicken to the frying pan. Add the pasta sauce. If the mixture seems dry, add some of the pasta water to the desired consistency. Heat, then divide into bowls. Serve immediately.
Nutrition:
Calories: 140, Protein: 34g, Carbohydrates: 52g, Fat: 17g, Sodium: 118mg, Potassium: 178mg.

Chapter 17. Fish and Seafood

822. Balsamic Salmon and Peaches Mix

Preparation Time: 10 minutes
Cooking Time: 10 minutes
Servings: 4
Ingredients:

- 1 tablespoon balsamic vinegar
- 1 teaspoon thyme, chopped
- 1 tablespoon ginger, grated
- 4 tablespoons olive oil
- Black pepper to taste
- 2 red onions, cut into wedges
- 2 peaches cut into wedges
- 3 lb. salmon steaks

Directions:

1. In a small bowl, combine vinegar with ginger, thyme, 3 tablespoons of olive oil and black pepper and whisk
2. In another bowl, mix onion with peaches, 1 tablespoon of oil and pepper and toss.
3. Season salmon with black pepper, place on preheated grill over medium heat, cook for 5 minutes on each side and divide between plates.
4. Put the peaches and onions on the same grill. Cook for 4 minutes on each side, divide next to the salmon, drizzle the vinegar mix and serve.
5. Enjoy!

Nutrition:
   Calories: 200, Fat: 2g, Fiber: 2g, Carbs: 3g, Protein: 2g, Sodium: 59mg, Potassium: 100mg.

823. Greek Style Salmon

Preparation Time: 10 minutes
Cooking Time: 10 minutes
Servings: 2
Ingredients:

- 4 medium salmon fillets, skinless and boneless
- 1 tablespoon lemon juice
- 1 tablespoon dried oregano
- 1 teaspoon dried thyme
- ¼ teaspoon onion powder
- 1 tablespoon olive oil

Directions:

1. Heat olive oil in the skillet.

2. Sprinkle the salmon with dried oregano, thyme, onion powder, and lemon juice.
3. Put the fish in the skillet and cook for 4 minutes per side.

Nutrition:
   Calories: 271, Protein: 34.7g, Carbohydrates: 1.1g, Fat: 14.7g, Fiber: 0.6g, Cholesterol: 78mg, Sodium: 80mg, Potassium: 34mg.

824. Spicy Ginger Sea Bass

Preparation Time: 5 minutes
Cooking Time: 10 minutes
Servings: 2
Ingredients:

- 1 tablespoon ginger, grated
- 2 tablespoons sesame oil
- ¼ teaspoon chili powder
- 4lb. sea bass fillets, boneless
- 1 tablespoon margarine

Directions:

1. Heat sesame oil and margarine in the skillet.
2. Add chili powder and ginger.
3. Then add sea bass and cook the fish for 3 minutes per side.
4. Then close the lid and simmer the fish for 3 minutes over low heat.

Nutrition:
   Calories: 216, Protein: 24g, Carbohydrates: 1.1g, Fat: 12.3g, Fiber: 0.2g, Cholesterol: 54mg, Sodium: 123mg, Potassium: 78mg.

825. Yogurt Shrimps

Preparation Time: 5 minutes
Cooking Time: 10 minutes
Servings: 2
Ingredients:

- 4 pound shrimp, peeled
- 1 tablespoon margarine
- ¼ cup low-fat yogurt
- 1 teaspoon lemon zest, grated
- 1 chili pepper, chopped

Directions:

1. Melt the margarine in the skillet, add chili pepper, and roast it for 1 minute.
2. Then add shrimps and lemon zest.

3. Roast the shrimps for 2 minutes per side.
4. After this, add yogurt, stir the shrimps well and cook for 5 minutes.

Nutrition:
   Calories: 137, Protein: 21.4g, Carbohydrates: 2.4g, Fat: 4g, Fiber: 0.1g, Cholesterol: 192mg, Sodium: 257mg, Potassium: 78mg.

826. Aromatic Salmon with Fennel Seeds

Preparation Time: 8 minutes
Cooking Time: 10 minutes
Servings: 2
Ingredients:

- 4 medium salmon fillets, skinless and boneless
- 1 tablespoon fennel seeds
- 3 tablespoons olive oil
- 1 tablespoon lemon juice
- 1 tablespoon water

Directions:

1. Heat olive oil in the skillet.
2. Add fennel seeds and roast them for 1 minute.
3. Add salmon fillets and sprinkle with lemon juice.
4. Add water and roast the fish for 4 minutes per side over medium heat.

Nutrition:
   Calories: 301, Protein: 4.8g, Carbohydrates: 0.8g, Fat: 18.2g, Fiber: 0.6g, Cholesterol: 78mg, Sodium: 81mg, Potassium: 89mg.

827. Shrimp Quesadillas

Preparation Time: 16 minutes
Cooking Time: 5 minutes
Servings: 2
Ingredients:

- 2 whole wheat tortillas
- ½ tsp. ground cumin
- 4 cilantro leaves
- 3 oz. diced cooked shrimp
- de-seeded plump tomato
- ¾ c. grated non-fat mozzarella cheese
- ¼ c. diced red onion

Directions:

1. In a medium bowl, combine the grated mozzarella cheese and the warm, cooked shrimp. Add the ground cumin, red onion, and tomato. Mix. Spread the mixture evenly on the tortillas.
2. Heat a non-stick frying pan. Place the tortillas in the pan, then heat until they are crisp.
3. Add the cilantro leaves. Fold over the tortillas.
4. Press down for 1 – 2 minutes. Slice the tortillas into wedges.
5. Serve immediately.

Nutrition:
Calories: 99, Fat: 9g, Carbs: 7.2g, Protein: 59g, Sugars: 4g, Sodium: 500mg, Potassium: 90mg.

828. The OG Tuna Sandwich

Preparation Time: 15 minutes
Cooking Time: 5 minutes
Servings: 2
Ingredients:
- 30 g olive oil
- peeled and diced medium cucumber
- ½ g pepper
- whole wheat bread slices
- 85 g diced onion
- 2 ½ g salt
- 1 can flavored tuna
- 85 g shredded spinach

Directions:
1. Grab your blender and add the spinach, tuna, onion, oil, salt and pepper in, and pulse for about 10 to 20 seconds.
2. In the meantime, toast your bread and add your diced cucumber to a bowl, which you can pour your tuna mixture in. Carefully mix and add the mixture to the bread once toasted.
3. Slice in half and serve while storing the remaining mixture in the fridge.

Nutrition:
Calories: 302, Fat: 5.8g, Carbs: 36.62g, Protein: 28g, Sugars: 3.22g, Sodium: 445mg, Potassium: 56mg.

829. Easy to Understand Mussels

Preparation Time: 10 minutes
Cooking Time: 10 minutes

Servings: 2
Ingredients:
- 2 lbs. cleaned mussels
- 4 minced garlic cloves
- 2 chopped shallots
- Lemon and parsley
- 2 tbsps. Butter
- ½ c. broth
- ½ c. white wine

Directions:
1. Clean the mussels and remove the beard.
2. Discard any mussels that do not close when tapped against a hard surface.
3. Set your pot to Sauté mode and add chopped onion and butter.
4. Stir and sauté onions.
5. Add garlic and cook for 1 minute.
6. Add broth and wine.
7. Lock up the lid and cook for 5 minutes on HIGH pressure.
8. Release the pressure naturally over 10 minutes.
9. Serve with a sprinkle of parsley and enjoy!

Nutrition:
Calories: 286, Fat: 14g, Carbs: 12g, Protein: 28g, Sugars: 0g, Sodium: 314mg, Potassium: 67mg.

830. Cheesy Shrimp Mix

Preparation Time: 10 minutes
Cooking Time: 30 minutes
Servings: 10
Ingredients:
- ½ pound shrimp, already peeled and deveined
- 1 cup avocado mayonnaise
- ½ cup low-fat mozzarella cheese, shredded
- 2 garlic cloves, minced
- ¼ teaspoon hot sauce
- 1 tablespoon lemon juice
- A drizzle of olive oil
- ½ cup scallions, sliced

Directions:
1. In a bowl, mix mozzarella with mayo, hot sauce, and garlic and lemon juice and whisk well.
2. Add scallions and shrimp, toss, pour into a baking dish greased with the olive oil, introduce in the oven at 350 degrees F and bake for 30 minutes.
3. Divide into bowls and serve.
4. Enjoy!

Nutrition:
Calories: 275, Fat: 3g, Fiber: 5g, Carbs: 10g, Protein: 12g,

Sodium: 223mg, Potassium: 124mg.

831. Smoked Salmon with Capers and Radishes

Preparation Time: 10 minutes
Cooking Time: 0 minutes
Servings: 8
Ingredients:
- 3 tablespoons beet horseradish, prepared
- 1-pound smoked salmon, skinless, boneless and flaked
- 2 teaspoons lemon zest, grated
- 4 radishes, chopped
- ½ cup capers, drained and chopped
- 1/3 cup red onion, roughly chopped
- 3 tablespoons chives, chopped

Directions:
1. In a bowl, combine the salmon with the beet horseradish, lemon zest, radish, capers, onions and chives, toss and serve cold.
2. Enjoy!

Nutrition:
Calories: 254, Fat: 2g, Fiber: 1g, Carbs: 7g, Protein: 7g, Sodium: 67mg, Potassium: 98mg.

832. Trout Spread

Preparation Time: 10 minutes
Cooking Time: 0 minutes
Servings: 8
Ingredients:
- 4 ounces smoked trout, skinless, boneless and flaked
- ¼ cup coconut cream
- 1 tablespoon lemon juice
- 1/3 cup non-fat yogurt
- 1 and ½ tablespoon parsley, chopped
- 2 tablespoons chives, chopped
- 1 tablespoon Black pepper to the taste
- A drizzle of olive oil

Directions:
1. In a bowl mix trout with yogurt, cream, black pepper, chives, lemon juice and the dill and stir.
2. Drizzle the olive oil at the end and serve.
3. Enjoy!

Nutrition:
Calories: 204, Fat: 2g, Fiber: 2g, Carbs: 8g, Protein: 15g, Sodium: 234mg, Potassium: 256mg.

833. Easy Shrimp and Mango

Preparation Time: 10 minutes
Cooking Time: 0 minutes
Servings: 4
Ingredients:
- 3 tablespoons balsamic vinegar
- 3 tablespoons coconut sugar
- 6 tablespoons avocado mayonnaise
- 3 mangos, peeled and cubed
- 3 tablespoons parsley, finely chopped
- 1 pound shrimp, peeled, deveined and cooked

Directions:
1. In a bowl, mix vinegar with sugar and mayo and whisk.
2. In another bowl, combine the mango with the parsley and shrimp, add the mayo mix, toss and serve.
3. Enjoy!

Nutrition:
Calories: 204, Fat: 3g, Fiber: 2g, Carbs: 8g, Protein: 8g, Sodium: 78mg, Potassium: 89mg.

834. Spring Salmon Mix

Preparation Time: 10 minutes
Cooking Time: 0 minutes
Servings: 4
Ingredients:
- 2 tablespoons scallions, chopped
- 2 tablespoons sweet onion, chopped
- 1 and ½ teaspoons lime juice
- 1 tablespoon chives, minced
- 1 Tablespoon olive oil
- 1-pound smoked salmon, flaked
- 1 cup cherry tomatoes, halved
- 1 tablespoon Black pepper to the taste
- 1 tablespoon parsley, chopped

Directions:
1. In a bowl, mix the scallions with sweet onion, lime juice, chives, oil, salmon, tomatoes, black pepper and parsley, toss and serve.
2. Enjoy!

Nutrition:
Calories: 200, Fat: 8g, Fiber: 3g, Carbs: 8g, Protein: 6g, Sodium: 34mg, Potassium: 78mg.

835. Smoked Salmon and Green Beans

Preparation Time: 10 minutes
Cooking Time: 0 minutes
Servings: 4
Ingredients:
- 3 tablespoons balsamic vinegar
- 2 tablespoons olive oil
- 1/3 cup Kalamata olives, pitted and minced
- 1 garlic clove, minced
- 1 tablespoon Black pepper to the taste
- ½ teaspoon lemon zest, grated
- 2 pound green beans, blanched and halved
- ½ pound cherry tomatoes, halved
- ½ fennel bulb, sliced
- ½ red onion, sliced
- 2 cups baby arugula
- ¾ pound smoked salmon, flaked

Directions:
1. In a bowl, combine the green beans with cherry tomatoes, fennel, onion, arugula and salmon and toss.
2. Add vinegar, oil, olives, garlic, black pepper and lemon zest, toss and serve.
3. Enjoy!

Nutrition:
Calories: 212, Fat: 3g, Fiber: 3g, Carbs: 6g, Protein: 4g, Sodium: 124mg, Potassium: 67mg.

836. Saffron Shrimp

Preparation Time: 10 minutes
Cooking Time: 30 minutes
Servings: 4
Ingredients:
- 1 Teaspoon lemon juice
- 1 tablespoon Black pepper to the taste
- ½ cup avocado mayo
- ½ teaspoon sweet paprika
- 2 Tablespoons olive oil
- 1 Fennel bulb, chopped
- 1 yellow onion, chopped
- 1 Garlic cloves, minced
- 1 cup canned tomatoes, no-salt-added and chopped
- 1 and ½ pounds big shrimp, peeled and deveined
- ¼ teaspoon saffron powder

Directions:

1. In a bowl, combine the garlic with lemon juice, black pepper, mayo and paprika and whisk.
2. Add the shrimp and toss.
3. Heat a pan with the oil over medium-high flame. Add the shrimp, fennel, onion and garlic mix, toss and cook for 4 minutes.
4. Add tomatoes and saffron, toss, divide into bowls and serve.
5. Enjoy!

Nutrition:
Calories: 210, Fat: 2g, Fiber: 5g, Carbs: 8g, Protein: 4g, Sodium: 89mg, Potassium: 79mg.

837. Crab, Zucchini and Watermelon Soup

Preparation Time: 4 hours
Cooking Time: 0 minutes
Servings: 4
Ingredients:
- ¼ cup basil, chopped
- 2 pounds tomatoes
- 5 cups watermelon, cubed
- ¼ cup red wine vinegar
- 1/3 cup olive oil
- 2 garlic cloves, minced
- zucchini, chopped
- Black pepper to the taste
- 1 cup crabmeat

Directions:
1. In your food processor, mix tomatoes with basil, vinegar, 4 cups watermelon, garlic, 1/3 cup oil and black pepper to the taste, pulse, pour into a bowl and keep in the fridge for 1 hour.
2. Divide this into bowls, add zucchini, crab and the rest of the watermelon and serve.
3. Enjoy!

Nutrition:
Calories: 231, Fat: 3g, Fiber: 3g, Carbs: 6g, Protein: 8g, Sodium: 56mg, Potassium: 78mg.

838. Shrimp and Orzo

Preparation Time: 10 minutes
Cooking Time: 30 minutes
Servings: 4
Ingredients:
- 1 Pound shrimp, peeled and deveined
- 1 tablespoon Black pepper to the taste
- 2 Garlic cloves, minced

- 1 Tablespoon olive oil
- ½ teaspoon oregano, dried
- 1 yellow onion, chopped
- 2 Cups low-sodium chicken stock
- 3 Ounces orzo
- ½ cup water
- 2 Ounces canned tomatoes, no-salt-added and chopped
- Juice of 1 lemon

Directions:
1. Heat a pan with the oil over medium-high flame. Add onion, garlic and oregano, stir and cook for 4 minutes.
2. Add orzo, stir and cook for 2 more minutes.
3. Add stock and the water, bring to a boil, cover, reduce heat to low and cook for 12 minutes.
4. Add lemon juice, tomatoes, black pepper and shrimp, introduce in the oven and bake at 400 degrees F for 15 minutes.
5. Divide between plates and serve.
6. Enjoy!

Nutrition:
Calories: 228, Fat: 4g, Fiber: 3g, Carbs: 7g, Protein: 8g, Sodium: 56mg, Potassium: 87mg.

839. Lemon and Garlic Scallops

Preparation Time: 10 minutes
Cooking Time: 5 minutes
Servings: 4
Ingredients:
- 1 Tablespoon olive oil
- ¼ pounds dried scallops
- 2 Tablespoons all-purpose flour
- ¼ teaspoon sunflower seeds
- 4-5 garlic cloves, minced
- 1 scallion, chopped
- 1 pinch of ground sage
- 1 lemon juice
- 2 Tablespoons parsley, chopped

Directions:
1. Take a nonstick skillet and place over medium-high heat.
2. Add oil and allow the oil to heat.
3. Take a medium-sized bowl and add scallops alongside sunflower seeds and flour.
4. Place the scallops in the skillet and add scallions, garlic, and sage.
5. Sauté for 3-4 minutes until they show an opaque texture.
6. Stir in lemon juice and parsley.
7. Remove heat and serve hot!

Nutrition:

Calories: 151, Fat: 4g, Carbohydrates: 10g, Protein: 18g, Sodium: 123mg, Potassium: 145mg.

840. Walnut Encrusted Salmon

Preparation Time: 10 minutes
Cooking Time: 14 minutes
Servings: 34
Ingredients:
- ½ cup walnuts
- 2 tablespoons stevia
- ½ tablespoon Dijon mustard
- ¼ teaspoon dill
- 2 salmon fillets (3 ounces each)
- 1 Tablespoon olive oil
- 1 tablespoon Sunflower seeds and pepper to taste

Directions:
1. Preheat your oven to 350 degrees F.
2. Add walnuts, mustard, stevia to a food processor and process until your desired consistency is achieved.
3. Take a frying pan and place it over medium heat.
4. Add oil and let it heat.
5. Add salmon and sear for 3 minutes.
6. Add walnut mix and coat well.
7. Transfer coated salmon to baking sheet, bake in the oven for 8 minutes.
8. Serve and enjoy!

Nutrition:
Calories: 373, Fat: 43g, Carbohydrates: 4g, Protein: 20g, Sodium: 145mg, Potassium: 167mg.

841. Roasted Lemon Swordfish

Preparation Time: 10 minutes
Cooking Time: 70-80 minutes
Servings: 4
Ingredients:
- ¼ cup parsley, chopped
- ½ teaspoon garlic, chopped
- ½ teaspoon canola oil
- 4 swordfish fillets, 6 ounces each
- ¼ teaspoon sunflower seeds
- 1 Tablespoon sugar
- 2 Lemons, quartered and seeds removed

Directions:

1. Preheat your oven to 375 degrees F.
2. Take a small-sized bowl and add sugar, sunflower seeds, lemon wedges.
3. Toss well to coat them.
4. Take a shallow baking dish and add lemons, cover with aluminum foil.
5. Roast for about 60 minutes until lemons are tender and browned (Slightly).
6. Heat your grill and place the rack about 4 inches away from the source of heat.
7. Take a baking pan and coat it with cooking spray.
8. Transfer fish fillets to the pan and brush with oil on top spread garlic on top.
9. Grill for about 5 minutes on each side until the fillet turns opaque.
10. Transfer fish to a serving platter, squeeze roasted lemon on top.
11. Sprinkle parsley serve with a lemon wedge on the side.
12. Enjoy!

Nutrition:
Calories: 280, Fat: 12g, Net Carbohydrates: 4g, Protein: 34g, Sodium: 156mg, Potassium: 167mg.

842. Especial Glazed Salmon

Preparation Time: 45 minutes
Cooking Time: 10 minutes
Servings: 4
Ingredients:
- 4 pieces salmon fillets, 5 ounces each
- 4 tablespoons coconut aminos
- 4 teaspoon olive oil
- 2 teaspoons ginger, minced
- 4 teaspoons garlic, minced
- 2 tablespoons sugar-free ketchup
- 4 tablespoons dry white wine
- 2 tablespoons red boat fish sauce, low sodium

Directions:
1. Take a bowl and mix in coconut aminos, garlic, ginger, fish sauce and mix.
2. Add salmon and let it marinate for 15-20 minutes.
3. Take a skillet/pan and place it over medium heat.
4. Add oil and let it heat.
5. Add salmon fillets and cook on High heat for 3-4 minutes per side.
6. Remove dish once crispy.

7. Add sauce and wine.
8. Simmer for 5 minutes on low heat.
9. Return salmon to the glaze and flip until both sides are glazed.
10. Serve and enjoy!

Nutrition:
Calories: 372, Fat: 24g, Carbohydrates: 3g, Protein: 35g, Sodium: 156mg, Potassium: 178mg.

843. Generous Stuffed Salmon Avocado

Preparation Time: 10 minutes
Cooking Time: 30 minutes
Servings: 2
Ingredients:

- 1 Ripe organic avocado
- 3 Ounces wild caught smoked salmon
- 1 Ounce cashew cheese
- 3 Tablespoons extra virgin olive oil
- 1 tablespoon Sunflower seeds as needed

Directions:
1. Cut avocado in half and deseed.
2. Add the rest of the ingredients to a food processor and process until coarsely chopped.
3. Place mixture into the avocado.
4. Serve and enjoy!

Nutrition:
Calories: 525, Fat: 48g, Carbohydrates: 4g, Protein: 19g, Sodium: 145mg, Potassium: 178mg.

844. Tilapia Broccoli Platter

Preparation Time: 4 minutes
Cooking Time: 14 minutes
Servings: 2
Ingredients:

- 6 ounces tilapia, frozen
- 1 Tablespoon almond butter
- 1 Tablespoon garlic, minced
- 1 teaspoon lemon pepper seasoning
- 1 cup broccoli florets, fresh

Directions:
1. Preheat your oven to 350 degrees F.
2. Add fish in aluminum foil packets.
3. Arrange broccoli around fish.
4. Sprinkle lemon pepper on top.
5. Close the packets and seal.

6. Bake for 14 minutes.
7. Take a bowl and add garlic and almond butter, mix well and keep the mixture on the side.
8. Remove the packet from the oven and transfer it to a platter.
9. Place almond butter on top of the fish and broccoli, serve and enjoy!

Nutrition:
Calories: 362, Fat: 25g, Carbohydrates: 2g, Protein: 29g, Sodium: 167mg, Potassium: 170mg.

845. Salmon with Peas and Parsley Dressing

Preparation Time: 15 minutes
Cooking Time: 15 minutes
Servings: 4
Ingredients:

- 16 ounces salmon fillets, boneless and skin-on
- 1 Tablespoon parsley, chopped
- 10 ounces peas
- 9 ounces vegetable stock, low sodium
- 2 Cups water
- ½ teaspoon oregano, dried
- ½ teaspoon sweet paprika
- 2 Garlic cloves, minced
- A pinch of black pepper

Directions:
1. Add garlic, parsley, paprika, oregano and stock to a food processor and blend.
2. Add water to your Instant Pot.
3. Add steam basket.
4. Add fish fillets inside the steamer basket.
5. Season with pepper.
6. Lock the lid and cook on HIGH pressure for 10 minutes.
7. Release the pressure naturally over 10 minutes.
8. Divide the fish amongst plates.
9. Add peas to the steamer basket and lock the lid again, cook on HIGH pressure for 5 minutes.
10. Quick release the pressure.
11. Divide the peas next to your fillets and serve with the parsley dressing drizzled on top
12. Enjoy!

Nutrition:
Calories: 315, Fat: 5g, Carbohydrates: 14g, Protein: 16g, Sodium: 123mg, Potassium: 176mg.

846. Mackerel and Orange Medley

Preparation Time: 10 minutes
Cooking Time: 10 minutes
Servings: 4
Ingredients:

- 4 mackerel fillets, skinless and boneless
- 4 spring onion, chopped
- 1 teaspoon olive oil
- 1-inch ginger piece, grated
- 1 tablespoon Black pepper as needed
- Juice and zest of 1 whole orange
- 1 cup low sodium fish stock

Directions:
1. Season the fillets with black pepper and rub olive oil.
2. Add stock, orange juice, ginger, orange zest and onion to Instant Pot.
3. Place a steamer basket and add the fillets.
4. Lock the lid and cook on HIGH pressure for 10 minutes.
5. Release the pressure naturally over 10 minutes.
6. Divide the fillets amongst plates and drizzle the orange sauce from the pot over the fish.
7. Enjoy!

Nutrition:
Calories: 200, Fat: 4g, Carbohydrates: 19g, Protein: 14g, Sodium: 178mg, Potassium: 176mg.

847. Spicy Chili Salmon

Preparation Time: 10 minutes
Cooking Time: 7 minutes
Servings: 4
Ingredients:

- 4 salmon fillets, boneless and skin-on
- 2 tablespoons assorted chili peppers, chopped
- Juice of 1 lemon
- lemon, sliced
- 1 cup water
- Black pepper

Directions:
1. Add water to the Instant Pot.
2. Add steamer basket and add salmon fillets. Season the fillets with salt and pepper.
3. Drizzle lemon juice on top.
4. Top with lemon slices.
5. Lock the lid and cook on HIGH pressure for 7 minutes.
6. Release the pressure naturally over 10 minutes.

7. Divide the salmon and lemon slices between serving plates.
8. Enjoy!

Nutrition:
Calories: 281, Fats: 8g, Carbs: 19g, Protein: 7g, Sodium: 198mg, Potassium: 167mg.

848. Simple One Pot Mussels

Preparation Time: 10 minutes
Cooking Time: 5 minutes
Servings: 4
Ingredients:
- 2 tablespoons butter
- 2 chopped shallots
- 4 minced garlic cloves
- ½ cup broth
- ½ cup white wine
- 2 pounds cleaned mussels
- Lemon and parsley for serving

Directions:
1. Clean the mussels and remove the beard.
2. Discard any mussels that do not close when tapped against a hard surface.
3. Set your pot to Sauté mode and add chopped onion and butter.
4. Stir and sauté onions.
5. Add garlic and cook for 1 minute.
6. Add broth and wine.
7. Lock the lid and cook for 5 minutes on HIGH pressure.
8. Release the pressure naturally over 10 minutes.
9. Serve with a sprinkle of parsley and enjoy!

Nutrition:
Calories: 286, Fats: 14g, Carbs: 12g, Protein: 28g, Sodium: 156mg, Potassium: 178mg.

849. Lemon Pepper and Salmon

Preparation Time: 5 minutes
Cooking Time: 6 minutes
Servings: 3
Ingredients:
- ¾ cup water
- Few sprigs of parsley, basil, tarragon, basil
- 1 pound of salmon, skin on
- 2 teaspoons ghee
- ¼ teaspoon salt
- ½ teaspoon pepper
- ½ lemon, thinly sliced
- 1 whole carrot, julienned

Directions:

1. Set your pot to Sauté mode; add water and herbs.
2. Place a steamer rack inside your pot and place salmon.
3. Drizzle the ghee on top of the salmon and season with salt and pepper.
4. Cover lemon slices.
5. Lock the lid and cook on HIGH pressure for 3 minutes.
6. Release the pressure naturally over 10 minutes.
7. Transfer the salmon to a serving platter.
8. Set your pot to Sauté mode and add vegetables.
9. Cook for 1-2 minutes.
10. Serve with vegetables and salmon.
11. Enjoy!

Nutrition:
Calories: 464, Fat: 34g, Carbohydrates: 3g, Protein: 34g, Sodium: 187mg, Potassium: 176mg.

850. Simple Sautéed Garlic and Parsley Scallops

Preparation Time: 5 minutes
Cooking Time: 25 minutes
Servings: 4
Ingredients:
- 8 tablespoons almond butter
- 2 garlic cloves, minced
- 16 large sea scallops
- Sunflower seeds and pepper to taste
- ½ tablespoons olive oil

Directions:
1. Season scallops with sunflower seeds and pepper.
2. Take a skillet, place it over medium heat. Add oil and let it heat.
3. Sauté scallops for 2 minutes per side. Repeat until all scallops are cooked.
4. Add almond butter to the skillet and let it melt.
5. Stir in garlic and cook for 15 minutes.
6. Return scallops to skillet and stir to coat.
7. Serve and enjoy!

Nutrition:
Calories: 417, Fat: 31g, Net Carbohydrates: 5g, Protein: 29g, Sodium: 176mg, Potassium: 197mg.

851. Salmon and Cucumber Platter

Preparation Time: 10 minutes
Cooking Time: 0 minutes
Servings: 4
Ingredients:
- 2 cucumbers, cubed
- 2 teaspoons fresh squeezed lemon juice
- 4 ounces non-fat yogurt
- 1 teaspoon lemon zest, grated
- 1 tablespoon Pepper to taste
- 2 teaspoons dill, chopped
- 8 ounces smoked salmon, flaked

Directions:
1. Take a bowl and add cucumbers, lemon juice, lemon zest, pepper, dill, salmon, and yogurt; toss well.
2. Serve cold.
3. Enjoy!

Nutrition:
Calories: 242, Fat: 3g, Carbohydrates: 3g, Protein: 3g, Sodium: 176mg, Potassium: 169mg.

852. Cinnamon Salmon

Preparation Time: 10 minutes
Cooking Time: 10 minutes
Servings: 4
Ingredients:
- 2 salmon fillets, boneless and skin on
- 1 tablespoon Pepper to taste
- 1 tablespoon cinnamon powder
- 1 tablespoon organic olive oil

Directions:
1. Take a pan and place it over medium heat. Add oil and let it heat.
2. Add pepper, cinnamon and stir.
3. Add salmon, skin side up and cook for 5 minutes on both sides.
4. Divide between plates and serve.
5. Enjoy!

Nutrition:
Calories: 220, Fat: 8g, Carbohydrates: 11g, Protein: 8g, Sodium: 145mg, Potassium: 123mg.

853. Salmon and Orange Dish

Preparation Time: 10 minutes
Cooking Time: 15 minutes

Servings: 4
Ingredients:
- 4 salmon fillets
- 1 Cup orange juice
- 2 Tablespoons arrowroot and water mixture
- 1 teaspoon orange peel, grated
- 1 teaspoon black pepper

Directions:
1. Add the listed ingredients to your pot.
2. Lock the lid and cook on HIGH pressure for 12 minutes.
3. Release the pressure naturally.
4. Serve and enjoy!

Nutrition:
Calories: 583, Fat: 20g, Carbohydrates: 71g, Protein: 33g, Sodium: 187mg, Potassium: 187mg.

854. Mesmerizing Coconut Haddock

Preparation Time: 10 minutes
Cooking Time: 12 minutes
Servings: 3
Ingredients:
- 4 haddock fillets, 5 ounces each, boneless
- 2 tablespoons coconut oil, melted
- 1 cup coconut, shredded and unsweetened
- ¼ cup hazelnuts, ground
- 1 tablespoon Sunflower seeds to taste

Directions:
1. Preheat your oven to 400 degrees F.
2. Line a baking sheet with parchment paper.
3. Keep it on the side.
4. Pat fish fillets with paper towels and season with sunflower seeds.
5. Take a bowl and stir in hazelnuts and shredded coconut.
6. Drag fish fillets through the coconut mix until both sides are coated well.
7. Transfer to baking dish.
8. Brush with coconut oil.
9. Bake for about 12 minutes until flaky.
10. Serve and enjoy!

Nutrition:
Calories: 299, Fat: 24g, Carbohydrates: 1g, Protein: 20g, Sodium: 176mg, Potassium: 198mg.

855. Asparagus and Lemon Salmon Dish

Preparation Time: 5 minutes
Cooking Time: 15 minutes
Servings: 3
Ingredients:
- 2 salmon fillets, 6 ounces each, skin on
- 1 tablespoon Sunflower seeds to taste
- 1 pound asparagus, trimmed
- 2 cloves garlic, minced
- 3 tablespoons almond butter
- ¼ cup cashew cheese

Directions:
1. Preheat your oven to 400 degrees F.
2. Line a baking sheet with oil.
3. Take a kitchen towel and pat your salmon dry, season as needed.
4. Put salmon onto the baking sheet and arrange asparagus around it.
5. Place a pan over medium heat and melt almond butter.
6. Add garlic and cook for 3 minutes until garlic browns slightly.
7. Drizzle sauce over salmon.
8. Sprinkle salmon with cheese and bake for 12 minutes until salmon looks cooked all the way and is flaky.
9. Serve and enjoy!

Nutrition:
Calories: 434, Fat: 26g, Carbohydrates: 6g, Protein: 42g, Sodium: 178mg, Potassium: 190mg.

856. Ecstatic "Foiled" Fish

Preparation Time: 20 minutes
Cooking Time: 40 minutes
Servings: 4
Ingredients:
- 2 rainbow trout fillets
- 1 Tablespoon olive oil
- 1 Teaspoon garlic salt
- 1 Teaspoon ground black pepper
- 1 Fresh jalapeno pepper, sliced
- 1 lemon, sliced

Directions:
1. Preheat your oven to 400 degrees F.
2. Rinse your fish and pat them dry.
3. Rub the fillets with olive oil, season with some garlic, salt and black pepper.

4. Place each of your seasoned fillets on a large-sized sheet of aluminum foil.
5. Top it with some jalapeno slices and squeeze the juice from your lemons over your fish.
6. Arrange the lemon slices on top of your fillets.
7. Carefully seal up the edges of your foil and form a nice, enclosed packet.
8. Place your packets on your baking sheet.
9. Bake them for about 20 minutes.
10. Once the flakes start to flake off with a fork, the fish is ready!

Nutrition:
Calories: 213, Fat: 10g, Carbohydrates: 8g, Protein: 24g, Sodium: 165mg, Potassium: 187mg.

857. Brazilian Shrimp Stew

Preparation Time: 20 minutes
Cooking Time: 25 minutes
Servings: 4
Ingredients:
- 4 tablespoons lime juice
- ½ tablespoons cumin, ground
- ½ tablespoons paprika
- ½ teaspoons garlic, minced
- 1 ½ teaspoons pepper
- 2 Pounds tilapia fillets, cut into bits
- 1 large onion, chopped
- 1 Large bell peppers, cut into strips
- 1 can (14 ounces) tomato, drained
- 1 can (14 ounces) coconut milk
- 1 Handful of cilantro, chopped

Directions:
1. Take a large-sized bowl and add lime juice, cumin, paprika, garlic, pepper and mix well.
2. Add tilapia and coat it up.
3. Cover and allow to marinate for 20 minutes.
4. Set your Instant Pot to Sauté mode and add olive oil.
5. Add onions and cook for 3 minutes until tender.
6. Add pepper strips, tilapia, and tomatoes to a skillet.
7. Pour coconut milk and cover, simmer for 20 minutes.
8. Add cilantro during the final few minutes.
9. Serve and enjoy!

Nutrition:
Calories: 471, Fat: 44g, Carbohydrates: 13g, Protein:

12g, Sodium: 190mg, Potassium: 154mg.

858. Inspiring Cajun Snow Crab

Preparation Time: 10 minutes
Cooking Time: 10 minutes
Servings: 2
Ingredients:
- 1 Lemon, fresh and quartered
- 2 Tablespoons Cajun seasoning
- 2 Bay leaves
- 4 Snow crab legs, precooked and defrosted
- 1 tablespoon Golden ghee

Directions:
1. Take a large pot and fill it about halfway with sunflower seeds and water.
2. Bring the water to a boil.
3. Squeeze lemon juice into the pot and toss in remaining lemon quarters.
4. Add bay leaves and Cajun seasoning.
5. Season for 1 minute.
6. Add crab legs and boil for 8 minutes (make sure to keep them submerged the whole time).
7. Melt ghee in microwave and use as a dipping sauce, enjoy!

Nutrition:
Calories: 643, Fat: 51g, Carbohydrates: 3g, Protein: 41g, Sodium: 189mg, Potassium: 109mg.

859. Grilled Lime Shrimp

Preparation Time: 25 minutes
Cooking Time: 5 minutes
Servings: 8
Ingredients:
- 1 pound medium shrimp, peeled and deveined
- 1 lime, juiced
- ½ cup olive oil
- 2 tablespoons Cajun seasoning

Directions:
1. Take a re-sealable zip bag and add lime juice, Cajun seasoning, and olive oil.
2. Add shrimp and shake it well, let it marinate for 20 minutes.
3. Preheat your outdoor grill to medium heat.
4. Lightly grease the grate.
5. Remove shrimp from marinade and cook for 2 minutes per side.

6. Serve and enjoy!
Nutrition:
Calories: 188, Fat: 3g, Net Carbohydrates: 1.2g, Protein: 13g, Sodium: 198mg, Potassium: 190mg.

860. Calamari Citrus

Preparation Time: 10 minutes
Cooking Time: 5 minutes
Servings: 4
Ingredients:
- 1 lime, sliced
- 1 lemon, sliced
- 2 pounds calamari tubes and tentacles, sliced
- 1 tablespoon Pepper to taste
- ¼ cup olive oil
- 2 garlic cloves, minced
- 2 tablespoons lemon juice
- 1 orange, peeled and cut into segments
- 2 tablespoons cilantro, chopped

Directions:
1. Take a bowl and add calamari, pepper, lime slices, lemon slices, orange slices, garlic, oil, cilantro, lemon juice and toss well.
2. Take a pan and place it over medium-high heat.
3. Add calamari mix and cook for 5 minutes.
4. Divide into bowls and serve.
5. Enjoy!

Nutrition:
Calories: 190, Fat: 2g, Net Carbohydrates: 11g, Protein: 14g, Sodium: 243mg, Potassium: 156mg.

861. Spanish Mussels Mix

Preparation Time: 10 minutes
Cooking Time: 23 minutes
Servings: 4
Ingredients:
- 3 tablespoons olive oil
- 2 pounds mussels, scrubbed
- 1 tablespoon Black pepper to the taste
- 3 cups canned tomatoes, crushed
- 1 lb. shallot, chopped
- 2 garlic cloves, minced
- 2 cups low-sodium veggie stock
- 1/3 cup cilantro, chopped

Directions:

1. Heat a pan with the oil over medium-high flame. Add shallot, stir and cook for 3 minutes.
2. Add garlic, stock, tomatoes and black pepper, stir, bring to a simmer and cook for 10 minutes.
3. Add mussels and cilantro, toss, cover the pan, cook for another 10 minutes, divide into bowls and serve.
4. Enjoy!

Nutrition:
Calories: 210, Fat: 2g, Fiber: 6g, Carbs: 5g, Protein: 8g, Sodium: 287mg, Potassium: 376mg.

862. Quinoa and Scallops Salad

Preparation Time: 10 minutes
Cooking Time: 20 minutes
Servings: 6
Ingredients:
- 12 ounces sea scallops
- 4 tablespoons olive oil + 2 teaspoons
- 4 teaspoons coconut aminos
- 1 and ½ cup quinoa, already cooked
- 2 teaspoons garlic, minced
- 1 cup snow peas, sliced
- 1/3 cup balsamic vinegar
- 1 cup scallions, sliced
- 1/3 cup red bell pepper, chopped
- ¼ cup cilantro, chopped

Directions:
1. In a bowl, mix scallops with half of the aminos and toss.
2. Heat a pan with 1 tablespoon olive oil over medium flame. Add quinoa, stir and cook for 8 minutes.
3. Add garlic and snow peas, stir, cook for 5 more minutes and take off the heat.
4. Meanwhile, in a bowl, mix 3 tablespoons of olive oil with the rest of the coconut aminos and vinegar. Whisk well, add the quinoa mix, scallions and bell pepper and toss.
5. Heat another pan with 2 teaspoons olive oil over medium-high flame. Add scallops and cook for 1 minute on each side. Add over the quinoa mix, toss a bit, sprinkle cilantro on top and serve.
6. Enjoy!

Nutrition:
Calories: 221, Fat: 5g, Fiber: 2g, Carbs: 7g, Protein: 8g, Sodium: 256mg, Potassium: 165mg.

863. Salmon and Veggies Soup

Preparation Time: 10 minutes
Cooking Time: 22 minutes
Servings: 6
Ingredients:

- 2 tablespoon olive oil
- 1 leek, chopped
- 1 red onion, chopped
- 1 tablespoon Black pepper to the taste
- 2 carrots, chopped
- 2 cups low-stock veggie stock
- 4 ounces salmon, skinless, boneless and cubed
- ½ cup coconut cream
- 1 tablespoon dill, chopped

Directions:

1. Heat a pan with the oil over medium flame. Add leek and onion, stir and cook for 7 minutes.
2. Add black pepper. Add carrots and stock, stir, bring to a boil and cook for 10 minutes.
3. Add salmon, cream and dill, stir, boil everything for 5-6 minutes more, ladle into bowls and serve.
4. Enjoy!

Nutrition:

Calories: 232, Fat: 3g, Fiber: 4g, Carbs: 7g, Protein: 12g, Sodium: 213mg, Potassium: 345mg.

864. Salmon Salsa

Preparation Time: 10 minutes
Cooking Time: 0 minutes
Servings: 12
Ingredients:

- 3 yellow tomatoes, seedless and chopped
- 1-pound smoked salmon, boneless, skinless and flaked
- 1 red tomato, seedless and chopped
- 1 tablespoon Black pepper to the taste
- 1 cup watermelon, seedless and chopped
- 1 red onion, chopped
- 1 mango, peeled, seedless and chopped
- 2 jalapeno peppers, chopped
- ¼ cup parsley, chopped
- 3 tablespoons lime juice

Directions:

1. In a bowl, mix all the tomatoes with mango, watermelon, onion, salmon, black pepper, jalapeno, parsley and lime juice, toss and serve cold.
2. Enjoy!

Nutrition:

Calories: 123, Fat: 2g, Fiber: 4g, Carbs: 5g, Protein: 5g, Sodium: 76mg, Potassium: 145mg.

865. Salmon and Easy Cucumber Salad

Preparation Time: 10 minutes
Cooking Time: 0 minutes
Servings: 4
Ingredients:

- 2 cucumbers, cubed
- 2 teaspoons lemon juice
- 4 ounces non-fat yogurt
- 1 teaspoon lemon zest, grated
- 1 tablespoon Black pepper to the taste
- 3 teaspoons dill, chopped
- 8 ounces smoked salmon, flaked

Directions:

1. In a bowl, add the cucumbers with the lemon juice, lemon zest, black pepper, dill, salmon and yogurt. Toss and serve cold.
2. Enjoy!

Nutrition:

Calories: 242, Fat: 3g, Fiber: 4g, Carbs: 8g, Protein: 3g, Sodium: 45mg, Potassium: 67mg.

866. Shrimp and Avocado Salad

Preparation Time: 10 minutes
Cooking Time: 0 minutes
Servings: 2
Ingredients:

- 2 green onions, chopped
- 2 avocados, pitted, peeled and cut into medium chunks
- 2 tablespoons cilantro, chopped
- 1 cup shrimp, already cooked, peeled and deveined
- A pinch of salt and black pepper

Directions:

1. In a salad bowl, mix shrimp with avocado, green onions, cilantro, salt and pepper. Toss and serve cold.
2. Enjoy!

Nutrition:

Calories: 160, Fat: 2g, Fiber: 3g, Carbs: 10g, Protein: 6g, Sodium: 67mg, Potassium: 98mg.

867. Shrimp with Cilantro Sauce

Preparation Time: 10 minutes
Cooking Time: 4 minutes

Servings: 2
Ingredients:

- 1 pound shrimp, peeled and deveined
- 2 tablespoons cilantro, chopped
- 3 tablespoons olive oil
- 1 tablespoon pine nuts
- Zest of 1 lemon, grated
- Juice of ½ lemon

Directions:

1. In your blender, combine the cilantro with 2 tablespoons of oil, pine nuts, lemon zest and lemon juice and pulse well.
2. Heat a pan with the rest of the oil over medium-high flame. Add the shrimp and cook for 3 minutes.
3. Add the cilantro mix, toss, cook for 1 minute, divide between plates and serve with a side salad.
4. Enjoy!

Nutrition:

Calories: 210, Fat: 5g, Fiber: 1g, Carbs: 8g, Protein: 12g, Sodium: 56mg, Potassium: 89mg.

868. Mussels Curry with Lime

Preparation Time: 10 minutes
Cooking Time: 10 minutes
Servings: 4
Ingredients:

- 2 and ½ pounds mussels, scrubbed
- 14 ounces canned coconut milk
- 3 tablespoons red curry paste
- 1 tablespoon olive oil
- 1 tablespoon Black pepper to the taste
- ½ cup low-sodium chicken stock
- Juice of 1 lime
- Zest of 1 lime, grated
- ¼ cup cilantro, chopped
- 3 tablespoons basil, chopped

Directions:

1. Heat a pan with the oil over medium-high flame. Add curry paste, stir and cook for 2 minutes.
2. Add stock, black pepper, coconut milk, lime juice, lime zest and mussels, toss, cover the pan and cook for 10 minutes.
3. Divide this into bowls, sprinkle cilantro and basil on top and serve.
4. Enjoy!

Nutrition:

Calories: 260, Fat: 12g, Fiber: 2g, Carbs: 10g, Protein: 12g,

Sodium: 56mg, Potassium: 178mg.

869. Salmon Casserole

Preparation Time: 10 minutes
Cooking Time: 1 hour
Servings: 4
Ingredients:
- 8 sweet potatoes, sliced
- 4 cups salmon, cooked and flaked
- 1 red onion, chopped
- 2 carrots, chopped
- 1 tablespoon Black pepper to the taste
- 1 celery stalk, chopped
- 3 cups coconut milk
- 2 tablespoons olive oil
- 4 tablespoons chives, chopped
- 2 garlic cloves, minced

Directions:
1. Heat a pan with the oil over medium flame. Add garlic, stir and cook for 1 minute.
2. Add coconut milk, black pepper, carrots, celery, chives, onion and salmon. Stir and take off the heat.
3. Arrange a layer of potatoes in a baking dish. Add the salmon mix, top with the rest of the potatoes, introduce in the oven and bake at 375 degrees F for 1 hour.
4. Slice, divide between plates and serve.
5. Enjoy!

Nutrition:
Calories: 220, Fat: 9g, Fiber: 6g, Carbs: 8g, Protein: 12g, Sodium: 123mg, Potassium: 45mg.

870. Scallops, Sweet Potatoes and Cauliflower Mix

Preparation Time: 10 minutes
Cooking Time: 10 minutes
Servings: 4
Ingredients:
- 12 sea scallops
- 3 garlic cloves, minced
- 1 tablespoon Black pepper to the taste
- 2 cups cauliflower florets, chopped
- 2 tablespoons olive oil
- 2 cups sweet potatoes, chopped
- 1 tablespoon thyme, chopped

- ¼ cup pine nuts, toasted
- 1 cup low-sodium veggie stock
- 2 tablespoons chives, finely chopped

Directions:
1. Heat a pan with the oil over medium-high flame. Add thyme and garlic, stir and cook for 2 minutes.
2. Add scallops and cook them for 2 minutes. Season them with black pepper, add cauliflower, sweet potatoes and the stock, toss and cook for 5 minutes more.
3. Divide the scallops mix between plates. Sprinkle chives and pine nuts on top and serve.
4. Enjoy!

Nutrition:
Calories: 200, Fat: 10g, Fiber: 4g, Carbs: 9g, Protein: 10g, Sodium: 230mg, Potassium: 176mg.

871. Spiced Salmon

Preparation Time: 10 minutes
Cooking Time: 10 minutes
Servings: 4
Ingredients:
- 4 salmon fillets
- 2 tablespoons olive oil
- 1 teaspoon cumin, ground
- 1 teaspoon sweet paprika
- 1 teaspoon onion powder
- 1 teaspoon chili powder
- ½ teaspoon garlic powder
- A pinch of salt and black pepper

Directions:
1. In a bowl, combine the cumin with paprika, onion powder, chili powder, garlic powder, salt and black pepper. Toss and rub the salmon with this mix.
2. Heat a pan with the oil over medium-high flame. Add the salmon, cook for 5 minutes on each side, divide between plates and serve with a side salad.
3. Enjoy!

Nutrition:
Calories: 220, Fat: 10g, Carbs: 8g, Fiber: 12g, Protein: 10g, Sodium: 234mg, Potassium: 56mg.

872. Salmon and Tomatoes Salad

Preparation Time: 10 minutes
Cooking Time: 0 minutes
Servings: 2

Ingredients:
- 4 cups cherry tomatoes, halved
- 1 red onion, sliced
- 8 ounces smoked salmon, thinly sliced
- 4 tablespoons olive oil
- ½ teaspoon garlic, minced
- 3 tablespoons lemon juice
- 1 tablespoon oregano, chopped
- 1 tablespoon Black pepper to the taste
- 1 teaspoon balsamic vinegar

Directions:
1. In a salad bowl, combine the tomatoes with the onion, salmon, oil, garlic, lemon juice, oregano, black pepper and vinegar, toss and serve cold.
2. Enjoy!

Nutrition:
Calories: 159, Fat: 8g, Fiber: 3g, Carbs: 7g, Protein: 7g, Sodium: 143mg, Potassium: 167mg.

873. Coconut Cream Shrimp

Preparation Time: 10 minutes
Cooking Time: 0 minutes
Servings: 2
Ingredients:
- 1 pound shrimp, cooked, peeled and deveined
- 1 tablespoon coconut cream
- ¼ teaspoon jalapeno, chopped
- ½ teaspoon lime juice
- 1 tablespoon parsley, chopped
- A pinch of black pepper

Directions:
1. In a bowl, mix the shrimp with the cream, jalapeno, lime juice, parsley and black pepper. Toss, divide into small bowls and serve.
2. Enjoy!

Nutrition:
Calories: 183, Fat: 5g, Fiber: 3g, Carbs: 12g, Protein: 8g, Sodium: 78mg, Potassium: 90mg.

874. Salmon with Mushroom

Preparation Time: 30 minutes
Cooking Time: 10 minutes
Servings: 4
Ingredients:
- 8 ounces salmon fillets, boneless
- 2 tablespoons olive oil
- Black pepper to the taste
- 2 ounces white mushrooms, sliced
- ½ shallot, chopped

- 2 tablespoons balsamic vinegar
- 2 teaspoons mustard
- 3 tablespoons parsley, chopped

Directions:
1. Brush salmon fillets with 1 tablespoon of olive oil. Season with black pepper, place on preheated grill over medium heat, cook for 4 minutes on each side and divide between plates.
2. Heat a pan with the rest of the oil over medium-high flame. Add mushrooms, shallot and some black pepper. Stir and cook for 5 minutes.
3. Add the mustard, the vinegar and the parsley. Stir, cook for 2-3 minutes more, add over the salmon and serve.
4. Enjoy!

Nutrition:
Calories: 220, Fat: 4g, Fiber: 8g, Carbs: 6g, Protein: 12g, Sodium: 98mg, Potassium: 90mg.

875. Cod Sweet Potato Chowder

Preparation Time: 10 minutes
Cooking Time: 20 minutes
Servings: 4
Ingredients:
- 3 cups sweet potatoes, cubed
- 4 cod fillets, skinless and boneless
- 1 cup celery, chopped
- 1 cup onion, chopped
- 1 tablespoon Black pepper to the taste
- 2 tablespoons garlic, minced
- 3 tablespoons olive oil
- 2 tablespoons tomato paste, no-salt-added
- 2 cups veggie stock
- 1 and ½ cups tomatoes, chopped
- 1 and ½ teaspoons thyme

Directions:
1. Heat a pot with the oil over medium flame. Add tomato paste, celery, onion and garlic, stir and cook for 5 minutes.
2. Add tomatoes, tomato paste, potatoes and pepper, stir, bring to a boil, reduce heat and cook for 10 minutes.
3. Add thyme and cod, stir, cook for 5 minutes more, ladle into bowls and serve.
4. Enjoy!

Nutrition:
Calories: 250, Fat: 6g, Fiber: 5g, Carbs: 7g, Protein: 12g, Sodium: 145mg, Potassium: 176mg.

876. Salmon with Cinnamon

Preparation Time: 10 minutes
Cooking Time: 10 minutes
Servings: 2
Ingredients:
- 2 salmon fillets, boneless and skin-on
- 1 tablespoon Black pepper to the taste
- 1 tablespoon cinnamon powder
- 1 tablespoon olive oil

Directions:
1. Heat a pan with the oil over medium flame. Add pepper and cinnamon and stir well.
2. Add salmon, skin side up, cook for 5 minutes on each side, divide between plates and serve with a side salad.
3. Enjoy!

Nutrition:
Calories: 220, Fat: 8g, Fiber: 4g, Carbs: 11g, Protein: 8g, Sodium: 154mg, Potassium: 187mg.

877. Scallops and Strawberry Mix

Preparation Time: 10 minutes
Cooking Time: 6 minutes
Servings: 2
Ingredients:
- 4 ounces scallops
- ½ cup Pico de Gallo
- ½ cup strawberries, chopped
- 1 tablespoon lime juice
- 1 tablespoon Black pepper to the taste

Directions:
1. Heat a pan over medium flame. Add scallops, cook for 3 minutes on each side and take off the heat.
2. In a bowl, mix strawberries with lime juice, Pico de Gallo, scallops and pepper. Toss and serve cold.
3. Enjoy!

Nutrition:
Calories: 169, Fat: 2g, Fiber: 2g, Carbs: 8g, Protein: 13g, Sodium: 165mg, Potassium: 128mg.

878. Baked Haddock with Avocado Mayonnaise

Preparation Time: 10 minutes
Cooking Time: 30 minutes
Servings: 4

Ingredients:
- 1 pound haddock, boneless
- 2 teaspoons water
- 3 tablespoons lemon juice
- A pinch of salt and black pepper
- 2 tablespoons avocado mayonnaise
- 1 teaspoon dill, chopped
- 1 tablespoon Cooking spray

Directions:
1. Spray a baking dish with some cooking oil. Add fish, water, lemon juice, salt, black pepper, mayo and dill. Toss, introduce in the oven and bake at 350 degrees F for 30 minutes.
2. Divide between plates and serve.
3. Enjoy!

Nutrition:
Calories: 264, Fat: 4g, Fiber: 5g, Carbs: 7g, Protein: 12g, Sodium: 176mg, Potassium: 198mg.

879. Basil Tilapia

Preparation Time: 10 minutes
Cooking Time: 10 minutes
Servings: 4
Ingredients:
- 4 tilapia fillets, boneless
- Black pepper to the taste
- ½ cup low-fat parmesan, grated
- 4 tablespoons avocado mayonnaise
- 2 teaspoons basil, dried
- 2 tablespoons lemon juice
- ¼ cup olive oil

Directions:
1. Grease a baking dish with the oil. Add the tilapia fillets, black pepper, spread the mayonnaise, basil, sprinkle with lemon juice and top with the Parmesan. Place on the preheated grill and cook over medium-high heat for 5 minutes on each side.
2. Divide between plates and serve with a side salad.
3. Enjoy!

Nutrition:
Calories: 215, Fat: 10g, Fiber: 5g, Carbs: 7g, Protein: 11g, Sodium: 254mg, Potassium: 165mg.

880. Salmon Meatballs with Garlic

Preparation Time: 10 minutes
Cooking Time: 30 minutes
Servings: 4
Ingredients:

- 1 tablespoon Cooking spray
- 2 garlic cloves, minced
- 1 yellow onion, chopped
- 1 pound wild salmon, boneless and minced
- ¼ cup chives, chopped
- 1 egg
- 2 tablespoons Dijon mustard
- 1 tablespoon coconut flour
- A pinch of salt and black pepper

Directions:
1. In a bowl, mix onion with garlic, salmon, chives, coconut flour, salt, pepper, mustard and egg. Stir well, shape medium meatballs, arrange them on a baking sheet and grease them with cooking spray. Introduce them in the oven at 350 degrees F and bake for 25 minutes.
2. Divide the meatballs between plates and serve with a side salad.
3. Enjoy!

Nutrition:
Calories: 211, Fat: 4g, Fiber: 1g, Carbs: 6g, Protein: 13g, Sodium: 127mg, Potassium: 198mg.

881. Spiced Cod Mix

Preparation Time: 10 minutes
Cooking Time: 25 minutes
Servings: 4
Ingredients:
- 4 cod fillets, skinless and boneless
- ½ teaspoon mustard seeds
- A pinch of black pepper
- 2 green chilies, chopped
- 1 teaspoon ginger, grated
- 1 teaspoon curry powder
- ¼ teaspoon cumin, ground
- 4 tablespoons olive oil
- 1 teaspoon turmeric powder
- 1 red onion, chopped
- ¼ cup cilantro, chopped
- 1 and ½ cups coconut cream
- 2 garlic cloves, minced

Directions:
1. Heat a pot with half of the oil over medium flame. Add mustard seeds, ginger, onion and garlic, stir and cook for 5 minutes.
2. Add turmeric, curry powder, chilies and cumin, stir and cook for 5 minutes more.
3. Add coconut milk, salt and pepper, stir, bring to a boil and cook for 15 minutes.
4. Heat another pan with the rest of the oil over medium flame. Add fish, stir, cook for 3

minutes, add over the curry mix, also add cilantro and toss. Cook for 5 minutes more, divide into bowls and serve.
5. Enjoy!

Nutrition:
Calories: 200, Fat: 14g, Fiber: 7g, Carbs: 6g, Protein: 9g, Sodium: 324mg, Potassium: 187mg.

882. Italian Shrimp

Preparation Time: 10 minutes
Cooking Time: 22 minutes
Servings: 4
Ingredients:
- 8 ounces mushrooms, chopped
- 1 asparagus bunch, cut into medium pieces
- 2 pound shrimp, peeled and deveined
- 1 tablespoon Black pepper to the taste
- 2 tablespoons olive oil
- 2 teaspoons Italian seasoning
- 1 yellow onion, chopped
- 1 teaspoon red pepper flakes, crushed
- 1 cup low-fat parmesan cheese, grated
- 2 garlic cloves, minced
- 1 cup coconut cream

Directions:
1. Put water in a pot, bring to a boil over medium heat. Add asparagus, steam for 2 minutes, transfer to a bowl with ice water, drain and put in a bowl.
2. Heat a pan with the oil over medium flame. Add onions and mushrooms, stir and cook for 7 minutes.
3. Add pepper flakes, Italian seasoning, black pepper and asparagus, stir and cook for 5 minutes more.
4. Add cream, shrimp, garlic and parmesan. Toss, cook for 7 minutes, divide into bowls and serve.
5. Enjoy!

Nutrition:
Calories: 225, Fat: 6g, Fiber: 5g, Carbs: 6g, Protein: 8g, Sodium: 187mg, Potassium: 156mg.

883. Shrimp, Snow Peas and Bamboo Soup

Preparation Time: 10 minutes

Cooking Time: 10 minutes
Servings: 4
Ingredients:
- 4 scallions, chopped
- and ½ tablespoons olive oil
- 1 teaspoon garlic, minced
- 8 cups low-sodium chicken stock
- ¼ cup coconut aminos
- 5 ounces canned bamboo shoots, no-salt-added sliced
- Black pepper to the taste
- 1 pound shrimp, peeled and deveined
- ½ pound snow peas

Directions:
1. Heat a pot with the oil over medium flame. Add scallions and ginger, stir and cook for 2 minutes.
2. Add coconut aminos, stock and black pepper, stir and bring to a boil.
3. Add shrimp, snow peas and bamboo shoots, stir, cook for 5 minutes, ladle into bowls and serve.
4. Enjoy!

Nutrition:
Calories: 200, Fat: 3g, Fiber: 2g, Carbs: 4g, Protein: 14g, Sodium: 100mg, Potassium: 140mg.

884. Lemony Mussels

Preparation Time: 5 minutes
Cooking Time: 5 minutes
Servings: 4
Ingredients:
- 2-pound mussels, scrubbed
- 2 garlic cloves, minced
- 1 tablespoon olive oil
- Juice of 1 lemon

Directions:
1. Put some water in a pot. Add mussels, bring to a boil over medium heat, cook for 5 minutes, discard unopened mussels and transfer them to a bowl.
2. In another bowl, mix the oil with garlic and lemon juice. Whisk well, and add over the mussels, toss and serve.
3. Enjoy!

Nutrition:
Calories: 140, Fat: 4g, Fiber: 4g, Carbs: 8g, Protein: 8g, Sodium: 234mg, Potassium: 167mg.

885. Citrus-Glazed Salmon with Zucchini Noodles

Preparation Time: 15 minutes
Cooking Time: 20 minutes
Servings: 4
Ingredients:

- 4 (5- to 6-ounce) pieces salmon
- ½ teaspoon kosher salt
- ¼ teaspoon freshly ground black pepper
- 1 tablespoon extra-virgin olive oil
- 1 cup freshly squeezed orange juice
- 1 teaspoon low-sodium soy sauce
- 2 zucchinis (about 16 ounces), spiralized
- 1 tablespoon fresh chives, chopped
- 1 tablespoon fresh parsley, chopped

Directions:

1. Preheat the oven to 350°F. Flavor the salmon with salt plus black pepper. Heat the olive oil in a large oven-safe skillet or sauté pan over medium-high heat. Add the salmon, skin-side down, and sear for 5 minutes, or until the skin is golden brown and crispy.
2. Flip the salmon over. Then transfer to the oven until your desired doneness is reached—about 5 minutes. Place the salmon on a cutting board to rest.
3. Place the same pan on the stove over medium-high heat. Add the orange juice and soy sauce to deglaze the pan. Bring to a simmer, scraping up any brown bits, and simmering 5 to 7 minutes.
4. Split or divide the zucchini noodles into 4 plates and place 1 piece of salmon on each. Pour the orange glaze over the salmon and zucchini noodles. Garnish with chives and parsley.

Nutrition:
Calories: 280, Fat: 13g, Sodium: 255mg, Carbohydrates: 11g, Protein: 30g, Potassium: 325mg.

886. Salmon Cakes with Bell Pepper plus Lemon Yogurt

Preparation Time: 15 minutes
Cooking Time: 15 minutes
Servings: 4
Ingredients:

- ¼ cup whole-wheat bread crumbs
- ¼ cup mayonnaise
- 1 large egg, beaten
- 1 tablespoon chives, chopped
- 1 tablespoon fresh parsley, chopped
- Zest of 1 lemon
- ¾ teaspoon kosher salt, divided
- ¼ teaspoon freshly ground black pepper
- (5- to 6-ounce) cans no-salt boneless/skinless salmon, drained and finely flaked
- ½ bell pepper, diced small tablespoons extra-virgin olive oil, divided
- 1 cup plain Greek yogurt
- Juice of 1 lemon

Directions:

1. Mix the bread crumbs, mayonnaise, egg, chives, parsley, lemon zest, ½ teaspoon of salt, and black pepper in a large bowl. Add the salmon and the bell pepper and stir gently until well combined. Shape the mixture into 8 patties.
2. Heat 1 tablespoon of the olive oil in a large skillet over medium-high flame. Cook half the cakes until the bottoms are golden brown, 4 to 5 minutes. Adjust the heat to medium if the bottoms start to burn.
3. Flip the cakes and cook until golden brown, an additional 4 to 5 minutes. Repeat the process with the rest of the 1 tablespoon olive oil and the rest of the cakes.
4. Mix the yogurt, lemon juice, and the remaining ¼ teaspoon salt in a small bowl. Serve with the salmon cakes.

Nutrition:
Calories: 330, Fat: 23g, Sodium: 385mg, Carbohydrates: 9g, Protein: 21g, Potassium: 127mg.

887. Halibut in Parchment with Zucchini, Shallots, and Herbs

Preparation Time: 15 minutes
Cooking Time: 15 minutes
Servings: 4
Ingredients:

- ½ cup zucchini, diced small
- shallot, minced
- 4 (5-ounce) halibut fillets (about 1-inch thick)
- 4 teaspoons extra-virgin olive oil
- ¼ teaspoon kosher salt
- 1/8 teaspoon freshly ground black pepper
- 1 lemon, sliced into 1/8 - inch-thick rounds
- 8 sprigs of thyme

Directions:

1. Preheat the oven to 450°F. Combine the zucchini and shallots in a medium bowl. Cut 4 (15-by-24-inch) pieces of parchment paper. Fold each sheet in half horizontally.
2. Draw a large half heart on one side of each folded sheet, with the fold along the heart center. Cut out the heart, open the parchment, and lay it flat.
3. Place a fillet near the center of each parchment heart. Drizzle 1 teaspoon olive oil on each fillet. Sprinkle with salt and pepper. Top each fillet with lemon slices and 2 sprigs of thyme. Sprinkle each fillet with one-quarter of the zucchini and shallot mixture. Fold the parchment over.
4. Starting at the top, fold the parchment edges over, and continue all the way around to make a packet. Twist the end tightly to secure. Arrange the 4 packets on a baking sheet. Bake for about 15 minutes. Place on plates; cut open. Serve immediately.

Nutrition:
Calories: 190, Fat: 7g, Sodium: 170mg, Carbohydrates: 5g, Protein: 27g, Potassium: 89mg.

888. Flounder with Tomatoes and Basil

Preparation Time: 15 minutes
Cooking Time: 20 minutes

Servings: 4
Ingredients:
- 1-pound cherry tomatoes
- 4 garlic cloves, sliced
- 2 tablespoons extra-virgin olive oil
- 2 tablespoons lemon juice
- 2 tablespoons basil, cut into ribbons
- ½ teaspoon kosher salt
- ¼ teaspoon freshly ground black pepper
- 4 (5- to 6-ounce) flounder fillets

Directions:
1. Preheat the oven to 425°F.
2. Mix the tomatoes, garlic, olive oil, lemon juice, basil, salt, and black pepper in a baking dish. Bake for 5 minutes.
3. Remove, then arrange the flounder on top of the tomato mixture. Bake until the fish is opaque and begins to flake, about 10 to 15 minutes, depending on thickness.

Nutrition:
Calories: 215, Fat: 9g, Sodium: 261mg, Carbohydrates: 6g, Protein: 28g, Potassium: 213mg.

889. Grilled Mahi-Mahi with Artichoke Caponata

Preparation Time: 15 minutes
Cooking Time: 30 minutes
Servings: 4
Ingredients:
- 2 tablespoons extra-virgin olive oil
- 2 celery stalks, diced
- 1 onion, diced
- 2 garlic cloves, minced
- ½ cup cherry tomatoes, chopped
- ¼ cup white wine
- 2 tablespoons white wine vinegar
- 1 can artichoke hearts, drained and chopped
- ¼ cup green olives, pitted and chopped
- 1 tablespoon capers, chopped
- ¼ teaspoon red pepper flakes
- 2 tablespoons fresh basil, chopped
- (5- to 6-ounces each) skinless mahi-mahi fillets
- ½ teaspoon kosher salt
- ¼ teaspoon freshly ground black pepper

- 1 tablespoon Olive oil cooking spray

Directions:
1. Heat olive oil in a skillet over medium heat, put the celery and onion and sauté for 4 to 5 minutes. Add the garlic and sauté for 30 seconds. Add the tomatoes and cook within 2 to 3 minutes. Add the wine and vinegar to deglaze the pan, increasing the heat to medium-high.
2. Add the artichokes, olives, capers, and red pepper flakes and simmer, reducing the liquid by half, about 10 minutes. Mix in the basil.
3. Season the mahi-mahi with salt and pepper. Heat a grill skillet or grill pan over medium-high flame and coat with olive oil cooking spray. Add the fish and cook within 4 to 5 minutes per side. Serve topped with the artichoke caponata.

Nutrition:
Calories: 245, Fat: 9g, Sodium: 570mg, Carbohydrates: 10g, Protein: 28g, Potassium: 130mg.

890. Cod and Cauliflower Chowder

Preparation Time: 15 minutes
Cooking Time: 40 minutes
Servings: 4
Ingredients:
- 2 tablespoons extra-virgin olive oil
- 1 leek, sliced thinly
- 4 garlic cloves, sliced
- 1 medium head cauliflower, coarsely chopped
- 1 teaspoon kosher salt
- ¼ teaspoon freshly ground black pepper
- 2 pints cherry tomatoes
- 2 cups no-salt-added vegetable stock
- ¼ cup green olives, pitted and chopped
- 1 to 1½ pounds cod
- ¼ cup fresh parsley, minced

Directions:
1. Heat the olive oil in a Dutch oven or large pot over medium heat. Add the leek and sauté until lightly golden brown, about 5 minutes.
2. Add the garlic and sauté within 30 seconds. Add the cauliflower,

salt, and black pepper and sauté for 2 to 3 minutes.
3. Add the tomatoes and vegetable stock, increase the heat to high and boil, then turn the heat to low and simmer within 10 minutes.
4. Add the olives and mix. Add the fish, cover, and simmer for 20 minutes or until the fish is opaque and flakes easily. Gently mix in the parsley.

Nutrition:
Calories: 270, Fat: 9g, Sodium: 545mg, Potassium: 1475mg, Carbohydrates: 19g, Protein: 30g.

891. Sardine Bruschetta with Fennel and Lemon Cream

Preparation Time: 15 minutes
Cooking Time: 0 minutes
Servings: 4
Ingredients:
- 1/3 cup plain Greek yogurt
- 2 tablespoons mayonnaise
- 2 tablespoons lemon juice, divided
- 2 teaspoons lemon zest
- ¾ teaspoon kosher salt, divided
- fennel bulb, cored and thinly sliced
- ¼ cup parsley, chopped, plus more for garnish
- ¼ cup fresh mint, chopped2 teaspoons extra-virgin olive oil
- 1/8 teaspoon freshly ground black pepper
- 8 slices multigrain bread, toasted
- (4.4-ounce) cans of smoked sardines

Directions:
1. Mix the yogurt, mayonnaise, 1 tablespoon of the lemon juice, the lemon zest, and ¼ teaspoon of the salt in a small bowl.
2. Mix the remaining ½ teaspoon of salt, the remaining 1 tablespoon of lemon juice, the fennel, parsley, mint, olive oil, and black pepper in a separate small bowl.
3. Spoon 1 tablespoon of the yogurt mixture on each piece of toast. Divide the fennel mixture evenly on top of the yogurt mixture. Divide the sardines among the toasts, placing them on top of the fennel mixture.

Garnish with more herbs, if desired.

Nutrition:
Calories: 400, Fat: 16g, Sodium: 565mg, Carbohydrates: 51g, Protein: 16g, Potassium: 230mg.

892. Chopped Tuna Salad

Preparation Time: 15 minutes
Cooking Time: 0 minutes
Servings: 4
Ingredients:
- 2 tablespoons extra-virgin olive oil
- 2 tablespoons lemon juice
- 2 teaspoons Dijon mustard
- ½ teaspoon kosher salt
- ¼ teaspoon freshly ground black pepper
- 12 olives, pitted and chopped
- ½ cup celery, diced
- ½ cup red onion, diced
- ½ cup red bell pepper, diced
- ½ cup fresh parsley, chopped
- 2 (6-ounce) cans no-salt-added tuna packed in water, drained
- 6 cups baby spinach

Directions:
1. Mix the olive oil, lemon juice, mustard, salt, and black pepper in a medium bowl. Add in the olives, celery, onion, bell pepper, and parsley and mix well. Add the tuna and gently incorporate. Divide the spinach evenly among 4 plates or bowls. Spoon the tuna salad evenly on top of the spinach.

Nutrition:
Calories: 220, Fat: 11g, Sodium: 396mg, Carbohydrates: 7g, Protein: 25g, Potassium: 128mg.

893. Monkfish with Sautéed Leeks, Fennel, and Tomatoes

Preparation Time: 15 minutes
Cooking Time: 35 minutes
Servings: 4
Ingredients:
- 1½ pounds monkfish
- 2 tablespoons lemon juice, divided
- 1 teaspoon kosher salt, divided
- 1/8 teaspoon freshly ground black pepper

- 2 tablespoons extra-virgin olive oil
- 1 leek, sliced in half lengthwise and thinly sliced
- ½ onion, julienned
- 2 garlic cloves, minced
- 2 bulbs fennel, cored and thinly sliced, plus ¼ cup fronds for garnish
- 1 (14.5-ounce) can no-salt-added diced tomatoes
- 2 tablespoons fresh parsley, chopped
- 2 tablespoons fresh oregano, chopped
- ¼ teaspoon red pepper flakes

Directions:
1. Place the fish in a medium baking dish and add 2 tablespoons of lemon juice, ¼ teaspoon of salt, plus the black pepper. Place in the refrigerator.
2. Heat olive oil in a large skillet over medium heat, then put the leek and onion and sauté until translucent, about 3 minutes. Add the garlic and sauté within 30 seconds. Add the fennel and sauté for 4 to 5 minutes. Add the tomatoes and simmer for 2 to 3 minutes.
3. Stir in the parsley, oregano, red pepper flakes, the remaining ¾ teaspoon of salt, and the remaining 1 tablespoon of lemon juice. Put the fish over the leek mixture, cover, and simmer for 20 to 25 minutes. Garnish with the fennel fronds.

Nutrition:
Calories: 220, Fat: 9g, Sodium: 345mg, Carbohydrates: 11g, Protein: 22g, Potassium: 169mg.

894. Caramelized Fennel and Sardines with Penne

Preparation Time: 15 minutes
Cooking Time: 30 minutes
Servings: 4
Ingredients:
- 8 ounces whole-wheat penne
- 2 tablespoons extra-virgin olive oil
- bulb fennel, cored and thinly sliced, plus ¼ cup fronds
- celery stalks, thinly sliced, plus ½ cup leaves
- garlic cloves, sliced
- ¾ teaspoon kosher salt

- ¼ teaspoon freshly ground black pepper
- Zest of 1 lemon
- Juice of 1 lemon
- 2 (4.4-ounce) cans boneless/skinless sardines packed in olive oil, undrained

Directions:
1. Cook the penne, as stated in the package directions. Drain, reserving 1 cup of pasta water. Heat olive oil in a large skillet over medium heat, then put the fennel and celery and cook within 10 to 12 minutes. Add the garlic and cook within 1 minute.
2. Add the penne, reserved pasta water, salt, and black pepper. Adjust the heat to medium-high and cook for 1 to 2 minutes.
3. Remove, then stir in the lemon zest, lemon juice, fennel fronds, and celery leaves. Break the sardines into bite-size pieces and gently mix them in, along with the oil they were packed in.

Nutrition:
Calories: 400, Fat: 15g, Sodium: 530mg, Carbohydrates: 46g, Protein: 22g, Potassium: 276mg.

895. Coppin

Preparation Time: 15 minutes
Cooking Time: 35 minutes
Servings: 4
Ingredients:
- 2 tablespoons extra-virgin olive oil
- 1 onion, diced
- 1 bulb fennel, chopped, plus ½ cup fronds for garnish
- 1-quart no-salt-added vegetable stock
- 4 garlic cloves, smashed
- 8 thyme sprigs
- 1 teaspoon kosher salt
- ¼ teaspoon red pepper flakes
- 1 tablespoon dried bay leaf
- 1 bunch kale, stemmed and chopped
- A dozen littleneck clams tightly closed, scrubbed
- 1-pound fish (cod, halibut, and bass are all good choices)
- ¼ cup fresh parsley, chopped

Directions:
1. Heat the olive oil in a large stockpot over medium heat. Add the onion and fennel and sauté for about 5 minutes. Add the vegetable stock, garlic, thyme, salt, red pepper flakes, and bay leaf. Adjust the heat to medium-

high, and simmer. Add the kale, cover, and simmer within 5 minutes.

2. Carefully add the clams, cover, and simmer for about 15 minutes until they open. Remove the clams and set them aside. Discard any clams that do not open.
3. Add the fish, cover, and simmer within 5 to 10 minutes, depending on the fish's thickness, until opaque and easily separated. Gently mix in the parsley. Divide the cioppino among 4 bowls. Place 3 clams in each bowl and garnish with the fennel fronds.

Nutrition:
Calories: 285, Fat: 9g, Sodium: 570mg, Carbohydrates: 19g, Protein: 32g, Potassium: 189mg.

896. Green Goddess Crab Salad with Endive

Preparation Time: 15 minutes
Cooking Time: 10 minutes
Servings: 4
Ingredients:
- 1-pound lump crabmeat
- 2/3 cup plain Greek yogurt
- 3 tablespoons mayonnaise
- 3 tablespoons fresh chives, chopped, plus additional for garnish
- 3 tablespoons fresh parsley, chopped, plus extra for garnish
- 3 tablespoons fresh basil, chopped, plus extra for garnish
- Zest of 1 lemon
- Juice of 1 lemon
- ½ teaspoon kosher salt
- ¼ teaspoon freshly ground black pepper
- 4 endives, ends cut off and leaves separated

Directions:
1. In a medium bowl, combine the crab, yogurt, mayonnaise, chives, parsley, basil, lemon zest, lemon juice, salt, plus black pepper, and mix until well combined.
2. Place the endive leaves on 4 salad plates. Divide the crab mixture evenly on top of the endive. Garnish with additional herbs, if desired.

Nutrition:

Calories: 200, Fat: 9g, Sodium: 570mg, Carbohydrates: 44g, Protein: 25g.

897. Seared Scallops with Blood Orange Glaze

Preparation Time: 15 minutes
Cooking Time: 20 minutes
Servings: 4
Ingredients:
- 3 tablespoons extra-virgin olive oil, divided
- 3 garlic cloves, minced
- ½ teaspoon kosher salt, divided
- 4 blood oranges, juiced
- 1 teaspoon blood orange zest
- ½ teaspoon red pepper flakes
- 1-pound scallops, small side muscle removed
- ¼ teaspoon freshly ground black pepper
- ¼ cup fresh chives, chopped

Directions:
1. Heat 1 tablespoon of the olive oil in a small saucepan over medium-high flame. Add the garlic and ¼ teaspoon of the salt and sauté for 30 seconds.
2. Add the orange juice and zest, bring to a boil, reduce the heat to medium-low, and cook within 20 minutes, or until the liquid reduces by half and becomes a thicker syrup consistency. Remove and mix in the red pepper flakes.
3. Pat the scallops dry with a paper towel and season with the remaining ¼ teaspoon salt and the black pepper. Heat the remaining 2 tablespoons of olive oil in a large skillet on medium-high heat. Add the scallops gently and sear.
4. Cook on each side within 2 minutes. If cooking in 2 batches, use 1 tablespoon of oil per batch. Serve the scallops with the blood orange glaze and garnish with the chives.

Nutrition:
Calories: 140, Fat: 4g, Sodium: 570mg, Carbohydrates: 12g, Protein: 15g, Potassium: 187mg.

898. Lemon Garlic Shrimp

Preparation Time: 15 minutes
Cooking Time: 10 minutes
Servings: 4

Ingredients:
- 2 tablespoons extra-virgin olive oil
- 3 garlic cloves, sliced
- ½ teaspoon kosher salt
- ¼ teaspoon red pepper flakes
- 1-pound large shrimp, peeled and deveined
- ½ cup white wine
- 3 tablespoons fresh parsley, minced
- Zest of ½ lemon
- Juice of ½ lemon

Directions:
1. Heat the olive oil in a wok or large skillet over medium-high heat. Add the garlic, salt, and red pepper flakes and sauté until the garlic starts to brown, 30 seconds to 1 minute.
2. Add the shrimp and cook within 2 to 3 minutes on each side. Pour in the wine and deglaze the wok, scraping up any flavorful brown bits, for 1 to 2 minutes. Turn off the heat; mix in the parsley, lemon zest, and lemon juice.

Nutrition:
Calories: 200, Fat: 9g, Sodium: 310mg, Carbohydrates: 3g, Protein: 23g, Potassium: 198mg.

899. Shrimp Fra Diavolo

Preparation Time: 15 minutes
Cooking Time: 10 minutes
Servings: 4
Ingredients:
- 2 tablespoons extra-virgin olive oil
- onion, diced small
- 1 fennel bulb, cored and diced small, plus ¼ cup fronds for garnish
- 1 bell pepper, diced small
- ½ teaspoon dried oregano
- ½ teaspoon dried thyme
- ½ teaspoon kosher salt
- ¼ teaspoon red pepper flakes
- 1 (14.5-ounce) can no-salt-added diced tomatoes
- 1-pound shrimp, peeled and deveined
- Juice of 1 lemon
- Zest of 1 lemon
- tablespoons fresh parsley, chopped for garnish

Directions:
1. Heat the olive oil in a large skillet or sauté pan over medium heat. Add the onion, fennel, bell pepper, oregano,

thyme, salt, and red pepper flakes. Sauté until translucent, about 5 minutes.
2. Drizzle the pan using the canned tomatoes' juice, scraping up any brown bits, and bringing to a boil. Add the diced tomatoes and the shrimp. Lower heat to a simmer within 3 minutes.
3. Turn off the heat. Add the lemon juice and lemon zest and toss well to combine. Garnish with the parsley and the fennel fronds.

Nutrition:
Calories: 240, Fat: 9g, Sodium: 335mg, Carbohydrates: 13g, Protein: 25g, Potassium: 276mg.

900. Fish Amandine
Preparation Time: 15 minutes
Cooking Time: 15 minutes
Servings: 4
Ingredients:
- 4-ounce skinless tilapia, trout, or halibut fillets, 1/2- to 1-inch thick
- ¼ cup buttermilk
- ½ teaspoon dry mustard
- 1/8 teaspoon crushed red pepper
- 1 tablespoon butter, melted
- ¼ teaspoon salt
- ½ cup panko breadcrumbs
- 1 tbsp. chopped fresh parsley
- ¼ cup sliced almonds, coarsely chopped
- 2 tablespoons grated Parmesan cheese

Directions:
1. Defrost fish if frozen. Preheat oven to 450F. Grease a shallow baking pan; set aside. Rinse fish; pat dry with paper towels.
2. Pour buttermilk into a shallow dish. In an extra shallow dish, mix bread crumbs, dry mustard, parsley, and salt. Soak fish into buttermilk, then into crumb mixture, turning to coat. Put coated fish in the ready baking pan.
3. Flavor the fish with almonds plus Parmesan cheese; drizzle with melted butter. Sprinkle with crinkled red pepper. Bake for 5 minutes per 1/2-inch thickness of fish or until fish flakes easily when checked with a fork.

Nutrition:
Calories: 209, Fat: 8.7g, Sodium: 302mg, Carbohydrates:

6.7g, Protein: 26.2g, Potassium: 258mg.

901. Air-Fryer Fish Cakes
Preparation Time: 15 minutes
Cooking Time: 10 minutes
Servings: 2
Ingredients:
- Cooking spray
- 10 oz. finely chopped white fish
- 2/3 cup whole-wheat panko breadcrumbs
- 3 tablespoons finely chopped fresh Cilantro
- 2 tablespoons Thai sweet chili sauce
- 2 tablespoons canola mayonnaise
- 1 large egg
- 1/8 teaspoon salt
- ¼ teaspoon ground pepper
- Lime wedges

Directions:
1. Grease the basket of an Air Fryer with cooking spray. Place fish, cilantro, panko, chili sauce, egg, mayonnaise, pepper and salt in a medium bowl; stir until well blended. Form mixture into four 3-inch-diameter cakes.
2. Brush cakes with cooking spray; place in basket. Bake at 400F until cakes are golden brown for 9 to 10 minutes. Serve with lime wedges.

Nutrition:
Calories: 399, Fat: 15.5g, Sodium: 537mg, Carbohydrates: 27.9g, Protein: 34.6g, Potassium: 187mg.

902. Pesto Shrimp Pasta
Preparation Time: 15 minutes
Cooking Time: 12 minutes
Servings: 4
Ingredients:
- 1/8 teaspoon freshly cracked pepper
- 1 cup dried orzo
- 4 tsp. packaged pesto sauce mix
- 1 lemon, halved
- 1/8 teaspoon coarse salt
- 1-pound medium shrimp, thawed
- 1 medium zucchini, halved lengthwise and sliced
- 2 tablespoons olive oil, divided
- 1-ounce shaved Parmesan cheese

Directions:

1. Prepare orzo pasta following package directions. Drain; reserving ¼ cup of the pasta cooking water. Mix 1 teaspoon of the pesto mix into the cooking water and set aside.
2. Mix 3 teaspoons of the pesto mix plus 1 tablespoon of the olive oil in a large plastic bag. Seal and shake to mix. Put the shrimp in the bag, seal and turn to coat. Set aside.
3. Sauté zucchini in a big skillet over moderate heat for 1 to 2 minutes, stirring repeatedly. Put the pesto-marinated shrimp in the skillet and cook for 5 minutes or until the shrimp is dense.
4. Put the cooked pasta in the skillet with the zucchini and shrimp combination. Stir in the kept pasta water until absorbed, grating up any seasoning in the bottom of the pan. Season with pepper and salt. Squeeze the lemon over the pasta. Top with Parmesan, then serve.

Nutrition:
Calories: 361, Fat: 10.1g, Sodium: 502mg, Carbohydrates: 35.8g, Protein: 31.6g, Potassium: 254mg.

903. Cod Salad with Mustard
Preparation Time: 12 minutes
Cooking Time: 12 minutes
Servings: 4
Ingredients:
- 4 medium cod fillets, skinless and boneless
- 2 tablespoons mustard
- 1 tablespoon tarragon, chopped
- 1 tablespoon capers, drained
- 4 tablespoons olive oil+ 1 teaspoon
- 1 tablespoon Black pepper to the taste
- 2 cups baby arugula
- 1 small red onion, sliced
- 1 small cucumber, sliced
- 2 tablespoons lemon juice

Directions:
1. In a bowl, mix mustard with 2 tablespoons of olive oil, tarragon and capers and whisk.
2. Heat a pan with 1 teaspoon oil over medium-high flame. Add fish, season with black pepper to the taste, and cook for 6 minutes on each side and cut into medium cubes.

3. In a salad bowl, combine the arugula with onion, cucumber, lemon juice, cod and mustard mix, toss and serve.

4. Enjoy!

Nutrition:
Calories: 258, Fat: 12g, Fiber: 6g, Carbs: 12g, Protein: 18g, Sodium: 49mg, Potassium: 134mg.

Chapter 18. Desserts

904. Green Tea and Banana Sweetening Mix

Preparation Time: 10 minutes
Cooking Time: 5 minutes
Servings: 3-4
Ingredients:
- 2 cups pitted avocados, chopped
- 1 cup coconut cream
- 2 peeled and chopped bananas
- 2 tablespoons green tea powder
- 1 tablespoon palm sugar
- 2 tablespoons grated lime zest

Directions:
1. Take all the ingredients in the Instant Pot.
2. Toss this, cover, and then cook on Low for 5 minutes. Do a manual, natural pressure release, divide and serve it cold.

Nutrition:
Calories: 207, Fat: 2g, Carbs: 11g, Net Carbs: 8g, Protein: 3g, Fiber: 8g, Sodium: 154mg, Potassium: 187mg.

905. Cheesecake Made Easy!

Preparation Time: 10 minutes
Cooking Time: 50 minutes
Servings: 8-10
Ingredients:
- 10 oz. crushed whole wheat crackers
- 16 oz., fat-free cream cheeses
- 2 teaspoons vanilla extract
- 5 tablespoons fat-free butter
- 1 cup coconut sugar
- 2 large eggs
- ¼ cup coconut cream
- 8 oz. sugar-free chocolate, melted
- 2 cups water
- cooking spray
- 2 tablespoons whole wheat flour

Directions:
1. In one bowl, mix crackers with butter and stir, then grease a cooking tin and push crackers into the bottom.
2. Mix the rest of the ingredients into another bowl, and then put it over the crust, then cover the pan with foil.
3. Put it in Instant Pot and cook on High for 45 minutes.

4. Chill cheesecake in the fridge before you serve it.

Nutrition:
Calories: 265, Fat: 9g, Carbs: 15g, Net Carbs: 12g, Protein: 4g, Fiber: 3g, Sodium: 135mg, Potassium: 243mg.

906. Grapefruit Compote

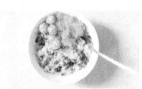

Preparation Time: 5 minutes
Cooking Time: 8 minutes
Servings: 4
Ingredients:
- 1 cup palm sugar
- 64 oz. Sugar-free red grapefruit juice
- ½ cup chopped mint
- 2 peeled and cubed grapefruits

Directions:
1. Take all ingredients and combine them into Instant Pot.
2. Cook on Low for 8 minutes, then divide into bowls and serve!

Nutrition:
Calories: 131, Fat: 1g, Carbs: 12g, Net Carbs: 11g, Protein: 2g, Fiber: 2g, Sodium: 175mg, Potassium: 198mg.

907. Instant Pot Applesauce

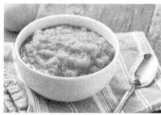

Preparation Time: 10 minutes
Cooking Time: 10 minutes
Servings: 8
Ingredients:
- 3 pounds of apples
- ½ cup water

Directions:

1. Core and peel the apples and then put them at the bottom of the Instant Pot and then secure the lid and seal the vent. Let it cook for 10 minutes; then do a natural pressure release.
2. From there, when it's safe to remove the lid, take the apples and juices and blend this till smooth.
3. Store it in jars or serve immediately.

Nutrition:
Calories: 88, Fat: 0g, Carbs: 23g, Net Carbs: 19g, Protein: 0g, Fiber: 4g, Sodium: 186mg, Potassium: 321mg.

908. Plum Cake

Preparation Time: 1 hour and 20 minutes
Cooking Time: 40 minutes
Servings: 8
Ingredients:
- 7 ounces whole wheat flour
- 1 teaspoon baking powder
- 1-ounce low-fat butter, soft
- 1 egg, whisked
- 5 tablespoons coconut sugar
- 3 ounces warm almond milk
- 1 and ¾ pounds plums, pitted and cut into quarters
- Zest of 1 lemon, grated
- 1-ounce almond flakes

Directions:
1. In a bowl, combine the flour with baking powder, butter, egg, sugar, milk and lemon zest. Stir well, transfer the dough to a lined cake pan, spread plums and almond flakes all over. Introduce in the oven and bake at 350 degrees F for 40 minutes.
2. Slice and serve cold.
3. Enjoy!

Nutrition:
Calories: 222, Fat: 4g, Fiber: 2g, Carbs: 7g, Protein: 7g, Sodium: 237mg, Potassium: 156mg.

909. Dates Brownies

Preparation Time: 10 minutes
Cooking Time: 15 minutes
Servings: 8
Ingredients:

- 28 ounces canned lentils, no-salt-added, rinsed and drained
- 12 dates
- 1 tablespoon coconut sugar
- 1 banana, peeled and chopped
- ½ teaspoon baking soda
- 4 tablespoons almond butter
- 2 tablespoons cocoa powder

Directions:
1. Put lentils in your food processor. Pulse, add dates, sugar, banana, baking soda, almond butter and cocoa powder. Pulse well, pour into a lined pan, spread, and bake in the oven at 375 degrees F for 15 minutes. Leave the mix aside to cool down a bit, cut into medium pieces and serve.
2. Enjoy!

Nutrition:
Calories: 202, Fat: 4g, Fiber: 2g, Carbs: 12g, Protein: 6g, Sodium: 168mg, Potassium: 354mg.

910. Rose Lentils Ice Cream

Preparation Time: 30 minutes
Cooking Time: 1 hour and 20 minutes
Servings: 4
Ingredients:
- ½ cup red lentils, rinsed
- Juice of ½ lemon
- 1 cup coconut sugar
- 1 and ½ cups water
- 3 cups almond milk
- Juice of 2 limes
- 2 teaspoons cardamom powder
- 1 teaspoon rose water

Directions:
1. Heat a pan over medium-high flame with the water and half of the sugar and lemon juice. Stir, bring to a boil, add lentils, stir, reduce heat to medium-low and cook for 1 hour and 20 minutes.
2. Drain lentils, transfer them to a bowl. Add coconut milk, the rest of the sugar, lime juice, cardamom and rose water, whisk everything, transfer to your ice cream machine, process for 30 minutes and serve.
3. Enjoy!

Nutrition:
Calories: 184, Fat: 4g, Fiber: 3g, Carbs: 8g, Protein: 5g, Sodium: 243mg, Potassium: 276mg.

911. Mandarin Almond Pudding

Preparation Time: 10 minutes
Cooking Time: 30 minutes
Servings: 8
Ingredients:
- 1 mandarin, peeled and sliced
- Juice of 2 mandarins
- 4 ounces low-fat butter, soft
- 2 eggs, whisked
- ¾ cup coconut sugar+ 2 tablespoons
- ¾ cup whole wheat flour
- ¾ cup almonds, ground

Directions:
1. Grease a loaf pan with some butter, sprinkle 2 tablespoons sugar on the bottom and arrange mandarin slices inside.
2. In a bowl, combine the butter with the rest of the sugar, eggs, almonds, flour and mandarin juice. Whisk using a mixer.
3. Spoon mix over mandarin slices. Introduce in the oven, bake at 350 degrees F for 30 minutes, divide into bowls and serve
4. Enjoy!

Nutrition:
Calories: 202, Fat: 3g, Fiber: 2g, Carbs: 12g, Protein: 6g, Sodium: 324mg, Potassium: 176mg.

912. Cherry Stew

Preparation Time: 10 minutes
Cooking Time: 10 minutes
Servings: 6
Ingredients:
- ½ cup cocoa powder
- 1 pound cherries, pitted
- ¼ cup coconut sugar
- 2 cups water

Directions:
1. In a pan, combine the cherries with the water, sugar and cocoa powder. Stir, cook over medium heat for 10 minutes, divide into bowls and serve cold.
2. Enjoy!

Nutrition:
Calories: 207, Fat: 1g, Fiber: 3g, Carbs: 8g, Protein: 6g, Sodium: 175mg, Potassium: 197mg.

913. Rice Pudding

Preparation Time: 10 minutes
Cooking Time: 45 minutes
Servings: 6
Ingredients:
- ½ cup basmati rice

- 4 cups almond milk
- ¼ cup raisins
- 3 tablespoons coconut sugar
- ½ teaspoon cardamom powder
- ¼ teaspoon cinnamon powder
- ¼ cup walnuts, chopped
- 1 tablespoon lemon zest, grated

Directions:
1. In a pan, mix sugar with milk. Stir, bring to a boil over medium-high heat. Add rice, raisins, cardamom, cinnamon, walnuts and lemon zest. Stir, cover the pan, reduce heat to low, cook for 40 minutes, divide into bowls and serve cold.
2. Enjoy!

Nutrition:
Calories: 200, Fat: 4g, Fiber: 5g, Carbs: 8g, Protein: 3g, Sodium: 254mg, Potassium: 195mg.

914. Apple Loaf

Preparation Time: 10 minutes
Cooking Time: 35 minutes
Servings: 6
Ingredients:
- 3 cups apples, cored and cubed
- 1 cup coconut sugar
- 1 tablespoon vanilla
- 2 eggs
- 1 tablespoon apple pie spice
- 2 cups almond flour
- 1 tablespoon baking powder
- 1 tablespoon coconut oil, melted

Directions:
1. In a bowl, mix apples with coconut sugar, vanilla, eggs, apple pie spice, almond flour, baking powder and oil. Whisk, pour into a loaf pan, introduce in the oven and bake at 350 degrees F for 35 minutes.
2. Serve cold.
3. Enjoy!

Nutrition:
Calories: 180, Fat: 6g, Fiber: 5g, Carbs: 12g, Protein: 4g, Sodium: 165mg, Potassium: 265mg.

915. Cauliflower Cinnamon Pudding

Preparation Time: 10 minutes
Cooking Time: 20 minutes
Servings: 6
Ingredients:
- 1 tablespoon coconut oil, melted
- 7 ounces cauliflower rice
- 4 ounces water
- 16 ounces coconut milk

- 3 ounces coconut sugar
- 1 egg
- 1 teaspoon cinnamon powder
- 1 teaspoon vanilla extract

Directions:
1. In a pan, combine the oil with the rice, water, milk, sugar, egg, cinnamon and vanilla, whisk well, bring to a simmer, cook for 20 minutes over medium heat. Divide into bowls and serve cold.
2. Enjoy!

Nutrition:
Calories: 202, Fat: 2g, Fiber: 6g, Carbs: 8g, Protein: 7g, Sodium: 213mg, Potassium: 276mg.

916. Rhubarb Stew

Preparation Time: 10 minutes
Cooking Time: 5 minutes
Servings: 3
Ingredients:
- Juice of 1 lemon
- 1 teaspoon lemon zest, grated
- 1 and ½ cup coconut sugar
- 4 and ½ cups rhubarbs, roughly chopped
- 1 and ½ cups water

Directions:
1. In a pan, combine the rhubarb with the water, lemon juice, lemon zest and coconut sugar. Toss, bring to a simmer over medium heat, cook for 5 minutes, divide into bowls and serve cold.
2. Enjoy!

Nutrition:
Calories: 108, Fat: 1g, Fiber: 4g, Carbs: 8g, Protein: 5g, Sodium: 254mg, Potassium: 187mg.

917. Pumpkin Pudding

Preparation Time: 1 hour
Cooking Time: 0 minutes
Servings: 4
Ingredients:
- 1 and ½ cups almond milk
- ½ cup pumpkin puree
- 2 tablespoons coconut sugar
- ½ teaspoon cinnamon powder
- ¼ teaspoon ginger, grated
- ¼ cup chia seeds

Directions:
1. In a bowl, combine the milk with pumpkin, sugar, cinnamon, ginger and chia seeds. Toss well, divide into small cups and keep them in the fridge for 1 hour before serving.
2. Enjoy!

Nutrition:
Calories: 145, Fat: 7g, Fiber: 7g, Carbs: 11g, Protein: 9g, Sodium: 176mg, Potassium: 287mg.

918. Cashew Lemon Fudge

Preparation Time: 2 hours
Cooking Time: 0 minutes
Servings: 4
Ingredients:
- 1/3 cup natural cashew butter
- 1 and ½ tablespoons coconut oil, melted
- 2 tablespoons coconut butter
- 5 tablespoons lemon juice
- ½ teaspoon lemon zest
- 1 tablespoon coconut sugar

Directions:
1. In a bowl, mix cashew butter with coconut butter, oil, lemon juice, lemon zest and sugar and stir well.
2. Line a muffin tray with some parchment paper. Scoop 1 tablespoon of lemon fudge mix in a lined muffin tray, keep in the fridge for 2 hours and serve.
3. Enjoy!

Nutrition:
Calories: 142, Fat: 4g, Fiber: 4g, Carbs: 8g, Protein: 5g, Sodium: 175mg, Potassium: 232mg.

919. Brown Cake

Preparation Time: 10 minutes
Cooking Time: 2 hours and 30 minutes
Servings: 8
Ingredients:
- 1 cup flour
- 1 and ½ cup stevia
- ½ cup chocolate almond milk
- 2 teaspoons baking powder
- 1 and ½ cups hot water
- ¼ cup cocoa powder+ 2 tablespoons
- 2 tablespoons canola oil
- 1 teaspoon vanilla extract
- Cooking spray

Directions:
1. In a bowl, mix flour with ¼-cup cocoa, baking powder, almond milk, oil and vanilla extract. Whisk well and spread on the bottom of the slow cooker greased with cooking spray.
2. In a separate bowl, mix stevia with the water and the rest of the cocoa. Whisk well, spread over the batter, cover, and cook your cake on High for 2 hours and 30 minutes.
3. Leave the cake to cool down, slice and serve.

Nutrition:
Calories: 150, Fat: 7.6g, Cholesterol: 1mg, Sodium: 7mg, Carbohydrates: 56.8g, Fiber: 1.8g, Sugars: 4.4g, Protein: 2.9g, Potassium: 185mg.

920. Delicious Berry Pie

Preparation Time: 10 minutes
Cooking Time: 1 hour
Servings: 6
Ingredients:
- ½ cup whole wheat flour
- Cooking spray
- 1/3 cup almond milk
- ¼ teaspoon baking powder
- ¼ teaspoon stevia
- ¼ cup blueberries
- 1 teaspoon olive oil
- 1 teaspoon vanilla extract
- ½ teaspoon lemon zest, grated

Directions:
1. In a bowl, mix flour with baking powder, stevia, blueberries, milk, oil, lemon zest and vanilla extract. Whisk, pour into your slow cooker lined with parchment paper and greased with the cooking spray, cover and cook on High for 1 hour.
2. Leave the pie to cool down, slice and serve.

Nutrition:
Calories: 82, Fat: 4.2g, Cholesterol: 0mg, Sodium: 3mg, Carbohydrates: 10.1g, Fiber: 0.7g, Sugars: 1.2g, Protein: 1.4g, Potassium: 74mg.

921. Cinnamon Peach Cobbler

Preparation Time: 10 minutes
Cooking Time: 4 hours
Servings: 4
Ingredients:
- 4 cups peaches, peeled and sliced
- Cooking spray
- ¼ cup coconut sugar
- 1 and ½ cups whole wheat sweet crackers, crushed
- ½ cup almond milk
- ½ teaspoon cinnamon powder
- ¼ cup stevia
- 1 teaspoon vanilla extract

- ¼ teaspoon nutmeg, ground

Directions:
1. In a bowl, mix peaches with sugar, cinnamon, and stir.
2. In a separate bowl, mix crackers with stevia, nutmeg, almond milk and vanilla extract and stir.
3. Grease your slow cooker with cooking spray. Spread peaches on the bottom, and add the crackers mix. Spread, cover and cook on Low for 4 hours.
4. Divide into bowls and serve.

Nutrition:
Calories: 249, Fat: 11.4g, Cholesterol: 0mg, Sodium: 179mg, Carbohydrates: 42.7g, Fiber: 3g, Sugars: 15.2g, Protein: 3.5g, Potassium: 366mg.

922. Resilient Chocolate Cream

Preparation Time: 10 minutes
Cooking Time: 1 hour and 30 minutes
Servings: 4
Ingredients:
- 1 cup dark and unsweetened chocolate, chopped
- ½ pound cherries, pitted and halved
- 1 teaspoon vanilla extract
- ½ cup coconut cream
- 3 tablespoons coconut sugar
- 2 teaspoons gelatin

Directions:
1. In the slow cooker, combine the chocolate with the cherries and the other ingredients. Toss, put the lid on and cook on Low for 1 hour and 30 minutes.
2. Stir the cream well, divide it into bowls and serve.

Nutrition:
Calories: 526, Fat: 39.9g, Cholesterol: 0mg, Sodium: 57mg, Carbohydrates: 47.2g, Fiber: 10.8g, Sugars: 1.1g, Protein: 13.4g, Potassium: 141mg.

923. Vanilla Poached Strawberries

Preparation Time: 10 minutes
Cooking Time: 3 hours
Servings: 10
Ingredients:
- 4 cups coconut sugar
- 2 tablespoons lemon juice

- 2 pounds strawberries
- 1 cup water
- 1 teaspoon vanilla extract
- 1 teaspoon cinnamon powder

Directions:
1. In your slow cooker, mix strawberries with water, coconut sugar, lemon juice, cinnamon and vanilla. Stir, cover, cook on Low for 3 hours, divide into bowls and serve cold.

Nutrition:
Calories: 69, Fat: 0.3g, Cholesterol: 0mg, Sodium: 18mg, Carbohydrates: 14.7g, Fiber: 1.8g, Sugars: 4.6g, Protein: 1g, Potassium: 143mg.

924. Lemon Bananas

Preparation Time: 10 minutes
Cooking Time: 2 hours
Servings: 4
Ingredients:
- 4 bananas, peeled and sliced
- Juice of ½ lemon
- 1 tablespoon coconut oil
- 3 tablespoons stevia
- ½ teaspoon cardamom seeds

Directions:
1. Arrange bananas in your slow cooker. Add stevia, lemon juice, oil and cardamom. Cover, cook on Low for 2 hours, divide everything into bowls and serve with.

Nutrition:
Calories: 137, Fat: 3.9g, Cholesterol: 0mg, Sodium: 2mg, Carbohydrates: 33.5g, Fiber: 3.2g, Sugars: 14.6g, Protein: 1.4g, Potassium: 433mg.

925. Pecans Cake

Preparation Time: 10 minutes
Cooking Time: 5 hours
Servings: 4
Ingredients:
- Cooking spray
- 1 cup almond flour
- 1 cup orange juice
- 1 cup coconut sugar
- 3 tablespoons coconut oil, melted
- 1 teaspoon baking powder
- ½ teaspoon cinnamon powder
- ½ cup almond milk
- ½ cup pecans, chopped
- ¾ cup water
- ½ cup orange peel, grated

Directions:

1. In a bowl, mix flour with half of the sugar, baking powder, cinnamon, 2 tablespoons oil, milk and pecans. Stir and pour this in your slow cooker greased with cooking spray.
2. Heat a small pan over medium flame. Add water, orange juice, orange peel, the rest of the oil and the rest of the sugar. Stir, bring to a boil, pour over the mix in the slow cooker, cover and cook on Low for 5 hours.
3. Divide into bowls and serve cold.

Nutrition:
Calories: 565, Fat: 48.8g, Cholesterol: 0mg, Sodium: 28mg, Carbohydrates: 26g, Fiber: 7.8g, Sugars: 7.1g, Protein: 10.2g, Potassium: 459mg.

926. Coconut Cream and Plums Cake

Preparation Time: 10 minutes
Cooking Time: 3 hours
Servings: 6
Ingredients:
- 2 cups whole wheat flour
- 1 teaspoon vanilla extract
- 1 and ½ cups plums, peeled and chopped
- ½ cup coconut cream
- 1 teaspoon baking powder
- ¾ cup coconut sugar
- 4 tablespoons avocado oil

Directions:
1. In the slow cooker lined with parchment paper, combine the flour with the plums and the other ingredients and whisk.
2. Put the lid on, cook on High for 3 hours, and leave the cake to cool down, slice and serve.

Nutrition:
Calories: 232, Fat: 6.4g, Cholesterol: 0mg, Sodium: 10mg, Carbohydrates: 38.3g, Fiber: 2.2g, Sugars: 2.7g, Protein: 5.1g, Potassium: 238mg.

927. Maple Syrup Poached Pears

Preparation Time: 10 minutes
Cooking Time: 4 hours
Servings: 4
Ingredients:
- 2 cups grapefruit juice

- 4 pears, peeled and cored
- ¼ cup maple syrup
- 1 tablespoon ginger, grated
- 2 teaspoons cinnamon powder

Directions:
1. In your slow cooker, mix pears with grapefruit juice, maple syrup, cinnamon and ginger. Cover, cook on Low for 4 hours, divide everything into bowls and serve.

Nutrition:
Calories: 214, Fat: 0.5g, Cholesterol: 0mg, Sodium: 5mg, Carbohydrates: 55.3g, Fiber: 7.9g, Sugars: 40.2g, Protein: 1.6g, Potassium: 461mg.

928. Ginger and Pumpkin Pie

Preparation Time: 10 minutes
Cooking Time: 2 hours
Servings: 10
Ingredients:
- 2 cups almond flour
- 1 egg, whisked
- 1 cup pumpkin puree
- 1 and ½ teaspoons baking powder
- Cooking spray
- 1 tablespoon coconut oil, melted
- 1 tablespoon vanilla extract
- ½ teaspoon baking soda
- 1 and ½ teaspoons cinnamon powder
- ¼ teaspoon ginger, ground
- 1/3 cup maple syrup
- 1 teaspoon lemon juice

Directions:
1. In a bowl, add flour with baking powder, baking soda, cinnamon, ginger, egg, oil, vanilla, pumpkin puree, maple syrup and lemon juice. Stir and pour in your slow cooker greased with cooking spray and lined with parchment paper. Cover the pot and cook on Low for 2 hours and 20 minutes.
2. Leave the pie to cool down, slice and serve.

Nutrition:
Calories: 91, Fat: 4.8g, Cholesterol: 16mg, Sodium: 74mg, Carbohydrates: 10.8g, Fiber: 1.3g, Sugars: 7.5g, Protein: 2g, Potassium: 157mg.

929. Cashew and Carrot Muffins

Preparation Time: 10 minutes

Cooking Time: 3 hours
Servings: 4
Ingredients:
- 4 tablespoons cashew butter, melted
- 4 eggs, whisked
- ½ cup coconut cream
- 1 cup carrots, peeled and grated
- 4 teaspoons maple syrup
- ¾ cup coconut flour
- ½ teaspoon baking soda

Directions:
1. In a bowl, mix the cashew butter with the eggs, cream and the other ingredients, whisk well and pour into a muffin pan that fits the slow cooker.
2. Put the lid on, cook the muffins on High for 3 hours, cool down and serve.

Nutrition:
Calories: 345, Fat: 21.7g, Cholesterol: 164mg, Sodium: 247mg, Carbohydrates: 28.6g, Fiber: 10.7g, Sugars: 6.7g, Protein: 12.3g, Potassium: 327mg.

930. Lemon Custard

Preparation Time: 10 minutes
Cooking Time: 3 hours
Servings: 10
Ingredients:
- 2 pounds lemons, washed, peeled and sliced
- 2 pounds coconut sugar
- 1 tablespoon vinegar

Directions:
1. In your slow cooker, mix lemons with coconut sugar and vinegar. Stir, cover, cook on High for 3 hours, blend using an immersion blender, divide into small bowls and serve.

Nutrition:
Calories: 46, Fat: 0.3g, Cholesterol: 0mg, Sodium: 10mg, Carbohydrates: 12.3g, Fiber: 2.5g, Sugars: 2.3g, Protein: 1.2g, Potassium: 126mg.

931. Rhubarb Dip

Preparation Time: 10 minutes
Cooking Time: 3 hours
Servings: 8
Ingredients:
- 1 cup coconut sugar
- 1/3 cup water
- 4 pounds rhubarb, chopped
- 1 tablespoon mint, chopped

Directions:
1. In your slow cooker, mix water with rhubarb, sugar and mint. Stir, cover, cook on High for 3 hours. Blend using an immersion blender, divide into cups and serve cold.

Nutrition:
Calories: 60, Fat: 0.5g, Cholesterol: 0mg, Sodium: 15mg, Carbohydrates: 12.7g, Fiber: 4.1g, Sugars: 2.5g, Protein: 2.2g, Potassium: 657mg.

932. Summer Jam

Preparation Time: 10 minutes
Cooking Time: 3 hours
Servings: 6
Ingredients:
- 2 cups coconut sugar
- 4 cups cherries, pitted
- 2 tablespoons lemon juice
- 3 tablespoons gelatin

Directions:
1. In your slow cooker, mix lemon juice with gelatin, cherries and coconut sugar. Stir, cover and cook on High for 3 hours. Divide into bowls and serve cold.

Nutrition:
Calories: 171, Fat: 0.1g, Cholesterol: 0mg, Sodium: 41mg, Carbohydrates: 37.2g, Fiber: 0.7g, Sugars: 0.1g, Protein: 3.8g, Potassium: 122mg.

933. Cinnamon Pudding

Preparation Time: 10 minutes
Cooking Time: 5 hours
Servings: 4
Ingredients:
- 2 cups white rice
- 1 cup coconut sugar
- 2 cinnamon sticks
- 6 and ½ cups water
- ½ cup coconut, shredded

Directions:
1. In your slow cooker, mix water with the rice, sugar, cinnamon and coconut, stir, cover, cook on High for 5 hours, discard cinnamon, divide the pudding into bowls and serve warm.

Nutrition:
Calories: 400, Fat: 4g, Cholesterol: 0mg, Sodium: 28mg, Carbohydrates: 81.2g, Fiber: 2.7g, Sugars: 0.8g, Protein: 7.2g, Potassium: 151mg.

934. Orange Compote

Preparation Time: 10 minutes
Cooking Time: 2 hours and 30 minutes
Servings: 4
Ingredients:

- ½ pound oranges, peeled and cut into segments
- ½ pound plums, pitted and halved
- 1 cup orange juice
- 3 tablespoons coconut sugar
- ½ cup water

Directions:

1. In the slow cooker, combine the oranges with the plums, orange juice and the other ingredients, put the lid on and cook on High for 2 hours and 30 minutes.
2. Stir, divide into bowls and serve cold.

Nutrition:
Calories: 130, Fat: 0.2g, Cholesterol: 0mg, Sodium: 31mg, Carbohydrates: 28.4g, Fiber: 1.6g, Sugars: 11.4g, Protein: 1.8g, Potassium: 240mg.

935. Chocolate Bars

Preparation Time: 10 minutes
Cooking Time: 2 hours and 30 minutes
Servings: 12
Ingredients:

- 1 cup coconut sugar
- ½ cup dark chocolate chips
- 1 egg white
- ¼ cup coconut oil, melted
- ½ teaspoon vanilla extract
- 1 teaspoon baking powder
- 1 and ½ cups almond meal

Directions:

1. In a bowl, mix the oil with sugar, vanilla extract, egg white, baking powder and almond flour and whisk well.
2. Fold in chocolate chips and stir gently.
3. Line your slow cooker with parchment paper, grease it, add cookie mix, press on the bottom, cover and cook on Low for 2 hours and 30 minutes.
4. Take the cookie sheet out of the slow cooker. Cut it into medium bars and serve.

Nutrition:
Calories: 141, Fat: 11.8g, Cholesterol: 0mg, Sodium: 7mg, Carbohydrates: 7.7g, Fiber: 1.5g, Sugars: 3.2g, Protein: 3.2g, Potassium: 134mg.

936. Lemon Zest Pudding

Preparation Time: 10 minutes
Cooking Time: 5 hours
Servings: 4
Ingredients:

- 1 cup pineapple juice, natural
- Cooking spray
- 1 teaspoon baking powder
- 1 cup coconut flour
- 3 tablespoons avocado oil
- 3 tablespoons stevia
- ½ cup pineapple, chopped
- ½ cup lemon zest, grated
- ½ cup coconut milk
- ½ cup pecans, chopped

Directions:

1. Grease your slow cooker with cooking spray.
2. In a bowl, mix flour with stevia, baking powder, oil, milk, pecans, pineapple, lemon zest and pineapple juice. Stir well, pour into your slow cooker greased with cooking spray; cover and cook on Low for 5 hours.
3. Divide into bowls and serve.

Nutrition:
Calories: 431, Fat: 29.7g, Cholesterol: 0mg, Sodium: 8mg, Carbohydrates: 47.1g, Fiber: 17g, Sugars: 10.9g, Protein: 8.1g, Potassium: 482mg.

937. Coconut Figs

Preparation Time: 6 minutes
Cooking Time: 5 minutes
Servings: 4
Ingredients:

- 2 tablespoons coconut butter
- 12 figs, halved
- ¼ cup coconut sugar
- 1 cup almonds, toasted and chopped

Directions:

1. Put butter in a pot, heat over medium flame. Add sugar, whisk well, also add almonds and figs. Toss, cook for 5 minutes, divide into small cups and serve cold.
2. Enjoy!

Nutrition:
Calories: 150, Fat: 4g, Fiber: 5g, Carbs: 7g, Protein: 4g, Sodium: 54mg, Potassium: 32mg.

938. Lemony Banana Mix

Preparation Time: 10 minutes
Cooking Time: 0 minutes
Servings: 4
Ingredients:

- 4 bananas, peeled and chopped
- 5 strawberries, halved
- Juice of 2 lemons
- 4 tablespoons coconut sugar

Directions:

1. In a bowl, combine the bananas with the strawberries, lemon juice and sugar, toss and serve cold.
2. Enjoy!

Nutrition:
Calories: 172, Fat: 7g, Fiber: 5g, Carbs: 5g, Protein: 5g, Sodium: 164mg, Potassium: 324mg.

939. Cocoa Banana Dessert Smoothie

Preparation Time: 5 minutes
Cooking Time: 0 minutes
Servings: 2
Ingredients:

- 2 medium bananas, peeled
- 2 teaspoons cocoa powder
- ½ big avocado, pitted, peeled and mashed
- ¾ cup almond milk

Directions:

1. In your blender, combine the bananas with the cocoa, avocado and milk. Pulse well, divide into 2 glasses and serve.
2. Enjoy!

Nutrition:
Calories: 155, Fat: 3g, Fiber: 4g, Carbs: 6g, Protein: 5g, Sodium: 324mg, Potassium: 187mg.

940. Kiwi Bars

Preparation Time: 30 minutes
Cooking Time: 0 minutes
Servings: 4
Ingredients:

- 1 cup olive oil
- 1 and ½ bananas, peeled and chopped
- 1/3 cup coconut sugar
- ¼ cup lemon juice
- 1 teaspoon lemon zest, grated
- 3 kiwis, peeled and chopped

Directions:

1. In your food processor, mix bananas with kiwis, almost all

the oil, sugar, lemon juice and lemon zest and pulse well.
2. Grease a pan with the remaining oil. Pour the kiwi mix, spread, keep in the fridge for 30 minutes, slice and serve,
3. Enjoy!
Nutrition:
Calories: 207, Fat: 3g, Fiber: 3g, Carbs: 4g, Protein: 4g, Sodium: 186mg, Potassium: 324mg.

941. Black Tea Bars

Preparation Time: 10 minutes
Cooking Time: 35 minutes
Servings: 12
Ingredients:
- 6 tablespoons black tea powder
- 2 cups almond milk
- ½ cup low-fat butter
- 2 cups coconut sugar
- 4 eggs
- 2 teaspoons vanilla extract
- ½ cup olive oil
- 3 and ½ cups whole wheat flour
- 1 teaspoon baking soda
- 3 teaspoons baking powder
Directions:
1. Put the milk in a pot, heat it over medium flame. Add tea, stir, take off the heat and cool down.
2. Add butter, sugar, eggs, vanilla, oil, flour, baking soda and baking powder. Stir well, pour into a square pan, spread and introduce in the oven. Bake at 350 degrees F for 35 minutes. Cool down, slice and serve. Enjoy!
Nutrition:
Calories: 220, Fat: 4g, Fiber: 4g, Carbs: 12g, Protein: 7g, Sodium: 324mg, Potassium: 187mg.

Green Pudding

Preparation Time: 2 hours
Cooking Time: 5 minutes
Servings: 6
Ingredients:
- 14 ounces almond milk
- 2 tablespoons green tea powder
- 14 ounces coconut cream
- 3 tablespoons coconut sugar
- 1 teaspoon gelatin powder
Directions:
1. Put the milk in a pan, add sugar, gelatin, coconut cream and green tea powder. Stir, bring to a simmer and cook for 5 minutes. Divide into cups and

keep in the fridge for 2 hours before serving.
2. Enjoy!
Nutrition:
Calories: 170, Fat: 3g, Fiber: 3g, Carbs: 7g, Protein: 4g, Sodium: 187mg, Potassium: 187mg.

942. Lemony Plum Cake

Preparation Time: 1 hour and 20 minutes
Cooking Time: 40 minutes
Servings: 8
Ingredients:
- 7 ounces whole wheat flour
- 1 teaspoon baking powder
- 1-ounce low-fat butter, soft
- 1 egg, whisked
- 5 tablespoons coconut sugar
- 3 ounces warm almond milk
- 1 and ¾ pounds plums, pitted and cut into quarters
- Zest of 1 lemon, grated
- 1-ounce almond flakes
Directions:
1. In a bowl, combine the flour with baking powder, butter, egg, sugar, milk and lemon zest. Stir well, transfer the dough to a lined cake pan, spread plums and almond flakes all over. Introduce in the oven and bake at 350 degrees F for 40 minutes.
2. Slice and serve cold.
3. Enjoy
Nutrition:
Calories: 222, Fat: 4g, Fiber: 2g, Carbs: 7g, Protein: 7g, Sodium: 176mg, Potassium: 342mg.

943. Lentils Sweet Bars

Preparation Time: 10 minutes
Cooking Time: 25 minutes
Servings: 14
Ingredients:
- 1 cup lentils, cooked, drained and rinsed
- 1 teaspoon cinnamon powder
- 2 cups whole wheat flour
- 1 teaspoon baking powder
- ½ teaspoon nutmeg, ground
- 1 cup low-fat butter
- 1 cup coconut sugar
- 1 egg
- 2 teaspoons almond extract
- 1 cup raisins
- 2 cups coconut, unsweetened and shredded
Directions:

1. Put the lentils in a bowl, mash them well using a fork, add cinnamon, flour, baking powder, nutmeg, butter, sugar, egg, almond extract, raisins and coconut. Stir, spread on a lined baking sheet and introduce in the oven. Bake at 350 degrees F for 25 minutes, cut into bars and serve cold.
2. Enjoy!
Nutrition:
Calories: 214, Fat: 4g, Fiber: 2g, Carbs: 5g, Protein: 7g, Sodium: 154mg, Potassium: 215mg.

944. Lentils and Dates Brownies

Preparation Time: 10 minutes
Cooking Time: 15 minutes
Servings: 8
Ingredients:
- 28 ounces canned lentils, no-salt-added, rinsed and drained
- 12 dates
- 1 tablespoon coconut sugar
- 1 banana, peeled and chopped
- ½ teaspoon baking soda
- 4 tablespoons almond butter
- 2 tablespoons cocoa powder
Directions:
1. Put lentils in your food processor, pulse, add dates, sugar, banana, baking soda, almond butter and cocoa powder. Pulse well, pour into a lined pan, spread and bake in the oven at 375 degrees F for 15 minutes. Leave the mix aside to cool down a bit, cut into medium pieces and serve.
2. Enjoy!
Nutrition:
Calories: 202, Fat: 4g, Fiber: 2g, Carbs: 12g, Protein: 6g, Sodium: 176mg, Potassium: 232mg.

945. Mandarin Pudding

Preparation Time: 10 minutes
Cooking Time: 30 minutes
Servings: 8
Ingredients:
- 1 mandarin, peeled and sliced
- Juice of 2 mandarins
- 4 ounces low-fat butter, soft
- 2 eggs, whisked
- ¾ cup coconut sugar + 2 tablespoons
- ¾ cup whole wheat flour
- ¾ cup almonds, ground

Directions:
1. Grease a loaf pan with some butter. Sprinkle 2 tablespoons of sugar on the bottom and arrange mandarin slices inside.
2. In a bowl, combine the butter with the rest of the sugar, eggs, almonds, flour and mandarin juice and whisk using a mixer.
3. Spoon mix over mandarin slices. Introduce in the oven, bake at 350 degrees F for 30 minutes, divide into bowls and serve
4. Enjoy!

Nutrition:
Calories: 202, Fat: 3g, Fiber: 2g, Carbs: 12g, Protein: 6g, Sodium: 176mg, Potassium: 187mg.

946. Walnut Apple Mix

Preparation Time: 10 minutes
Cooking Time: 4 hours
Servings: 4
Ingredients:
- 6 big apples, roughly chopped
- Cooking spray
- ½ cup almond flour
- ½ cup walnuts, chopped
- ¼ cup coconut oil, melted
- 2 teaspoons lemon juice
- 3 tablespoons stevia
- ¼ teaspoon ginger, grated
- ¼ teaspoon cinnamon powder

Directions:
1. Grease your slow cooker with cooking spray.
2. In a bowl, mix stevia with lemon juice, ginger, apples and cinnamon. Stir and pour into your slow cooker.
3. In another bowl, mix flour with walnuts and oil. Stir, pour into the slow cooker, cover, and cook on Low for 4 hours.
4. Divide into bowls and serve.

Nutrition:
Calories: 474, Fat: 30.3g, Cholesterol: 0mg, Sodium: 9mg, Carbohydrates: 58.4g, Fiber: 10.7g, Sugars: 35g, Protein: 7.7g, Potassium: 444mg.

947. Vanilla and Grapes Compote

Preparation Time: 10 minutes
Cooking Time: 2 hours
Servings: 4
Ingredients:

- 4 tablespoons coconut sugar
- 1 and ½ cups water
- 1 pound green grapes
- 1 teaspoon vanilla extract

Directions:
1. In your slow cooker, combine the grapes with the sugar and the other ingredients. Put the lid on and cook on High for 2 hours, divide into bowls and serve.

Nutrition:
Calories: 227, Fat: 1.5g, Cholesterol: 0mg, Sodium: 45mg, Carbohydrates: 47.6g, Fiber: 2.3g, Sugars: 18.8g, Protein: 3.6g, Potassium: 271mg.

948. Soft Pudding

Preparation Time: 6 minutes
Cooking Time: 1 hour
Servings: 4
Ingredients:
- ½ cup coconut water
- 2 teaspoons lime zest, grated
- 2 tablespoons green tea powder
- 1 and ½ cup avocado, pitted, peeled and chopped
- 1 tablespoon stevia

Directions:
1. In your slow cooker, mix the coconut water with avocado, green tea powder, lime zest and stevia. Stir, cover and cook on Low for 1 hour. Divide into bowls and serve.

Nutrition:
Calories: 120, Fat: 10.7g, Cholesterol: 0mg, Sodium: 35mg, Carbohydrates: 8.5g, Fiber: 4.4g, Sugars: 1.1g, Protein: 1.5g, Potassium: 362mg.

949. Ginger and Cinnamon Pudding

Preparation Time: 10 minutes
Cooking Time: 1 hour
Servings: 4
Ingredients:
- ½ cup pumpkin puree
- 2 tablespoons maple syrup
- 1 and ½ cup coconut milk
- ½ cup chia seeds
- ¼ teaspoon ginger, grated
- ½ teaspoon cinnamon powder

Directions:
1. In your slow cooker, mix the milk with the pumpkin puree,

maple syrup, chia, cinnamon and ginger. Stir, cover, cook on High for 1 hour, divide into bowls and serve.

Nutrition:
Calories: 366, Fat: 29.3g, Cholesterol: 0mg, Sodium: 20mg, Carbohydrates: 24.8g, Fiber: 11.5g, Sugars: 10g, Protein: 6.6g, Potassium: 423mg.

950. Honey Compote

Preparation Time: 10 minutes
Cooking Time: 2 hours
Servings: 6
Ingredients:
- 64 ounces red grapefruit juice
- 1 cup honey
- ½ cup mint, chopped
- 1 cup water
- 2 grapefruits, peeled and chopped

Directions:
1. In your slow cooker, mix grapefruit with water, honey, mint and grapefruit juice. Stir, cover, cook on High for 2 hours, divide into bowls and serve cold.

Nutrition:
Calories: 364, Fat: 0.1g, Cholesterol: 0mg, Sodium: 52mg, Carbohydrates: 94.9g, Fiber: 1.1g, Sugars: 49.4g, Protein: 0.7g, Potassium: 124mg.

951. Dark Cherry and Stevia Compote

Preparation Time: 10 minutes
Cooking Time: 2 hours
Servings: 6
Ingredients:
- 1-pound dark cherries, pitted and halved
- ¾ cup red grape juice
- ¼ cup maple syrup
- ½ cup dark cocoa powder
- 2 tablespoons stevia
- 2 cups water

Directions:
1. In your slow cooker, mix cocoa powder with grape juice, maple syrup, cherries, water and stevia. Stir, cover, cook on High for 2 hours, divide into bowls and serve cold.

Nutrition:

Calories: 132, Fat: 1.4g,
Cholesterol: 0mg, Sodium:
179mg, Carbohydrates: 37.9g,
Fiber: 7g, Sugars: 23g, Protein:
3.2g, Potassium: 28mg.

952. Vanilla Grapes Bowls

Preparation Time: 10 minutes
Cooking Time: 2 hours
Servings: 4
Ingredients:
- 1-pound green grapes
- 3 tablespoons coconut sugar
- 1 and ½ cups coconut cream
- 2 teaspoons vanilla extract

Directions:
1. In the slow cooker, combine the grapes with the cream and the other ingredients. Put the lid on and cook on High for 2 hours.
2. Divide into bowls and serve.

Nutrition:
Calories: 360, Fat: 21.9g,
Cholesterol: 0mg, Sodium:
46mg, Carbohydrates: 39g,
Fiber: 3g, Sugars: 21.7g, Protein:
3.5g, Potassium: 456mg.

953. Pears Mix

Preparation Time: 10 minutes
Cooking Time: 1 hour
Servings: 6
Ingredients:
- 1 quart water
- 5 star anise
- 2 tablespoons stevia
- ½ pound pears, cored and cut into wedges
- ½ pound apple, cored and cut into wedges
- Zest of 1 orange, grated
- Zest of 1 lemon, grated
- 2 cinnamon sticks

Directions:
1. Put the water, stevia, apples, pears, star anise, and cinnamon, orange and lemon zest in your slow cooker. Cover, cook on High for 1 hour, divide into bowls and serve cold.

Nutrition:
Calories: 43, Fat: 0.4g,
Cholesterol: 0mg, Sodium: 6mg,
Carbohydrates: 14.3g, Fiber:
2.7g, Sugars: 5.9g, Protein: 0.7g,
Potassium: 109mg.

954. Pork Beef Bean Nachos

Preparation Time: 15 minutes
Cooking Time: 40 minutes
Servings: 10
Ingredients:
- 1 package beef jerky
- 4 cans black beans, drained and rinsed
- 6 bacon strips, crumbled
- 3 pounds pork spareribs
- 1 cup chopped onion
- 4 teaspoons minced garlic
- 4 cups divided beef broth
- optional toppings such as cheddar, sour cream, green onions, jalapeno slices
- 1 teaspoon crushed red pepper flakes
- Tortilla chips

Directions:
1. Pulse jerky in the processor till ground. Working in batches, put the ribs in the Instant Pot, topping with half jerky, two beans, and ½ cup onion, three pieces of bacon, 2 teaspoons of garlic, 2 cups of broth, and half teaspoon of red pepper flakes. Cook on High for forty minutes.
2. Do a natural pressure release for 10 minutes, then quick release what's next, and do the same with the second batch.
3. Discard bones, and shred meat and then sauté it. Next, strain the mixture, and finally discard juice. Serve with chips and your desired toppings.

Nutrition:
Calories: 469, Fat: 24g, Carbs:
27g Net Carbs: 20g, Protein:
33g, Fiber: 7g, Sodium: 126mg,
Potassium: 365mg.

955. Pressure Cooker Cranberry Hot Wings

Preparation Time: 45 minutes
Cooking Time: 35 minutes
Servings: 4 dozen
Ingredients:
- 1 can jellied cranberry sauce
- ¼ cup Louisiana-style hot sauce
- 2 tablespoons honey
- 1 tablespoon Dijon mustard
- ½ cup sugar-free orange juice
- 2 tablespoons soy sauce
- 2 teaspoons garlic powder
- 1 minced garlic clove

- 1 teaspoon dried minced onion
- 5 pounds chicken wings
- 1 teaspoon salt
- 2 tablespoons cold water
- 4 teaspoons cornstarch

Directions:
1. Whisk the ingredients together but discard wing tips.
2. Put the wins in your Instant Pot, and then put cranberry mixture over the top.
3. Lock lid, and then adjust the pressure to high for 10 minutes.
4. Next, do a natural pressure release and then a quick release.
5. Preheat the grill, remove the fat and, then let it roast for 20-25 minutes.
6. When browned, brush with the glaze before serving

Nutrition:
Calories: 71 per piece, Fat: 4g,
Carbs: 5g, Net Carbs: 5g,
Protein: 5g, Fiber: 0g, Sodium:
187mg, Potassium: 346mg.

956. Bacon hot Dog Bites

Preparation Time: 5 minutes
Cooking Time: 10 minutes
Servings: 12
Ingredients:
- 1 pack of hot dogs
- ½ bottle cocktail sauce
- 4 slices smoked bacon

Directions:
1. Slice the meat, set the hot dogs aside and cook the bacon until done.
2. Separate the bacon from the fat and place the hot dogs and bacon in the pot, and then add the cocktail sauce until it heats. Next. cook on High pressure 5 minutes. Do a quick release.
3. Turn off the pot and place on a serving platter, it will thicken over time.

Nutrition:
Calories: 83, Fat: 10g, Carbs: 2g,
Net Carbs: 2g, Protein: 10g,
Fiber: 0g, Sodium: 265mg,
Potassium: 324mg.

957. Instant Pot Cocktail Wieners

Preparation Time: 2 minutes
Cooking Time: 1 minute
Servings: 12
Ingredients:

- 1 package 12 cocktail wieners
- ¼ teaspoon brown sugar
- ½ cup chicken or veggie broth
- 1 jar jalapeno jelly
- ¼ cup chili sauce
- 1 diced jalapeno

Directions:
1. Put ½ cup of chicken broth into Instant Pot. Then add wieners and rest of ingredients, till everything is coated.
2. Cook on high pressure for a minute, do a quick release pressure and then serve!

Nutrition:
Calories: 92, Fat: 5g, Carbs: 6g, Net Carbs: 5g, Protein: 10g, Fiber: 1g, Sodium: 218mg, Potassium: 187mg.

958. Pressure Cooker Braised Pulled Ham

Preparation Time: 10 minutes
Cooking Time: 25 minutes
Servings: 16
Ingredients:
- 2 bottles beer, or nonalcoholic beer
- ½ teaspoon coarse ground pepper
- 1 cup Dijon mustard, divided
- 1 cooked bone-in ham
- 16 split pretzel hamburger buns
- 4 rosemary sprigs
- dill pickle slices

Directions:
1. Whisk the beer, pepper and mustard. Then add ham and rosemary, lock lid, and set pressure to high for 20 minutes. Do a natural pressure release.
2. Let it cool, discard rosemary, and skim the fat. Let it boil for 5 minutes.
3. When the ham is cool, shred with forks, discard bone and heat it again. Put the ham on the pretzel buns, adding Dijon mustard at the end and the dill pickle slices.

Nutrition:
Calories: 378, Fat: 9g, Carbs: 50g, Net Carbs: 2g, Protein: 25g, Fiber: 2g, Sodium: 286mg, Potassium: 176mg.

959. Mini Teriyaki Turkey Sandwiches

Preparation Time: 20 minutes

Cooking Time: 30 minutes
Servings: 20
Ingredients:
- 2 chicken breast halves
- 1 cup soy sauce, low-salt
- ¼ cup cider vinegar
- 3 minced garlic cloves
- 1 tablespoon fresh ginger root
- 2 tablespoons cornstarch
- 20 Hawaiian sweet rolls
- ½ teaspoon pepper
- 2 tablespoons melted butter

Directions:
1. Put turkey in the pressure cooker and combine the first six ingredients over it.
2. Cook it on manual for 25 minutes, and when finished, do a natural pressure release.
3. Push sauté after removing the turkey. Then mix cornstarch and water, stirring into cooking juices, and cook until sauce is thickened. Shred meat and stir to heat.
4. You can split the rolls, buttering each side, and bake till golden brown, adding the meat mixture to the top.

Nutrition:
Calories: 252, Fat: 5g, Carbs: 25g, Net Carbs: 24g, Protein: 26g, Fiber: 1g, Sodium: 198mg, Potassium: 197mg.

960. Elegant Cranberry Muffins

Preparation Time: 10 minutes
Cooking Time: 20 minutes
Servings: 24 muffins
Ingredients:
- 2 cups almond flour
- 2 teaspoons baking soda
- ¼ cup avocado oil
- 1 whole egg
- ¾ cup almond milk
- ½ cup Erythritol
- ½ cup apple sauce
- Zest of 1 orange
- 2 teaspoons ground cinnamon
- 2 cup fresh cranberries

Directions:
1. Preheat your oven to 350 degrees F.
2. Line a muffin tin with paper muffin cups and keep them on the side.
3. Add flour, baking soda and keep it on the side.

4. Take another bowl and whisk in the remaining ingredients. Add flour and mix well.
5. Pour batter into prepared muffin tin and bake for 20 minutes.
6. Once done, let it cool for 10 minutes.
7. Serve and enjoy!

Nutrition:
Total Carbs: 7g, Fiber: 2g, Protein: 2.3g, Fat: 7g, Sodium: 186mg, Potassium: 198mg.

961. Apple and Almond Muffins

Preparation Time: 10 minutes
Cooking Time: 20 minutes
Servings: 6 muffins
Ingredients:
- 6 ounces ground almonds
- 1 teaspoon cinnamon
- ½ teaspoon baking powder
- 1 pinch sunflower seeds
- 1 whole egg
- 1 teaspoon apple cider vinegar
- 2 tablespoons Erythritol
- 1/3 cup apple sauce

Directions:
1. Preheat your oven to 350 degrees F.
2. Line muffin tin with paper muffin cups, keep them on the side.
3. Mix in almonds, cinnamon, baking powder, sunflower seeds and keep it on the side.
4. Take another bowl and beat in eggs, apple cider vinegar, apple sauce and Erythritol.
5. Add the mix to dry ingredients and mix well until you have a smooth batter.
6. Pour batter into the tin and bake for 20 minutes.
7. Once done, let them cool.
8. Serve and enjoy!

Nutrition:
Total Carbs: 10, Fiber: 4g, Protein: 13g, Fat: 17g, Sodium: 154mg, Potassium: 216mg.

962. Stylish Chocolate Parfait

Preparation Time: 2 hours
Cooking Time: 0 minutes
Servings: 4
Ingredients:
- 2 tablespoons cocoa powder
- 1 cup almond milk

- 1 tablespoon chia seeds
- Pinch of sunflower seeds
- ½ teaspoon vanilla extract

Directions:
1. Take a bowl and add cocoa powder, almond milk, chia seeds, vanilla extract and stir.
2. Transfer to dessert glass and place in your fridge for 2 hours.
3. Serve and enjoy!

Nutrition:
Calories: 130, Fat: 5g, Carbohydrates: 7g, Protein: 16g, Sodium: 176mg, Potassium: 534mg.

963. Supreme Matcha Bomb

Preparation Time: 100 minutes
Cooking Time: 0 minutes
Servings: 10
Ingredients:
- 3/4 cup hemp seeds
- ½ cup coconut oil
- 2 tablespoons coconut almond butter
- 1 teaspoon Matcha powder
- 2 tablespoons vanilla bean extract
- ½ teaspoon mint extract
- Liquid stevia

Directions:
1. Take your blender/food processor and add hemp seeds, coconut oil, Matcha, vanilla extract and stevia.
2. Blend until you have a nice batter and divide into silicon molds.
3. Melt coconut almond butter and drizzle on top.
4. Let the cups chill and enjoy!

Nutrition:
Calories: 200, Fat: 20g, Carbohydrates: 3g, Protein: 5g, Sodium: 176mg, Potassium: 325mg.

964. Mesmerizing Avocado and Chocolate Pudding

Preparation Time: 30 minutes
Cooking Time: 0 minutes
Servings: 2
Ingredients:
- 1 avocado, chunked
- 1 tablespoon natural sweetener such as stevia
- 2 ounces cream cheese, at room temp

- ¼ teaspoon vanilla extract
- 4 tablespoons cocoa powder, unsweetened

Directions:
1. Blend listed ingredients in a blender until smooth.
2. Divide the mix between dessert bowls, chill for 30 minutes.
3. Serve and enjoy!

Nutrition:
Calories: 281, Fat: 27g, Carbohydrates: 12g, Protein: 8g, Sodium: 234mg, Potassium: 187mg.

965. Hearty Pineapple Pudding

Preparation Time: 10 minutes
Cooking Time: 5 hours
Servings: 4
Ingredients:
- 1 teaspoon baking powder
- 1 cup coconut flour
- 3 tablespoons stevia
- 3 tablespoons avocado oil
- ½ cup coconut milk
- ½ cup pecans, chopped
- ½ cup pineapple, chopped
- ½ cup lemon zest, grated
- 1 cup pineapple juice, natural

Directions:
1. Grease Slow Cooker with oil.
2. Take a bowl and mix in flour, stevia, baking powder, oil, milk, pecans, pineapple, lemon zest, pineapple juice and stir well.
3. Pour the mix into the Slow Cooker.
4. Place lid and cook on LOW for 5 hours.
5. Divide between bowls and serve.
6. Enjoy!

Nutrition:
Calories: 188, Fat: 3g, Carbohydrates: 14g, Protein: 5g, Sodium: 324mg, Potassium: 276mg.

966. Healthy Berry Cobbler

Preparation Time: 10 minutes
Cooking Time: 2 hours 30 minutes
Servings: 8
Ingredients:
- 1 ¼ cups almond flour
- 1 cup coconut sugar
- 1 teaspoon baking powder
- ½ teaspoon cinnamon powder
- 1 whole egg
- ¼ cup low-fat milk

- 2 tablespoons olive oil
- 2 cups raspberries
- 2 cups blueberries

Directions:
1. Take a bowl and add almond flour, coconut sugar, baking powder and cinnamon.
2. Stir well.
3. Take another bowl and add egg, milk, oil, raspberries, blueberries and stir.
4. Combine both of the mixtures.
5. Grease your Slow Cooker.
6. Pour the combined mixture into your Slow Cooker and cook on HIGH for 2 hours 30 minutes.
7. Divide between serving bowls and enjoy!

Nutrition:
Calories: 250, Fat: 4g, Carbohydrates: 30g, Protein: 3g, Sodium: 231mg, Potassium: 198mg.

967. Tasty Poached Apples

Preparation Time: 10 minutes
Cooking Time: 2 hours 30 minutes
Servings: 8
Ingredients:
- 6 apples, cored, peeled and sliced
- 1 cup apple juice, natural
- 1 cup coconut sugar
- 1 tablespoon cinnamon powder

Directions:
1. Grease Slow Cooker with cooking spray.
2. Add apples, sugar, juice, cinnamon to your Slow Cooker.
3. Stir gently.
4. Place lid and cook on HIGH for 4 hours.
5. Serve cold and enjoy!

Nutrition:
Calories: 180, Fat: 5g, Carbohydrates: 8g, Protein: 4g, Sodium: 213mg, Potassium: 276mg.

968. Home Made Trail Mix for the Trip

Preparation Time: 10 minutes
Cooking Time: 55 minutes
Servings: 4
Ingredients:
- ¼ cup raw cashews
- ¼ cup almonds
- ¼ cup walnuts
- 1 teaspoon cinnamon

- 2 tablespoons melted coconut oil
- Sunflower seeds as needed

Directions:
1. Put the nuts in a large bowl and add the cinnamon and melted coconut oil.
2. Stir. Line a baking sheet with parchment paper.
3. Preheat your oven to 275 degrees F.
4. Melt coconut oil and keep it on
5. Sprinkle sunflower seeds.
6. Place in oven and brown for 6 minutes.
7. Enjoy!

Nutrition:
Calories: 363, Fat: 22g, Carbohydrates: 41g, Protein: 7g, Sodium: 175mg, Potassium: 234mg.

969. Heart Warming Cinnamon Rice Pudding

Preparation Time: 10 minutes
Cooking Time: 5 hours
Servings: 4
Ingredients:
- 6 ½ cups water
- 1 cup coconut sugar
- 2 cups white rice
- 2 cinnamon sticks
- ½ cup coconut, shredded

Directions:
1. Add water, rice, sugar, cinnamon and coconut to your Slow Cooker.
2. Gently stir.
3. Place lid and cook on HIGH for 5 hours.
4. Discard cinnamon.
5. Divide pudding between dessert dishes and enjoy!

Nutrition:
Calories: 173, Fat: 4g, Carbohydrates: 9g, Protein: 4g, Sodium: 216mg, Potassium: 342mg.

970. Pure Avocado Pudding

Preparation Time: 3 hours
Cooking Time: 0 minutes
Servings: 4
Ingredients:
- 1 cup almond milk
- 2 avocados, peeled and pitted

- ¾ cup cocoa powder
- 1 teaspoon vanilla extract
- 2 tablespoons stevia
- ¼ teaspoon cinnamon
- Walnuts, chopped for serving

Directions:
1. Add avocados to a blender and pulse well.
2. Add cocoa powder, almond milk, stevia, vanilla bean extract and pulse the mixture well.
3. Pour into serving bowls and top with walnuts.
4. Chill for 2-3 hours and serve!

Nutrition:
Calories: 221, Fat: 8g, Carbohydrates: 7g, Protein: 3g, Sodium: 234mg, Potassium: 433mg.

971. Spicy Popper Mug Cake

Preparation Time: 5 minutes
Cooking Time: 5 minutes
Servings: 2
Ingredients:
- 2 tablespoons almond flour
- 1 tablespoon flaxseed meal
- 1 tablespoon almond butter
- 1 tablespoon cream cheese
- 1 large egg
- 1 bacon, cooked and sliced
- ½ jalapeno pepper
- ½ teaspoon baking powder
- ¼ teaspoon sunflower seeds

Directions:
1. Take a frying pan and place it over medium heat.
2. Add a slice of bacon and cook until it has a crispy texture.
3. Take a microwave proof container and mix all the listed ingredients (including cooked bacon), clean the sides.
4. Microwave for 75 seconds, making to put your microwave to high power.
5. Take out the cup and tap it against a surface to take the cake out.
6. Garnish with a bit of jalapeno and serve!

Nutrition:
Calories: 429, Fat: 38g, Carbohydrates: 6g, Protein: 16g, Sodium: 138mg, Potassium: 124mg.

972. The Most Elegant Parsley Soufflé Ever

Preparation Time: 5 minutes
Cooking Time: 6 minutes
Servings: 5
Ingredients:
- 2 whole eggs
- 1 fresh red chili pepper, chopped
- 2 tablespoons coconut cream
- 1 tablespoon fresh parsley, chopped
- Sunflower seeds to taste

Directions:
1. Preheat your oven to 390 degrees F.
2. Almond butter 2 soufflé dishes.
3. Add the ingredients to a blender and mix well.
4. Divide batter into soufflé dishes and bake for 6 minutes.
5. Serve and enjoy!

Nutrition:
Calories: 108, Fat: 9g, Carbohydrates: 9g, Protein: 6g, Sodium: 154mg, Potassium: 324mg.

973. Fennel and Almond Bites

Preparation Time: 10 minutes
Cooking Time: 0 minutes
Freeze Time: 3 hours
Servings: 12
Ingredients:
- 1 teaspoon vanilla extract
- ¼ cup almond milk
- ¼ cup cocoa powder
- ½ cup almond oil
- A pinch of sunflower seeds
- 1 teaspoon fennel seeds

Directions:
1. Take a bowl and mix the almond oil and almond milk.
2. Beat until smooth and glossy using an electric beater.
3. Mix in the rest of the ingredients.
4. Take a piping bag and pour it into a parchment paper-lined baking sheet.
5. Freeze for 3 hours and store in the fridge.

Nutrition:
Total Carbs: 1g, Fiber: 1g, Protein: 1g, Fat: 20g, Sodium: 213mg, Potassium: 216mg.

974. Feisty Coconut Fudge

Preparation Time: 20 minutes
Cooking Time: 0 minutes
Freeze Time: 2 hours
Servings: 12
Ingredients:

- ¼ cup coconut, shredded
- 2 cups coconut oil
- ½ cup coconut cream
- ¼ cup almonds, chopped
- 1 teaspoon almond extract
- A pinch of sunflower seeds
- Stevia to taste

Directions:

1. Take a large bowl and pour coconut cream and coconut oil into it.
2. Whisk using an electric beater.
3. Whisk until the mixture becomes smooth and glossy.
4. Add the cocoa powder slowly and mix well.
5. Add in the rest of the ingredients.
6. Pour into a bread pan lined with parchment paper.
7. Freeze until set.
8. Cut them into squares and serve.

Nutrition:
Total Carbs: 1g, Fiber: 1g, Protein: 0g, Fat: 20g, Sodium: 213mg, Potassium: 324mg.

975. No Bake Cheesecake

Preparation Time: 120 minutes
Cooking Time: 0 minutes
Servings: 10
Ingredients:
For Crust:

- 2 tablespoons ground flaxseeds
- 2 tablespoons desiccated coconut
- 1 teaspoon cinnamon

For Filling:

- 4 ounces vegan cream cheese
- 1 cup cashews, soaked
- ½ cup frozen blueberries
- 2 tablespoons coconut oil
- 1 tablespoon lemon juice
- 1 teaspoon vanilla extract
- Liquid stevia

Directions:

1. Take a container and mix in the crust ingredients, mix well.
2. Flatten the mixture at the bottom to prepare the crust of your cheesecake.

3. Take a blender/ food processor and add the filling ingredients, blend until smooth.
4. Gently pour the batter on top of your crust and chill for 2 hours.
5. Serve and enjoy!

Nutrition:
Calories: 182, Fat: 16g, Carbohydrates: 4g, Protein: 3g, Sodium: 213mg, Potassium: 165mg.

976. Easy Chia Seed Pumpkin Pudding

Preparation Time: 10-15 minutes/ overnight chill time
Cooking Time: 0 minutes
Servings: 4
Ingredients:

- 1 cup maple syrup
- 2 teaspoons pumpkin spice
- 1 cup pumpkin puree
- 1 ¼ cup almond milk
- ½ cup chia seeds

Directions:

1. Add all the ingredients to a bowl and gently stir.
2. Let it refrigerate overnight or at least 15 minutes.
3. Top with your desired ingredients, such as blueberries, almonds, etc.
4. Serve and enjoy!

Nutrition:
Calories: 230, Fat: 10g, Carbohydrates: 22g, Protein: 11g, Sodium: 176mg, Potassium: 234mg.

977. Lovely Blueberry Pudding

Preparation Time: 20 minutes
Cooking Time: 0 minutes
Servings: 4
Ingredients:

- 2 cups frozen blueberries
- 2 teaspoons lime zest, grated freshly
- 20 drops liquid stevia
- 2 small avocados, peeled, pitted and chopped
- ½ teaspoon fresh ginger, grated freshly
- 4 tablespoons fresh lime juice
- 10 tablespoons water

Directions:

1. Add all the listed ingredients to a blender (except blueberries) and pulse the mixture well.

2. Transfer the mix into small serving bowls and chill the bowls.
3. Serve with a topping of blueberries.
4. Enjoy!

Nutrition:
Calories: 166, Fat: 13g, Carbohydrates: 13g, Protein: 1.7g, Sodium: 216mg, Potassium: 187mg.

978. Decisive Lime and Strawberry Popsicle

Preparation Time: 2 hours
Cooking Time: 0 minutes
Servings: 4
Ingredients:

- 1 tablespoon lime juice, fresh
- ¼ cup strawberries, hulled and sliced
- ¼ cup coconut almond milk, unsweetened and full fat
- 2 teaspoons natural sweetener

Directions:

1. Blend the listed ingredients in a blender until smooth.
2. Pour mix into Popsicle molds and let them chill for 2 hours.
3. Serve and enjoy!

Nutrition:
Calories: 166, Fat: 17g, Carbohydrates: 3g, Protein: 1g, Sodium: 187mg, Potassium: 179mg.

979. Ravaging Blueberry Muffin

Preparation Time: 10 minutes
Cooking Time: 30 minutes
Servings: 4
Ingredients:

- 1 cup almond flour
- Pinch of sunflower seeds
- 1/8 teaspoon baking soda
- 1 whole egg
- 2 tablespoons coconut oil, melted
- ½ cup coconut almond milk
- ¼ cup fresh blueberries

Directions:

1. Preheat your oven to 350 degrees F.
2. Line a muffin tin with paper muffin cups.

3. Add almond flour, sunflower seeds, baking soda to a bowl and mix, keep it on the side.
4. Take another bowl and add egg, coconut oil, coconut almond milk and mix.
5. Add mix to flour mix and gently combine until incorporated.
6. Mix in blueberries and fill the cupcake tins with batter.
7. Bake for 20-25 minutes.
8. Enjoy!

Nutrition:
Calories: 167, Fat: 15g, Carbohydrates: 2.1g, Protein: 5.2g, Sodium: 186mg, Potassium: 187mg.

980. The Coconut Loaf

Preparation Time: 15 minutes
Cooking Time: 40 minutes
Servings: 4
Ingredients:
- 1 ½ tablespoons coconut flour
- ¼ teaspoon baking powder
- 1/8 teaspoon sunflower seeds
- 1 tablespoon coconut oil, melted
- 1 whole egg

Directions:
1. Preheat your oven to 350 degrees F.
2. Add coconut flour, baking powder, sunflower seeds.
3. Add coconut oil, eggs and stir well until mixed.
4. Leave the batter for several minutes.
5. Pour half batter onto the baking pan.
6. Spread it to form a circle, repeat with the remaining batter.
7. Bake in the oven for 10 minutes.
8. Once you have a golden-brown texture, let it cool and serve.
9. Enjoy!

Nutrition:
Calories: 297, Fat: 14g, Carbohydrates: 15g, Protein: 15g, Sodium: 198mg, Potassium: 243mg.

981. Fresh Figs with Walnuts and Ricotta

Preparation Time: 5 minutes
Cooking Time: 2-3 minutes
Servings: 4
Ingredients:
- 8 dried figs, halved
- ¼ cup ricotta cheese
- 16 walnuts, halved

- 1 tablespoon honey

Directions:
1. Take a skillet and place it over medium heat. Add walnuts and toast for 2 minutes.
2. Top figs with cheese and walnuts.
3. Drizzle honey on top.
4. Enjoy!

Nutrition:
Calories: 142, Fat: 8g, Carbohydrates: 10g, Protein: 4g, Sodium: 187mg, Potassium: 187mg.

982. Authentic Medjool Date Truffles

Preparation Time: 10-15 minutes
Cooking Time: 0 minutes
Servings: 4
Ingredients:
- 2 tablespoons peanut oil
- ½ cup popcorn kernels
- 1/3 cup peanuts, chopped
- 1/3 cup peanut almond butter
- ¼ cup wildflower honey

Directions:
1. Take a pot and add popcorn kernels, peanut oil.
2. Place it over medium heat and shake the pot gently until all corn has popped.
3. Take a saucepan and add honey, gently simmer for 2-3 minutes.
4. Add peanut almond butter and stir.
5. Coat popcorn with the mixture and enjoy!

Nutrition:
Calories: 430, Fat: 20g, Carbohydrates: 56g, Protein: 9g, Sodium: 236mg, Potassium: 187mg.

983. Tasty Mediterranean Peanut Almond Butter Popcorns

Preparation Time: 5 minutes + 20 minutes chill time
Cooking Time: 2-3 minutes
Servings: 4
Ingredients:
- 3 cups Medjool dates, chopped
- 12 ounces brewed coffee
- 1 cup pecans, chopped
- ½ cup coconut, shredded
- ½ cup cocoa powder

Directions:
1. Soak dates in warm coffee for 5 minutes.
2. Remove dates from coffee and mash them, making a fine smooth mixture.
3. Stir in the remaining ingredients (except cocoa powder) and form small balls out of the mixture.
4. Coat with cocoa powder, serve and enjoy!

Nutrition:
Calories: 265, Fat: 12g, Carbohydrates: 43g, Protein: 3g, Sodium: 234mg, Potassium: 176mg.

984. Just a Minute Worth Muffin

Preparation Time: 5 minutes
Cooking Time: 1 minute
Servings: 2
Ingredients:
- Coconut oil for grease
- 2 teaspoons coconut flour
- 1 pinch baking soda
- 1 pinch sunflower seeds
- 1 whole egg

Directions:
1. Grease ramekin dish with coconut oil and keep it on the side.
2. Add ingredients to a bowl and combine until no lumps.
3. Pour batter into the ramekin.
4. Microwave for 1 minute on HIGH.
5. Slice in half and serve.
6. Enjoy!

Nutrition:
Total Carbs: 5.4, Fiber: 2g, Protein: 7.3g, Sodium: 187mg, Potassium: 323mg.

985. Hearty Almond Bread

Preparation Time: 15 minutes
Cooking Time: 60 minutes
Servings: 8
Ingredients:
- 3 cups almond flour
- 1 teaspoon baking soda
- 2 teaspoons baking powder
- ¼ teaspoon sunflower seeds
- ¼ cup almond milk
- ½ cup + 2 tablespoons olive oil
- 3 whole eggs

Directions:
1. Preheat your oven to 300 degrees F.

2. Take a 9x5 inch loaf pan and grease, keep it on the side.
3. Add listed ingredients to a bowl and pour the batter into the loaf pan.
4. Bake for 60 minutes.
5. Once baked, remove from the oven and let it cool.
6. Slice and serve!

Nutrition:
Calories: 277, Fat: 21g, Carbohydrates: 7g, Protein: 10g, Sodium: 186mg, Potassium: 165mg.

986. Mixed Berries Smoothie

Preparation Time: 4 minutes
Cooking Time: 0 minutes
Servings: 2
Ingredients:
- ¼ cup frozen blueberries
- ¼ cup frozen blackberries
- 1 cup unsweetened almond milk
- 1 teaspoon vanilla bean extract
- 3 teaspoons flaxseeds
- 1 scoop chilled Greek yogurt
- Stevia as needed

Directions:
1. Mix everything in a blender and emulsify.
2. Pulse the mixture until you have your desired thickness.
3. Pour the mixture into a glass and enjoy!

Nutrition:
Calories: 221, Fat: 9g, Protein: 21g, Carbohydrates: 10g, Sodium: 187mg, Potassium: 123mg.

987. Satisfying Berry and Almond Smoothie

Preparation Time: 10 minutes
Cooking Time: 0 minutes
Servings: 4
Ingredients:
- 1 cup blueberries, frozen
- 1 whole banana
- ½ cup almond milk
- 1 tablespoon almond butter
- Water as needed

Directions:
1. Add the listed ingredients to your blender and blend well until you have a smoothie-like texture.
2. Chill and serve.
3. Enjoy!

Nutrition:
Calories: 321, Fat: 11g, Carbohydrates: 55g, Protein: 5g, Sodium: 185mg, Potassium: 187mg.

988. Refreshing Mango and Pear Smoothie

Preparation Time: 10 minutes
Cooking Time: 0 minutes
Servings: 1
Ingredients:
- 1 ripe mango, cored and chopped
- ½ mango, peeled, pitted and chopped
- 1 cup kale, chopped
- ½ cup plain Greek yogurt
- 2 ice cubes

Directions:
1. Add pear, mango, yogurt, kale, and mango to a blender and puree.
2. Add ice and blend until you have a smooth texture.
3. Serve and enjoy!

Nutrition:
Calories: 293, Fat: 8g, Carbohydrates: 53g, Protein: 8g, Sodium: 186mg, Potassium: 276mg.

989. Epic Pineapple Juice

Preparation Time: 10 minutes
Cooking Time: 0 minutes
Servings: 4
Ingredients:
- 4 cups fresh pineapple, chopped
- 1 pinch sunflower seeds
- 1 ½ cups water

Directions:
1. Add the listed ingredients to your blender and blend well until you have a smoothie-like texture.
2. Chill and serve.
3. Enjoy!

Nutrition:
Calories: 82, Fat: 0.2g, Carbohydrates: 21g, Protein: 21 Sodium: 343mg, Potassium: 298mg.

990. Choco Lovers Strawberry Shake

Preparation Time: 10 minutes

Cooking Time: 0 minutes
Servings: 1
Ingredients:
- ½ cup heavy cream, liquid
- 1 tablespoon cocoa powder
- 1 pack stevia
- ½ cup strawberry, sliced
- 1 tablespoon coconut flakes, unsweetened
- 1 ½ cups water

Directions:
1. Add listed ingredients to a blender.
2. Blend until you have a smooth and creamy texture.
3. Serve chilled and enjoy!

Nutrition:
Calories: 470, Fat: 46g, Carbohydrates: 15g, Protein: 4g, Sodium: 324mg, Potassium: 278mg.

991. Healthy Coffee Smoothie

Preparation Time: 10 minutes
Cooking Time: 0 minutes
Servings: 1
Ingredients:
- 1 tablespoon chia seeds
- 2 cups strongly brewed coffee, chilled
- 1 ounce Macadamia nuts
- 1-2 packets stevia, optional
- 1 tablespoon MCT oil

Directions:
1. Add all the listed ingredients to a blender.
2. Blend on high until smooth and creamy.
3. Enjoy your smoothie.

Nutrition:
Calories: 395, Fat: 39g, Carbohydrates: 11g, Protein: 5.2g, Sodium: 329mg, Potassium: 231mg.

992. Blackberry and Apple Smoothie

Preparation Time: 5 minutes
Cooking Time: 0 minutes
Servings: 2
Ingredients:
- 2 cups frozen blackberries
- ½ cup apple cider
- 1 apple, cubed
- 2/3 cup non-fat lemon yogurt

Directions:

1. Add the listed ingredients to your blender and blend until smooth.
2. Serve chilled!

Nutrition:
Calories: 200, Fat: 10g, Carbohydrates: 14g, Protein: 2g, Sodium: 165mg, Potassium: 170mg.

993. The Mean Green Smoothie

Preparation Time: 5 minutes
Cooking Time: 0 minutes
Servings: 2
Ingredients:
- 1 avocado
- 1 handful spinach, chopped
- Cucumber, 2-inch slices, peeled
- 1 lime, chopped
- Handful of grapes, chopped
- 5 dates, stoned and chopped
- 1 cup apple juice (fresh)

Directions:
1. Add all the listed ingredients to your blender.
2. Blend until smooth.
3. Add a few ice cubes and serve the smoothie.
4. Enjoy!

Nutrition:
Calories: 200, Fat: 10g, Carbohydrates: 14g, Protein: 2g, Sodium: 175mg, Potassium: 187mg.

994. Mint Flavored Pear Smoothie

Preparation Time: 5 minutes
Cooking Time: 0 minutes
Servings: 2
Ingredients:
- ¼ honey dew
- 2 green pears, ripe
- ½ apple, juiced
- 1 cup ice cubes
- ½ cup fresh mint leaves

Directions:
1. Add the listed ingredients to your blender and blend until smooth.
2. Serve chilled!

Nutrition:
Calories: 200, Fat: 10g, Carbohydrates: 14g, Protein: 2g, Sodium: 186mg, Potassium: 186mg.

995. Chilled Watermelon Smoothie

Preparation Time: 5 minutes
Cooking Time: 0 minutes
Servings: 2
Ingredients:
- 1 cup watermelon chunks
- ½ cup coconut water
- 1 ½ teaspoons lime juice
- 4 mint leaves
- 4 ice cubes

Directions:
1. Add the listed ingredients to your blender and blend until smooth.
2. Serve chilled!

Nutrition:
Calories: 200, Fat: 10g, Carbohydrates: 14g, Protein: 2g, Sodium: 544mg, Potassium: 234mg.

996. Banana Ginger Medley

Preparation Time: 5 minutes
Cooking Time: 0 minutes
Servings: 2
Ingredients:
- 1 banana, sliced
- ¾ cup vanilla yogurt
- 1 tablespoon honey
- ½ teaspoon ginger, grated

Directions:
1. Add the listed ingredients to your blender and blend until smooth.
2. Serve chilled!

Nutrition:
Calories: 200, Fat: 10g, Carbohydrates: 14g, Protein: 2g, Sodium: 134mg, Potassium: 255mg.

997. Banana and Almond Flax Glass

Preparation Time: 5 minutes
Cooking Time: 0 minutes
Servings: 2
Ingredients:
- 1 ripe frozen banana, diced
- 2/3 cup unsweetened almond milk
- 1/3 cup fat-free plain Greek Yogurt
- 1 ½ tablespoons almond butter
- 1 tablespoon flaxseed meal
- 1 teaspoon honey
- 2-3 drops almond extract

Directions:
1. Add the listed ingredients to your blender and blend until smooth
2. Serve chilled!

Nutrition:
Calories: 200, Fat: 10g, Carbohydrates: 14g, Protein: 2g, Sodium: 534mg, Potassium: 265mg.

998. Sensational Strawberry Medley

Preparation Time: 5 minutes
Cooking Time: 0 minutes
Servings: 2
Ingredients:
- 1-2 handful baby greens
- 3 medium kale leaves
- 5-8 mint leaves
- 1-inch piece ginger, peeled
- 1 avocado
- 1 cup strawberries
- 6-8 ounces coconut water + 6-8 ounces filtered water
- Fresh juice of one lime
- 1-2 teaspoon olive oil

Directions:
1. Add all the listed ingredients to your blender.
2. Blend until smooth.
3. Add a few ice cubes and serve the smoothie.
4. Enjoy!

Nutrition: Calories: 200, Fat: 10g, Carbohydrates: 14g, Protein: 2g, Sodium: 234mg, Potassium: 176mg.

999. Healthy Tahini Buns

Preparation Time: 10 minutes
Cooking Time: 15-20 minutes
Servings: 3 buns
Ingredients:
- 1 whole egg
- 5 tablespoons Tahini paste
- ½ teaspoon baking soda
- 1 teaspoon lemon juice
- 1 pinch salt

Directions:
1. Preheat your oven to 350 degrees F.
2. Line a baking sheet with parchment paper and keep it on the side.
3. Add the listed ingredients to a blender and blend until you have a smooth batter.

4. Scoop batter onto prepared sheet forming buns.
5. Bake for 15-20 minutes.
6. Once done, remove from the oven and let them cool.
7. Serve and enjoy!

Nutrition:
Total Carbs: 7g, Fiber: 2g, Protein: 6g, Fat: 14g, Calories: 172, Sodium: 234mg, Potassium: 125mg.

1000. Spicy Pecan Bowl

Preparation Time: 10 minutes
Cooking Time: 120 minutes
Servings: 3
Ingredients:
- 1 pound pecans, halved
- 2 tablespoons olive oil
- 1 teaspoon basil, dried
- 1 tablespoon chili powder
- 1 teaspoon oregano, dried
- ¼ teaspoon garlic powder
- 1 teaspoon rosemary, dried
- ½ teaspoon onion powder

Directions:
1. Add pecans, oil, basil, chili powder, oregano, garlic powder, onion powder, rosemary and toss well.
2. Transfer to Slow Cooker and cook on LOW for 2 hours.
3. Divide between bowls and serve.

Enjoy!

Nutrition: Calories: 152, Fat: 3g, Carbohydrates: 11g, Protein: 2g, Sodium: 56mg, Potassium: 125mg.

Chapter 19. Meal Plan

Week 1

Days	Breakfast	Snacks	Lunch	Snacks	Dinner	Total
1	Blueberry Waffles	Herb-Marinated Feta and Artichokes	Zucchini Zoodles with Chicken and Basil	Spinach and Endives Salad	Shrimp Cocktail	770mg
2	Apple Pancakes	Yellowfin Croquettes	Parmesan Baked Chicken	Basil Olives Mix	Squid and Shrimp Salad	1271mg
3	Super-Simple Granola	Spiced Salmon Crudités	Crazy Japanese Potato and Beef Croquettes	Arugula Salad	Parsley Seafood Cocktail	502mg
4	Savory Yogurt Bowls	All-Spiced Olives	Golden Eggplant Fries	Spanish rice	Shrimp and Onion Ginger Dressing	1269mg
5	Energy Sunrise Muffins	Pitted Olives and Anchovies	Very Wild Mushroom Pilaf	Sweet Potatoes and Apples	Fruit Shrimp Soup	551mg
6	Spinach, Egg, and Cheese Breakfast Quesadillas	Medi Deviled Eggs	Sporty Baby Carrots	Roasted Turnips	Mussels and Chickpea Soup	1434mg
7	Simple Cheese and Broccoli Omelets	Cheese Crackers	Garden Salad	No-Mayo Potato Salad	Fish Stew	844mg

Week 2

Days	Breakfast	Snacks	Lunch	Snacks	Dinner	
1	Creamy Avocado and Egg Salad Sandwiches	Cheesy Caprese Stack	Baked Smoky Broccoli and Garlic	Zucchini Tomato Bake	Shrimp and Broccoli Soup	1267mg
2	Breakfast Hash	Zucchini-Cheese Fritters with Aioli	Roasted Cauliflower and Lima Beans	Creamy Broccoli Cheddar Rice	Coconut Turkey Mix	1166mg
3	Hearty Breakfast Casserole	Cucumbers Filled with Salmon	Thai Roasted Spicy Black Beans and Choy Sum	Smashed Brussels sprouts	Lime Shrimp and Kale	1387mg
4	Creamy Apple-Avocado Smoothie	Smoked Mackerel Pâté	Simple Roasted Broccoli and Cauliflower	Cilantro Lime Rice	Parsley Cod Mix	1028mg
5	Strawberry, Orange,	Medi Fat: Bombs	Roasted Napa Cabbage	Corn Salad with Lime Vinaigrette	Salmon and	993mg

	and Beet Smoothie		and Turnips Extra		Cabbage Mix	
6	Blueberry-Vanilla Yogurt Smoothie	Avocado Cold Soup	Simple Roasted Kale Artichoke Heart and Choy Sum Extra	Mediterranean Chickpea Salad	Decent Beef and Onion Stew	506mg
7	Greek Yogurt Oat Pancakes	Crab Cake Lettuce Cups	Roasted Kale and Bok Choy Extra	Italian Roasted Cabbage	Clean Parsley and Chicken Breast	967mg

Week 3

Days	Breakfast	Snacks	Lunch	Snacks	Dinner	
1	Scrambled Egg and Veggie Breakfast Quesadillas	Orange-Tarragon Chicken Salad Wrap	Roasted Soy Beans and Winter Squash	Tex-Mex Cole Slaw	Zucchini Beef Sauté with Coriander Greens	816mg
2	Stuffed Breakfast Peppers	Feta and Quinoa Stuffed Mushrooms	Roasted Button Mushrooms and Squash	Roasted Okra	Hearty Lemon and Pepper Chicken	621mg
3	Sweet Potato Toast Three Ways	Five-Ingredient Falafel with Garlic-Yogurt Sauce	Roasted Tomatoes Rutabaga and Kohlrabi Main	Brown Sugar Glazed Carrots	Walnuts and Asparagus Delight	595mg
4	Apple-Apricot Brown Rice Breakfast Porridge	Lemon Shrimp with Garlic Olive Oil	Roasted Brussels sprouts and Broccoli	Oven-Roasted Beets with Honey Ricotta	Healthy Carrot Chips	680mg
5	Carrot Cake Overnight Oats	Crispy Green Bean Fries with Lemon-Yogurt Sauce	Roasted Broccoli Sweet Potatoes & Bean Sprouts	Easy Carrots Mix	Beef Soup	632mg
6	Steel-Cut Oatmeal with Plums and Pear	Homemade Sea Salt Pita Chips	Roasted Sweet Potato and Red Beets	Tasty Grilled Asparagus	Amazing Grilled Chicken and Blueberry Salad	1014mg
7	French toast with Applesauce	Baked Spanakopita Dip	Sichuan Style Baked Chioggia Beets and Broccoli Florets	Roasted Carrots	Clean Chicken and Mushroom Stew	502mg

Week 4

Days	Breakfast	Snacks	Lunch	Snacks	Dinner	
1	Banana-Peanut Butter and	Roasted Pearl	Baked Enoki and Mini Cabbage	Oven Roasted Asparagus	Elegant Pumpkin Chili Dish	509mg

	Greens Smoothie	Onion Dip				
2	Baking Powder Biscuits	Red Pepper Tapenade	Roasted Triple Mushrooms	Baked Potato with Thyme	Tasty Roasted Broccoli	553mg
3	Oatmeal Banana Pancakes with Walnuts	Greek Potato Skins with Olives and Feta	Roasted Mini Cabbage and Sweet Potato	Spicy Brussels sprouts	The Almond Breaded Chicken Goodness	821mg
4	Creamy Oats, Greens & Blueberry Smoothie	Artichoke and Olive Pita Flatbread	Tofu & Green Bean Stir-Fry	Baked Cauliflower with Chili	South-Western Pork Chops	691mg
5	Banana & Cinnamon Oatmeal	Mini Crab Cakes	Peanut Vegetable Pad Thai	Baked Broccoli	Almond butter Pork Chops	739mg
6	Bagels Made Healthy	Zucchini Feta Roulades	Spicy Tofu Burrito Bowls with Cilantro Avocado Sauce	Slow Cooked Potatoes with Cheddar	Chicken Salsa	802mg
7	Cereal with Cranberry-Orange Twist	Garlic-Roasted Tomatoes and Olives	Sweet Potato Cakes with Classic Guacamole	Squash Salad with Orange	Healthy Mediterranean Lamb Chops	648mg

Week 5

Days	Breakfast	Snacks	Lunch	Snacks	Dinner	
1	No Cook Overnight Oats	Chocolate Oatmeal	Chickpea Cauliflower Tikka Masala	Colored Iceberg Salad	Amazing Sesame Breadsticks	688mg
2	Avocado Cup with Egg	Goat Cheese and Garlic Crostini	Eggplant Parmesan Stacks	Fennel Salad with Arugula	Brown Butter Duck Breast	776mg
3	Mediterranean Toast	Rosemary-Roasted Red Potatoes	Roasted Vegetable Enchiladas	Corn Mix	Generous Garlic Bread Stick	812mg
4	Instant Banana Oatmeal	Guaca Egg Scramble	Lentil Avocado Tacos	Persimmon Salad	Cauliflower Bread Stick	812mg
5	Almond Butter-Banana Smoothie	Morning Tostadas	Tomato & Olive Orecchiette with Basil Pesto	Avocado Side Salad	Bacon and Chicken Garlic Wrap	875mg
6	Brown Sugar Cinnamon Oatmeal	Cheese Omelet	Italian Stuffed Portobello Mushroom Burgers	Spiced Broccoli Florets	Chipotle Lettuce Chicken	976mg
7	Buckwheat Pancakes with Vanilla Almond Milk	Fruity Pizza	Gnocchi with Tomato Basil Sauce	Lima Beans Dish	Balsamic Chicken and Vegetables	946mg

Week 6

Days	Breakfast	Snacks	Lunch	Snacks	Dinner	
1	Salmon and Egg Scramble	Morning Sprouts Pizza	Creamy Pumpkin Pasta	Soy Sauce Green Beans	Exuberant Sweet Potatoes	628mg
2	Pumpkin Muffins	Quinoa with Banana and Cinnamon	Mexican-Style Potato Casserole	Butter Corn	The Vegan Lovers Refried Beans	902mg
3	weet Berries Pancake	Egg Casserole	Black Bean Stew with Cornbread	Stevia Peas with Marjoram	Cool Apple and Carrot Harmony	655mg
4	Zucchini Pancakes	Cheese-Cauliflower Fritters	Mushroom Florentine	Pilaf with Bella Mushrooms	Mac and Chokes	211mg
5	Breakfast Banana Split	Creamy Oatmeal Figs	Hassel back Eggplant	Parsley Fennel	Black Eyed Peas and Spinach Platter	212mg
6	Easy Veggie Muffins	Baked Cinnamon Oatmeal	Vegetarian Kebabs	Sweet Butternut	Humble Mushroom Rice	224mg
7	Carrot Muffins	Chia and Nut Porridge	White Beans Stew	Mushroom Sausages	Sweet and Sour Cabbage and Apples	704mg

Week 7

Days	Breakfast	Snacks	Lunch	Snacks	Dinner	
1	Pineapple Oatmeal	Cinnamon Roll Oats	Vegetarian Lasagna	Parsley Red Potatoes	Delicious Aloo Palak	670mg
2	Spinach Muffins	Pumpkin Oatmeal with Spices	Pan-Fried Salmon with Salad	Jalapeno Black-Eyed Peas Mix	Orange and Chili Garlic Sauce	564mg
3	Chia Seeds Breakfast Mix	Turmeric Endives	Veggie Variety	Sour Cream Green Beans	Tantalizing Mushroom Gravy	426mg
4	Breakfast Fruits Bowls	Parmesan Endives	Vegetable Pasta	Cumin Brussels sprouts	Everyday Vegetable Stock	261mg
5	Pumpkin Cookies	Lemon Asparagus	Vegetable Noodles with Bolognese	Peach and Carrots	Grilled Chicken with Lemon and Fennel	632mg
6	Veggie Scramble	Lime Carrots	Harissa Bolognese with Vegetable Noodles	Baby Spinach and Grains Mix	Caramelized Pork Chops and Onion	750mg
7	Mushrooms and Turkey Breakfast	Garlic Potato Pan	Curry Vegetable Noodles with Chicken	Quinoa Curry	Hearty Pork Belly Casserole	958mg

Week 8

Days	Breakfast	Snacks	Lunch	Snacks	Dinner	
1	Mushrooms and Cheese Omelet	Balsamic Cabbage	Sweet and Sour Vegetable Noodles	Lemon and Cilantro Rice	Apple Pie Crackers	795mg
2	Egg White Breakfast Mix	Chili Broccoli	Tuna Sandwich	Chili Beans	Paprika Lamb Chops	1055mg
3	Pesto Omelet	Hot Brussels sprouts	Fruited Quinoa Salad	Bean Spread	Fennel Sauce Tenderloin	1462mg
4	Quinoa Bowls	Paprika Brussels sprouts	Turkey Wrap	Stir-Fried Steak, Shiitake, and Asparagus	Beefy Fennel Stew	1188mg
5	Strawberry Sandwich	Creamy Cauliflower Mash	Chicken Wrap	Chickpeas and Curried Veggies	Currant Pork Chops	683mg
6	Apple Quinoa Muffins	Avocado, Tomato, and Olives Salad	Veggie Wrap	Brussels sprouts Casserole	Spicy Tomato Shrimp	1175mg
7	Very Berry Muesli	Radish and Olives Salad	Salmon Wrap	Lemon and Cilantro Rice	Beef Stir Fry	1296mg

Conclusion

The Dash diet has gained popularity in recent years as it is extremely helpful in strengthening metabolism and controlling hypertension. Contrary to popular belief that by following the Dash diet you only eat vegetarian foods, you get a balanced diet that includes fresh fruits, vegetables, nuts, low-fat dairy products and whole grains. You don't have to stop eating meat completely, just reduce the sodium and fat content of your daily diet.

The diet also has many health benefits, helping to reduce hypertension and obesity, decreasing osteoporosis and preventing cancer. This balanced diet boosts metabolism, which helps break down fat deposits stored in the body. This improves a person's overall health.

This book provides an 8-week meal plan with morning and afternoon snack options. However, you can consult experts in case you suffer from contemporary health conditions or follow certain exercise routines as this will help you customize the diet as per your requirement.

This diet is easy to follow as you get everything but in a healthier way and in limited quantity.

Talking about the DASH diet out of theory and more in practice reveals more of its efficiency as a diet. Besides the excess of research and experiments, the real reasons people look into this diet are its certain characteristics. It gives the feeling of ease and comfort, which makes users more comfortable with its rules and regulations. Here are some of the reasons why the DASH diet works amazingly:

1. Easy to Adopt:

The broad range of options available under the label of the DASH diet makes it more flexible for all. This is the reason why people find it easier to switch to and harness its true health benefits. It makes adaptability easier for its users.

2. Promotes Exercise:

It is most effective than all the other factors because not only does it focus on the food and its intake, but it also duly stresses daily exercises and routine physical activities. This is the reason why it produces quick, visible results.

3. All Inclusive:

With few limitations, this Diet has taken every food item into its fold with certain modifications. It rightly guides about the Dos and Don'ts of all the ingredients and prevents us from consuming those which are harmful to the body and its health.

4. A Well-Balanced Approach:

One of its biggest advantages is that it maintains balance in our diet, in our routine, our caloric intake, and our nutrition.

5. Good Caloric Check:

Every meal we plan on the DASH diet is pre-calculated in terms of calories. We can easily keep track of the daily caloric intake and consequently restrict them easily by cutting off certain food items.

6. Prohibits Bad Food:

The DASH diet suggests the use of more organic and fresh food and discourages the use of processed food and junk items available in stores. So, it creates better eating habits in the users.

7. Focused on Prevention:

Though it is proven to be a cure for many diseases, it is described as more of a preventive strategy.

8. Slow, Yet Progressive Changes:

The diet is not highly restrictive and accommodates gradual changes towards achieving the ultimate health goal. You can set up your daily, weekly, or even monthly targets at your own convenience.

9. Long Term Effects:

The results of the DASH diet are not just incredible, but they are also long-lasting. It is considered slow in progress, but the effects last longer.

10. Accelerates Metabolism:

With its healthy approach to life, the DASH diet has the ability to activate our metabolism and boost it for better functioning of the body.

Recipe Index

Made in the USA
Monee, IL
02 November 2021